Application of Nanomaterials in Biomedical Imaging and Cancer Therapy

Application of Nanomaterials in Biomedical Imaging and Cancer Therapy

Editor

James C. L. Chow

MDPI • Basel • Beijing • Wuhan • Barcelona • Belgrade • Manchester • Tokyo • Cluj • Tianjin

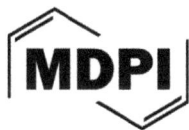

Editor
James C. L. Chow
University Health Network and
University of Toronto
Canada

Editorial Office
MDPI
St. Alban-Anlage 66
4052 Basel, Switzerland

This is a reprint of articles from the Special Issue published online in the open access journal *Nanomaterials* (ISSN 2079-4991) (available at: https://www.mdpi.com/journal/nanomaterials/special_issues/Cancer_Therapy_Nanomaterials).

For citation purposes, cite each article independently as indicated on the article page online and as indicated below:

LastName, A.A.; LastName, B.B.; LastName, C.C. Article Title. *Journal Name* **Year**, *Volume Number*, Page Range.

ISBN 978-3-0365-3513-5 (Hbk)
ISBN 978-3-0365-3514-2 (PDF)

© 2022 by the authors. Articles in this book are Open Access and distributed under the Creative Commons Attribution (CC BY) license, which allows users to download, copy and build upon published articles, as long as the author and publisher are properly credited, which ensures maximum dissemination and a wider impact of our publications.

The book as a whole is distributed by MDPI under the terms and conditions of the Creative Commons license CC BY-NC-ND.

Contents

About the Editor vii

James C. L. Chow
Special Issue: Application of Nanomaterials in Biomedical Imaging and Cancer Therapy
Reprinted from: *Nanomaterials* 2022, 12, 726, doi:10.3390/nano12050726 1

Sarkar Siddique and James C. L. Chow
Application of Nanomaterials in Biomedical Imaging and Cancer Therapy
Reprinted from: *Nanomaterials* 2020, 10, 1700, doi:10.3390/nano10091700 5

Costica Caizer
Computational Study Regarding $Co_xFe_{3-x}O_4$ Ferrite Nanoparticles with Tunable Magnetic Properties in Superparamagnetic Hyperthermia for Effective Alternative Cancer Therapy
Reprinted from: *Nanomaterials* 2021, 11, 3294, doi:10.3390/nano11123294 45

Mehwish Jabeen and James C. L. Chow
Gold Nanoparticle DNA Damage by Photon Beam in a Magnetic Field: A Monte Carlo Study
Reprinted from: *Nanomaterials* 2021, 11, 1751, doi:10.3390/nano11071751 65

Yunfeng Yan and Hangwei Ding
pH-Responsive Nanoparticles for Cancer Immunotherapy: A Brief Review
Reprinted from: *Nanomaterials* 2020, 10, 1613, doi:10.3390/nano10081613 73

Thais P. Pivetta, Caroline E. A. Botteon, Paulo A. Ribeiro, Priscyla D. Marcato and Maria Raposo
Nanoparticle Systems for Cancer Phototherapy: An Overview
Reprinted from: *Nanomaterials* 2021, 11, 3132, doi:10.3390/nano11113132 89

Paolo Emidio Costantini, Matteo Di Giosia, Luca Ulfo, Annapaola Petrosino, Roberto Saporetti, Carmela Fimognari, Pier Paolo Pompa, Alberto Danielli, Eleonora Turrini, Luca Boselli and Matteo Calvaresi
Spiky Gold Nanoparticles for the Photothermal Eradication of Colon Cancer Cells
Reprinted from: *Nanomaterials* 2021, 11, 1608, doi:10.3390/nano11061608 127

Yunying Zhao, Zheng He, Qiang Zhang, Jing Wang, Wenying Jia, Long Jin, Linlin Zhao and Yan Lu
880 nm NIR-Triggered Organic Small Molecular-Based Nanoparticles for Photothermal Therapy of Tumor
Reprinted from: *Nanomaterials* 2021, 11, 773, doi:10.3390/nano11030773 143

Oscar Knights, Steven Freear and James R. McLaughlan
Improving Plasmonic Photothermal Therapy of Lung Cancer Cells with Anti-EGFR Targeted Gold Nanorods
Reprinted from: *Nanomaterials* 2020, 10, 1307, doi:10.3390/nano10071307 155

Sreekar Babu. Marpu, Brian Leon. Kamras, Nooshin MirzaNasiri, Oussama Elbjeirami, Denise Perry. Simmons, Zhibing Hu and Mohammad A. Omary
Single-Step Photochemical Formation of Near-Infrared-Absorbing Gold Nanomosaic within PNIPAm Microgels: Candidates for Photothermal Drug Delivery
Reprinted from: *Nanomaterials* 2020, 10, 1251, doi:10.3390/nano10071251 169

Masfer Alkahtani, Anfal Alfahd, Najla Alsofyani, Anas A. Almuqhim, Hussam Qassem, Abdullah A. Alshehri, Fahad A. Almughem and Philip Hemmer
Photostable and Small YVO$_4$:Yb,Er Upconversion Nanoparticles in Water
Reprinted from: *Nanomaterials* **2021**, *11*, 1535, doi:10.3390/nano11061535 . . . . **195**

Neeraj Prabhakar, Ilya Belevich, Markus Peurla, Xavier Heiligenstein, Huan-Cheng Chang, Cecilia Sahlgren, Eija Jokitalo and Jessica M. Rosenholm
Cell Volume (3D) Correlative Microscopy Facilitated by Intracellular Fluorescent Nanodiamonds as Multi-Modal Probes
Reprinted from: *Nanomaterials* **2021**, *11*, 14, doi:10.3390/nano11010014 . . . . **205**

About the Editor

James C. L. Chow is a Medical Physicist working in the Princess Margaret Cancer Centre, University Health Network, Canada, and an Associate Professor at the Department of Radiation Oncology, University of Toronto, Canada. He is also a Scientist of the Cancer Clinical Research Unit in the Princess Margaret Cancer Centre; an Affiliated Scientist of the TECHNA Institute for the Advancement of Technology for Health, University Health Network, Canada; and a member of Temerty Centre for Artificial Intelligence Research and Education in Medicine, University of Toronto, Canada.

As a Clinical Physicist specializing in radiation dosimetry and treatment planning, he uses the Monte Carlo method to develop a precise and accurate dose-delivery process in radiation treatment. He is especially interested in the DNA dosimetry and damage of cancer cells in nanoparticle-enhanced radiotherapy. Moreover, his work includes the use of machine learning to predict dose–volume variables in radiation treatment plan QA, and generating radiation-beam segments for a photon-fluence map used in intensity-modulated radiotherapy. Chow has published over 175 peer-reviewed research papers, 15 book chapters and has delivered over 190 presentations at national and international conferences. He is a senior member of the Institute of Electrical and Electronics Engineers in USA, a fellow of the Institute of Physics in the UK, and a fellow of the Canadian College of Physicists in Medicine in Canada. He is also an editor of international, peer-reviewed journals such as Biomedical Physics & Engineering Express, Biomedical Engineering Online, IOP SciNotes, Practical Radiation Oncology and Frontiers in Oncology

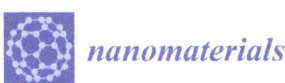

Editorial

Special Issue: Application of Nanomaterials in Biomedical Imaging and Cancer Therapy

James C. L. Chow [1,2]

[1] Radiation Medicine Program, Princess Margaret Cancer Centre, University Health Network, Toronto, ON M5G 1X6, Canada; james.chow@rmp.uhn.ca
[2] Department of Radiation Oncology, University of Toronto, Toronto, ON M5T 1P5, Canada

Citation: Chow, J.C.L. Special Issue: Application of Nanomaterials in Biomedical Imaging and Cancer Therapy. *Nanomaterials* **2022**, *12*, 726. https://doi.org/10.3390/nano12050726

Received: 11 February 2022
Accepted: 16 February 2022
Published: 22 February 2022

Publisher's Note: MDPI stays neutral with regard to jurisdictional claims in published maps and institutional affiliations.

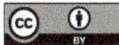

Copyright: © 2022 by the author. Licensee MDPI, Basel, Switzerland. This article is an open access article distributed under the terms and conditions of the Creative Commons Attribution (CC BY) license (https://creativecommons.org/licenses/by/4.0/).

Nanomaterials of different types—namely, inorganic-based, organic-based, carbon-based, and composite-based ones, with various structures such as nanoparticles, nanofibers, nanorods, nanoshells, and nanostars, all have demonstrated a wide range of medical biophysical and chemical properties. Taking advantage of recent advanced synthetic and drug delivery techniques, nanomaterials become superior candidates for a wide range of usages, including dose enhancers, contrast agents, and drug delivery vehicles in biomedical imaging and cancer therapy. To celebrate the rapid application development of nanomaterials in biomedical imaging and cancer therapy, this Special Issue entitled "Application of Nanomaterials in Biomedical Imaging and Cancer Therapy" is an innovative collection of nanomaterial studies on various types of cancer therapy such as hyperthermia, radiotherapy, immunotherapy, photothermal therapy, and photodynamic therapy, as well as medical imaging such as high-contrast and deep-tissue imaging, quantum sensing, super-resolution microscopy, and three-dimensional correlative light and electron microscopy.

This Special Issue begins with a review of nanomaterial applications in biomedical imaging and cancer therapy [1]. This topical review focuses on the latest studies of nanotechnology on theranostic applications and explores the role of nanomaterials in biomedical imaging and cancer therapy. Studying hyperthermia, Caizer carried out a computational study on the magnetic properties of $Co_xFe_{3-x}O_4$ ferrite nanoparticles used in superparamagnetic hyperthermia [2]. Through computational simulations on the Co_x^{2+} ion concentration with x = 0 to 1, the efficiency of hyperthermia of tumours can be optimized to maximum using the $Co_xFe_{3-x}O_4$ nanoparticles. Focusing on radiotherapy, Jabeen et al. performed a Monte Carlo simulation to investigate the DNA dosimetry and damage when photon beams irradiated a DNA molecule with a gold nanoparticle under a magnetic field [3]. The simulation results provided significant information regarding dose enhancement at the DNA in gold nanoparticle-enhanced radiotherapy, using magnetic resonance imaging-guided linear accelerator. Examining immunotherapy, Yan et al. provided a comprehensive review on the pH-responsive nanoparticles in cancer treatment [4]. The review investigated the challenges of immunotherapy on inadequate efficacy and toxic side effects. They concluded that using pH-responsive nanoparticles in immunotherapy could manage these challenges. This is because the nanoparticles can target tumour tissues and organelles of antigen-presenting cells, which have an acidic microenvironment.

Pivetta et al. reviewed the nanoparticle systems for photodynamic and photothermal therapy [5]. They highlighted the technical developments of drug encapsulation and surfaces' functionalization of organic- and inorganic-based nanoparticles to improve the effectiveness of phototherapy. In photothermal therapy, spiky gold nanoparticles were synthesized by carefully controlling the nanoparticle growth process [6]. These branched gold nanoparticles demonstrated large absorption in the first near-infrared (NIR) window and efficient light-to-heat conversion capability under 880 nm lasers. It is, therefore, possible to use these gold nanoparticles in photothermal therapy for colon cancer. At the same time, Zhao et al. developed organic molecular-based nanoparticles, which were novel 880 nm

NIR laser-triggered agents for photothermal therapy of tumour [7]. The in vitro results showed that these organic-based nanoparticles had superior biocompatibility and phototoxicity. Moreover, the nanoparticles exhibited good photothermal stability and conversion efficiency. To treat lung cancer using photothermal therapy, plasmonic gold nanorods were developed and functionalized with anti-EGFR antibodies [8]. The performance of nanorods was tested by the pulsed lasers and continuous-wave lasers based on lung cancer cells (A549). The in vitro results demonstrated that the combination of pulse wave laser illumination of nanorods could produce about a 93% reduction in cell viability, compared with control exposures. In studying drug delivery, Marpu et al. proposed a one-step method for the photochemical formation of NIR-absorbing gold nanomosaic using thermoresponsive poly(N-isopropylacrylamide) microgels [9]. This nanomosaic was generated based on photochemical reduction of a gold precursor, without reducing agent or growth-assisting surfactants. In a drug release model, photothermal shrinkage in microgels was shown by the release of a model luminescent dye.

For biomedical imaging, a silica coating method was reported for upconversion nanoparticles that did not agglomerate post-annealing [10]. These photostable, YVO_4:Yb,Er nanoparticles produced bright visible emission reacting to NIR light and had potential in many imaging applications such as quantum sensing, super-resolution microscopy, and deep-tissue imaging. Furthermore, Prabhakar et al. proposed a method for executing three-dimensional correlative light and electron microscopy using fluorescent nanodiamonds as multimodal probes [11]. Nanodiamonds are fluorescent, nanosized, and electron-dense materials, which are biocompatible and easily identified in living cell fluorescence imaging and serial block-face scanning electron microscopy.

This Special Issue covered a wide spectrum of most recent nanomaterial applications in biomedical imaging and cancer therapy. The results and findings in this issue are expected to be useful for researchers who are working in medical nanotechnology. Finally, I would like to express my heartfelt gratitude to all authors who contributed their innovative research to this Special Issue.

Funding: This research received no external funding.

Acknowledgments: I would like to thank all authors and reviewers who have contributed to this Special Issue.

Conflicts of Interest: The author declares no conflict of interest.

References

1. Siddique, S.; Chow, J.C.L. Application of nanomaterials in biomedical imaging and cancer therapy. *Nanomaterials* **2020**, *10*, 1700. [CrossRef] [PubMed]
2. Caizer, C. Computational Study Regarding $Co_xFe_{3-x}O_4$ Ferrite Nanoparticles with Tunable Magnetic Properties in Superparamagnetic Hyperthermia for Effective Alternative Cancer Therapy. *Nanomaterials* **2021**, *11*, 3294. [CrossRef] [PubMed]
3. Jabeen, M.; Chow, J.C.L. Gold Nanoparticle DNA Damage by Photon Beam in a Magnetic Field: A Monte Carlo Study. *Nanomaterials* **2021**, *11*, 1751. [CrossRef] [PubMed]
4. Yan, Y.; Ding, H. pH-responsive nanoparticles for cancer immunotherapy: A brief review. *Nanomaterials* **2020**, *10*, 1613. [CrossRef] [PubMed]
5. Pivetta, T.P.; Botteon, C.E.; Ribeiro, P.A.; Marcato, P.D.; Raposo, M. Nanoparticle Systems for Cancer Phototerapy: An Overview. *Nanomaterials* **2021**, *11*, 3132. [CrossRef] [PubMed]
6. Costantini, P.E.; Di Giosia, M.; Ulfo, L.; Petrosino, A.; Saporetti, R.; Fimognari, C.; Pompa, P.P.; Danielli, A.; Turrini, E.; Boselli, L.; et al. Spiky Gold Nanoparticles for the Photothermal Eradication of Colon Cancer Cells. *Nanomaterials* **2021**, *11*, 1608. [CrossRef] [PubMed]
7. Zhao, Y.; He, Z.; Zhang, Q.; Wang, J.; Jia, W.; Jin, L.; Zhao, L.; Lu, Y. 880 nm NIR-Triggered Organic Small Molecular-Based Nanoparticles for Photothermal Therapy of Tumor. *Nanomaterials* **2021**, *11*, 773. [CrossRef] [PubMed]
8. Knights, O.; Freear, S.; McLaughlin, J.R. Improving plasmonic photothermal therapy of lung cancer cells with anti-EGFR targeted gold nanorods. *Nanomaterials* **2020**, *10*, 1307. [CrossRef] [PubMed]
9. Marpu, S.B.; Kamras, B.L.; MirzaNasiri, N.; Elbjeirami, O.; Simmons, D.P.; Hu, Z.; Omary, M.A. Single-Step Photochemical Formation of Near-Infrared-Absorbing Gold Nanomosaic within PNIPAm Microgels: Candidates for Photothermal Drug Delivery. *Nanomaterials* **2020**, *10*, 1251. [CrossRef] [PubMed]

10. Alkahtani, M.; Alfahd, A.; Alsofyani, N.; Almuqhim, A.A.; Qassem, H.; Alshehri, A.A.; Almughem, F.A.; Hemmer, P. Photostable and Small YVO$_4$: Yb, Er Upconversion Nanoparticles in Water. *Nanomaterials* **2021**, *11*, 1535. [CrossRef] [PubMed]
11. Prabhakar, N.; Belevich, I.; Peurla, M.; Heiligenstein, X.; Chang, H.C.; Sahlgren, C.; Jokitalo, E.; Rosenholm, J.M. Cell Volume (3D) Correlative Microscopy Facilitated by Intracellular Fluorescent Nanodiamonds as Multi-Modal Probes. *Nanomaterials* **2021**, *11*, 14. [CrossRef] [PubMed]

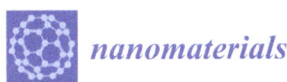

Review

Application of Nanomaterials in Biomedical Imaging and Cancer Therapy

Sarkar Siddique [1] and James C.L. Chow [2,3,*]

1 Department of Physics, Ryerson University, Toronto, ON M5B 2K3, Canada; sarkar.siddique@ryerson.ca
2 Radiation Medicine Program, Princess Margaret Cancer Centre, University Health Network, Toronto, ON M5G 1X6, Canada
3 Department of Radiation Oncology, University of Toronto, Toronto, ON M5T 1P5, Canada
* Correspondence: james.chow@rmp.uhn.ca; Tel.: +1-416-946-4501

Received: 12 August 2020; Accepted: 27 August 2020; Published: 29 August 2020

Abstract: Nanomaterials, such as nanoparticles, nanorods, nanosphere, nanoshells, and nanostars, are very commonly used in biomedical imaging and cancer therapy. They make excellent drug carriers, imaging contrast agents, photothermal agents, photoacoustic agents, and radiation dose enhancers, among other applications. Recent advances in nanotechnology have led to the use of nanomaterials in many areas of functional imaging, cancer therapy, and synergistic combinational platforms. This review will systematically explore various applications of nanomaterials in biomedical imaging and cancer therapy. The medical imaging modalities include magnetic resonance imaging, computed tomography, positron emission tomography, single photon emission computerized tomography, optical imaging, ultrasound, and photoacoustic imaging. Various cancer therapeutic methods will also be included, including photothermal therapy, photodynamic therapy, chemotherapy, and immunotherapy. This review also covers theranostics, which use the same agent in diagnosis and therapy. This includes recent advances in multimodality imaging, image-guided therapy, and combination therapy. We found that the continuous advances of synthesis and design of novel nanomaterials will enhance the future development of medical imaging and cancer therapy. However, more resources should be available to examine side effects and cell toxicity when using nanomaterials in humans.

Keywords: nanoparticles; application; biomedical imaging; cancer therapy

1. Introduction

In the past 10 years, there have been advances in nanomaterials, such as the development of hundreds of nanoparticles (NPs)-based probes for molecular imaging. The use of NPs has enhanced almost all major imaging techniques, particularly magnetic resonance imaging (MRI), positron emission tomography (PET), and optical imaging. Some of the important milestones are the use of iron oxide NPs in T_1 weighted and/or T_2 weighted MRI, the design of radioisotope chelator free (use of radioactive metals that form a stable interaction directly with the surface or core of the NP) particles for PET, and the development of fluorescent NPs such as carbon dots and upconverting NPs [1]. On the other hand, novel types of optical nanoprobes, such as persistent luminescence nanoparticles (PLNPs), are being developed to take advantage of long lasting near-infrared (NIR) luminescence capability [2]. This allows optical imaging without constant excitation and autofluorescence [3].

The latest research and advancement in nanotechnology lead to the development of various NPs for diagnostic and therapeutic applications. Even though clinically, the number of usages of NPs is limited by the complex demands on their pharmacokinetic properties, nanodiagnostics improve the understanding of important physiological principles of various diseases and treatments. On the other hand, NPs are widely used in the clinic for therapeutic purposes. Therapeutic NPs improve the accumulation and release of pharmacologically active agents at the pathological site, which overall, increases therapeutic efficacy and reduces the incidence and intensity of the side effects. NPs hold great promise for integrating diagnostic and therapeutic agents into a single NP for theranostic purposes. A good example would be monitoring biodistribution and target site accumulation, quantifying and visualizing drug release, and longitudinally assessing therapeutic efficacy. Theranostic NPs can be used for personalized nanomedicine-based therapies [4]. Nanoparticles' intrinsic unique magnetic or optical properties make their application ideal for various imaging modalities. Nanoparticles make excellent contrast agents due to their high sensitivity, small size, and composition. Nanoparticles are often conjugated with suitable targeting ligands on the surface of the particles. Multifunctional NPs can be developed by incorporating various functional materials, and this enables multimodal imaging and therapy simultaneously, also known as theranostics [5].

Although each of the imaging and therapy modalities has improved significantly over the past few years, there are caveats in nanomaterial application that are impeding its application. For example, no single molecular imaging modality can offer all the required data fully characterizing the properties of an administered agent. Each imaging modality has a major shortcoming, such as MRI has high-resolution but low sensitivity, optical techniques have limited tissue penetration, and radioisotope imaging techniques have relatively poor resolution but high sensitivity. Combining multiple imaging techniques can enable these applications to complement one another, and a multimodal imaging agent becomes the key to enhancing those imaging systems [6].

This review analyzed the different roles of nanomaterials, such as contrast agent and dose enhancer, in biomedical imaging and cancer therapy. Moreover, the review discussed the underlying mechanisms of nanomaterials including physical, chemical, and biological mechanisms. Some new applications of nanomaterials as theranostic agents are explored. Through a thorough understanding of the recent advances in nanomaterial application in biomedical imaging and cancer therapy, we identified new directions for the optimization and clinical transformation of nanomaterials.

2. Medical Imaging

Medical imaging has improved significantly in recent decades and allows us to precisely obtain anatomical information via different modalities. Nanoparticles play a significant part in medical imaging, as discussed below:

2.1. Magnetic Resonance Imaging

Magnetic resonance imaging is a noninvasive imaging technique that can provide multiparametric and comprehensive information [7]. In 1980s, magnetic resonance imaging was introduced, and it revolutionized modern medical imaging technology. It quickly became one of the best paraclinical diagnostic and monitoring tools available [8]. In 2015, an estimate of 17 million MRI examinations were performed in the United States with the use of contrast agents. The contrast agent enhances the image and plays an important role in MRI. An ideal contrast agent should be injected and eliminated from the body without any adverse effects; however, many of the current contrast agents show side effects such as allergic reactions, nephrotoxicity, gadolinium deposition, and physiologic reactions [9]. Recent advances in NPs show their potential to be used as a contrast agent in MRI and minimize many of the side effects.

2.1.1. Gadolinium (Gd)

Gadolinium-based contrast agents have been used for diagnostic MRI for the last 30 years and have continued to be studied for more functional and improved applications. Recent advances in Gd show that when it is exposed to Zn^{+2} ions, they have increased r_1 relaxivity [10]. This characteristic has multiple advantages in various applications. Since Zn^{+2} ions are important in the biological process involving enzyme catalyst reaction, they can be used as a biomarker for insulin secretion in β-cells. The prostate contains a high volume of Zn^{+2}, which can be used to enhance the image contrast in MRI.

Collagen is dysregulated in the diseased cell or cancer cells, and excess production of collagen is seen in common liver conditions such as alcohol and/or drug abuse. Magnetic resonance imaging can be used to detect excess collagen with Gd NPs-based contrast agents. With increased r_1 relaxivity, Gd can covalently attach to a larger molecule, which does not involve water exchange. Multiple Gd can be attached to a target molecule, along with enhanced permeation and retention effects, which increases MRI contrast significantly [11]. Gadolinium can also be used as a contrast agent and carrier for IL-13 liposome to bypass the blood–brain barrier and use the interleukin-13 receptor as a targeting moiety in the detection of glioma [12].

Dendrimers have great potential in nanomedical imaging and MRI applications. They have very adventitious properties such as their rigidity, low polydispersity, and ease of surface modification. Some applications of dendrimers in MRI are cell tracking, lymph node imaging, blood pool imaging, and tumour-targeted theranostic. Gadolinium is a paramagnetic agent with one of the highest relaxivities due to the high rotational correlation time of the large dendrimer molecules. The relaxivity per Gd (III) ion of the dendrimer is enhanced up to six-fold compared to that of a single Gd (III) chelate. Dendrimer-based Gd contrast agents provide excellent contrast on 3D time of flight MR angiograms. Target-specific bindings of Gd dendrimer can significantly enhance cellular uptake, for example, a cyclic peptide specifically binds to fibrin fibronectin in conjugation with the Gd dendrimer. In one study, Arg-Gly-Asp-Phe-Lys (mpa)(RGD) peptide complex was used as a targeting moiety in combination with a multimodal Gd dendrimer contrast agent and gold nanoparticles (Au NPs) as carriers. It was able to visualize alpha V beta 3-integrin overexpressing tumour cells on both computed tomography (CT) and MRI. Targeted dendrimers can also be used as a therapeutic agent. In neutron capture therapy, dendrimers are irradiated with an external neutron beam; then, the dendrimer-bound Gd generates auger electrons that are highly cytotoxic to tumour cells. This method requires a high accumulation of Gd in the target cell and has been tested on SHIN3 ovarian carcinomas. Recently, Gd-based dendrimers have been even further optimized and provided us with Gd-17, which is based on a poly-L-Lysine dendrimer scaffold, glycodendrimers, and self-assembled dendritic-like NPs. In one study, a manganese-chelating hexametric dendrimer containing six tyrosine-derived [Mn(EDTA)(H_2O)](-2) moieties exhibited relaxivities ranging from 8.2 to 3.8 $nM^{-1} s^{-1}$ under 0.47 to 11.7 T, which was six-fold higher on a per molecule basis compared to a single moiety. This study also showed in a targeted manganese dendrimer, when conjugated with antibody-specific malondialdehyde lysine epitopes, observed enhancement larger than 60% compared to the untargeted counterpart. Along with MRI, manganese dendrimer can also be used as a dual-mode agent for CT-MRI [13]. Another study showed gadolinium oxide with diethylene glycol polymer and magneto liposome NPs in Hepa 1–6 cell lines could be used as a positive MRI contrast agent and marker for cell tracking [14]. Gadolinium chelates have been used in clinical use for a long time and were primarily considered safe. However, recent studies showed an association between a clinically approved Gd-based contrast agent and the development of nephrogenic systemic fibrosis [15]. A few other studies showed a Gd-based contrast agent can potentially result in Gd deposition in human bone and brain tissue, even in the presence of normal renal function [16,17].

2.1.2. Super Paramagnetic Iron Oxide Nano Particles (SPIONs)

Magnetic resonance imaging contrast agents are classified as either T_1 (positive) or T_2 (negative). Radiologists primarily prefer the T_1 positive contrast due to the ease of distinguishability of internal bleeding and air tissue boundaries. Gadolinium-based contrast agents are T_1 contrast agents, and even though they provide good image enhancement, they have a small risk of adverse side effects. Superparamagnetic iron oxide nanoparticles are a good alternative to Gd. They have a hydrodynamic diameter ranging from 1 to 100 nm. In general, large SPIONs function as T_2 contrast agents, whereas small SPIONs function as T_1 [18]. Superparamagnetic iron oxide nanoparticles are particles formed by small crystals of iron oxide, and the coating can be made of organic compounds. Three different types of iron oxide may make up the SPIONs core: hematite (α-Fe_2O_3), magnetite (Fe_3O_4), and maghemite

(γ-Fe_2O_3). Superparamagnetic iron oxide nanoparticles can be conjugated to a variety of particles, such as antibodies, and can also be used as a drug carrier in cancer therapy [19]. A study was conducted to observe the efficiency and viability of SPIONs' tracking ability of stem cells. In one study, FereTRack Direct, a SPION was used in various stem cells. Magnetic resonance imaging was used to monitor the homing-labelled stem cell and cytotoxicity was observed. The study results showed that it was effective at tracking the stem cells in glioma-bearing mice [20]. Clinical translation was greatly increased with the improvement in the delivery system and the ability to track and monitor injected cells. Superparamagnetic iron oxide nanoparticles can be used to label cells and can easily be monitored using MRI [21]. Clustering SPIONs into a raspberry shape within a polymeric envelope outputs a vastly superior image contrast. A study was conducted to observe the effect of increased transverse relaxivity in ultra-small superparamagnetic iron oxide NPs used in MRI contrast agents. Spherical magnetic iron oxide NPs with 12 ± 2 nm size exhibited having superior T_2 relaxation rate and high relaxivities. Due to strong relaxation properties of the NPs before and after NP administration, MRI analysis shows the clear distinguished signal intensity of specific organ imaging, tumour imaging, and whole-body imaging [22]. Superparamagnetic iron oxide nanoparticles have gained considerable attention as a T_2 contrast agent due to their unique magnetic properties. However, several SPIONs have recently been discontinued due to a variety of reasons, such as poor contrast enhancement when compared with Gd-based contrast agents. Gadolinium-based contrast agents still need to be investigated thoroughly due to toxicity concerns [23].

Molecular imaging combines multidisciplinary knowledge and expertise from several disciplines such as medical physics, imaging technology, molecular biology, bioinformatics, and mathematics. Molecular imaging allows the study of biochemical processes of disease without disturbing the integrity of the living subject (noninvasive imaging). Magnetic resonance imaging is well-suited to molecular imaging due to its inherent noninvasive properties and excellent spatial resolution. Inflammation is a process that prepares the ground for tissue healing. Due to the involvement of inflammation in the pathogenesis of various human conditions including infection, ischemia, atherosclerosis, and formation of tumour metastasis, monitoring the inflammatory process is clinically important. Misdirected leukocytes may damage healthy tissue by inducing inflammation, where molecular methods and markers can monitor such processes. Target inflammatory cells can be tagged with SPIONs through the internalization of the NPs. Superparamagnetic iron oxide nanoparticles-tagged macrophages can invade tissues through inflammatory processes. In one study, this method was tested on a model of inflammation in the central nervous system. Upon internalization of SPIONs, microglial cells were detected by MRI. In tumour targeting and imaging, macromolecular antibodies with cancer cell surface receptors are the most favoured targeting moieties for the functionalization of NPs due to their high specificity. A well-known tumour target, human epidermal growth factor receptor 2 (Her-2/neu receptor), was attached to poly (amino acid)-coated NPs, where approximately eight Her-2/neu antibodies attached per particle. T_2 weighted MRI confirmed that the functionalized NPs could specifically target the Her-2/neu receptors on the cell surface. Drawbacks to antibody-targeted NPs are their large hydrodynamic size and poor diffusion through biological barriers. Nanoparticles functionalized with single-chain antibody fragments (scFvs) can help to solve that problem, since they are smaller in size and can more easily cross the biological membrane. In the case of breast cancer, more than half of human breast cancers express receptors for luteinizing hormone-releasing hormone (LHRH). Nanoparticles functionalized with LHRH can selectively accumulate in primary tumour cells and metastatic cells. Some of the tumour cells overexpress transferrin receptors (TfRs), so Tf-SPIONs can be used for specific labelling and detection of gliosarcoma and breast carcinoma. Folate receptors are generally overexpressed in cancerous tissues. Folate molecules as a targeting ligand can be grafted on SPIONs with different coatings such as PEG, Dextran, and 2-carboxyethyl phosphoric acid target-specific binding [24].

2.1.3. Carbon

Carbon-13 (^{13}C)

Carbon-13 (^{13}C) MRI is a very useful metabolic imaging technique because carbon is the backbone for all organic molecules. It can observe a wide range of biological processes relevant to human disease. The MRI signal of carbon-13 is very low due to its natural abundance (1.1%). However, hyperpolarization of ^{13}C increases the signal significantly (more than 10,000-fold) and allows nonradioactive, real-time, safe, and pathway-specific investigation of dynamic metabolism and physiologic processes, which were previously not possible in imaging. The most used hyperpolarized carbon probe is [1-^{13}C] pyruvate. Its polarization reached up to 50% polarization level in current clinical polarizers and it has a long T_1 relaxation (approximately 67 sec in solution at 3.0 T). Pyruvate has been used to study metabolism in a variety of diseases such as ischemia inflammation and cancer. Pyruvate is also useful for monitoring early anticancer therapies and study energy metabolism involving cardiovascular disease. It can also be used to investigate metabolic changes related to hypoxia and oxidative stress [25]. Pyruvate can be used as a tool to predict cancer progression, characterize cancer biology, and be used as a biological marker [26]. The Warburg effect is where cancer cells exhibit elevated levels of glycolysis and lactic acid fermentation. Hyperpolarized pyruvate can be used to quantify the flux. Lactate dehydrogenase-mediated conversion of pyruvate to lactate is elevated in malignant cells as a result of the Warburg effect. The high concentration of glutathione, which correlates to the increased reduction in 1-^{13}C dehydroascorbate to 1-^{13}C vitamin C, can be associated with malignancy, and can be used as a detection tool [27]. A NP-based pyruvate biosensor was developed that can detect total pyruvate level in sera [28].

Nanodiamonds

Nanodiamond is a nontoxic substrate that can be used for drug delivery and cellular tracking (fluorescent marker). The Overhauser effect is a proton–electron polarization transfer technique that can enable high contrast MRI of nanodiamond in water at room temperature and in an ultra-low magnetic field. Magnetic resonance imaging cannot efficiently detect nanodiamond directly due to low abundance and the small gyromagnetic ratio of spin $\frac{1}{2}$ ^{13}C nuclei, which compromise the carbon lattice. At ultra-low magnetic field, efficient Overhauser polarization transfer between electronic and nuclear spins in a compatible radiofrequency is possible. Radiofrequency pulsing of the electron paramagnetic resonance transition between MRI signals continually transfers spin polarization from the paramagnetic centers at the surface of nanodiamond to ^1H nuclei in the surrounding water. Therefore, the presence of nanodiamond in water produces an enhancement in the ^1H MRI signal, which can produce images with contrast sensitivity to nanodiamond concentrations [29].

Carbon Nanotubes

Carbon nanotubes can be synthesized single-walled or multiwalled commercially and have diameters in the nm range and length in the μm range. Since carbon nanotubes can easily be internalized by living cells, they are expected to have a wide range of applications in biomedicine such as imaging and therapy. However, carbon nanotubes are insoluble in most solvents. Therefore, noncovalent coating of amphiphilic molecules or functionalization of various chemical groups on the nanotube surface are carried out to make the nanotubes soluble in biologically compatible buffers. The unique electromagnetic property of carbon nanotubes makes them highly sensitive in various imaging modalities such as photoacoustic molecular imaging and NIR imaging [30]. Photoacoustic imaging allows higher resolution and deeper imaging depth than optical imaging. It is found that a single-walled carbon nanotube conjugated with cyclic ArgGly-Asp (RGD) peptides can be used as an effective contrast agent for tumours. A preclinical study showed that eight times the photoacoustic signal in the tumour could be acquired with mice injected with targeted nanotubes compared to mice with nontargeted nanotubes [31]. For NIR imaging, another preclinical study showed that single-walled carbon nanotubes with sodium cholate could be used as in vivo imaging agents to produce high-resolution imaging with deep tissue penetration and low autofluorescence in the NIR region beyond 1 μm [32].

Graphene

Graphene is a single layer of carbon atoms arranged in a 2D honeycomb lattice. Due to its excellent physicochemical, surface engineering, and biological properties such as small hydrodynamic size, low toxicity, and biocompatibility, graphene-based nanomaterials, namely, graphene–dye conjugates, graphene–antibody conjugates, graphene–NP composites, and graphene quantum dots can act as an in vitro and in vivo imaging agent for molecular imaging [33]. In an in vitro and in vivo study, carboxylated photoluminescent graphene nanodots were synthesized for photoluminescent experiments. It was found that the nanodots could enhance the visualization of tumour in mice and therefore, was proved to be an effective optical imaging agent for detecting cancer in deep tissue noninvasively [34].

2.1.4. Manganese (Mn)

Manganese-based contrast agents have good biocompatibility and ideal characteristics for MRI, such as the short circulation time of Mn(II) ion chelate in the T_1 weighted image. Manganese oxide NPs have negligible toxicity and good T_1 weighted contrast effects. If manganese oxide NPs are retained by the reticuloendothelial system and stored up in the liver and spleen, it will lead to Mn^{2+} induced toxicity. Pegylated bis-phosphonate dendrons are attached to the surface of the manganese oxide NPs, which can solve the problem. This improves colloidal stability, excretion ability, and relaxation performance. Manganese oxide NPs with a hydrodynamic diameter of 13.4 ± 1.6 nm will eventually be discharged through the hepatobiliary pathway as feces or urinary excretion. Polyethylene glycol coating also has a high potential to reduce toxicity with manganese oxide NPs [35].

2.1.5. Silicon (^{29}Si)

Hyperpolarized silicon particles can be used in MRI applications. Large silicon particles with an average size of 2.2 μm generally have larger polarization than NPs. However, a recent study showed that a much smaller silicon-29 particle (APS = 55 ± 12 nm) can be hyperpolarized. For MRI application, a silicon-based contrast agent can be produced by incorporating transition metal ions into a particle's body. This contrast agent shortens the nuclear spin-lattice relaxation time (T_1) of the protons of nearby tissues, and ultimately, amplifies the signal in T_1 weighted proton imaging. Direct detection of the silicon signal is not possible due to its low sensitivity of ^{29}Si nuclei, which leads to long acquisition times. However, this limitation can be solved via hyperpolarization. Utilizing this technique, the imaging window span lasts around 60–120 s, which allows rapid enzymatic reactions and anaerobic metabolism to be studied and further be used to characterize the pathology of the tissue. One of the advantages of using a silicon-based contrast agent is its versatility of surface chemistry; the attachment of functional organic molecules on the surface of the particles does not significantly reduce any of the desired nuclear magnetic resonance properties [36].

2.1.6. Peptide

Atherosclerosis contributes to cardiovascular disease and is the leading cause of morbidity and mortality in the United States. Atherosclerosis is characterized as a chronic and inflammatory disease. Early detection of unstable plaques improves treatment success rate significantly. Magnetic resonance imaging is an important imaging modality for cases such as this, due to its ability to image and characterize the blood vessel wall and plaque in a noninvasive manner and without any ionizing radiation. Peptide-based NPs are useful for enhancing MRI images due to their biodegradable properties and inherent biocompatibility. Super molecular peptide amphiphile micelles can be used to target unstable atherosclerotic plaques displaying microthrombi. The peptide amphiphile micelles can be functionalized using two types of amphiphilic molecules containing Gd chelator. This target-specific NP compound enhances the image and detection probability. It can be used in dual optical imaging-MRI [37].

2.2. Computed Tomography

Computed tomography works by making use of an x-ray source and a detector array to form images. It has been widely used in clinical imaging for a long time and can produce an image with high spatial and temporal resolution. It can provide 3D anatomical information of specific tissues and organs such as the cardiovascular track, gastrointestinal track, liver, and lung noninvasively. One drawback to CT is that it lacks sensitivity toward contrast agents, where other modalities such as MRI shine. However, there are still few promising contrast agents available for CT [38].

2.2.1. Gold Nanoparticles

Gold nanoparticles have unique x-ray attenuation properties and easy surface modification. Au NPs can be functionalized with glucosamine to be an effective contrast agent [39]. Gold nanoparticles have a high x-ray absorption coefficient and can specifically image tumours using CT with an enhanced permeability and retention effect (EPR). In a breast cancer experiment, Au NPs were conjugated with PEG chains and tumour biomarkers (human epidermal growth factor 2). They were able to provide an enhanced image in CT due to their specific targeting ability [40]. A mesenchymal stem cell is a type of adult stem cell that has high potential in cellular-based regenerative therapy and is able to treat various medical conditions such as autoimmune, neurodegenerative, and cardiovascular disease. They can also be used to repair cartilage and bones. Their most adventitious property is being able to migrate into different tissue, and monitoring this migration is very beneficial for studying metastases. A study was done to observe such migration of mesenchymal cells using Au NPs as a marker, and a micro CT was used to obtain movement information from the Au NP marker [41]. The study observed the comparison between porous and solid Au NPs as a contrast agent and their effect on the liver and kidney. Porous Au NPs show brighter contrast of 45 HU, where solid AuNPs show almost half less (26 HU). Computed tomography scans of porous Au NPs show significantly enhanced contrast as compared to solid Au NPs [42]. A new approach to Au NP-based contrast agents for CT was developed, where they encapsulated biodegradable poly-di (carboxylatophenoxy) phosphazene into gold nanospheres. They can function as a contrast agent, then, subsequently break down into harmless by-products, and the Au NPs can be released through excretion. The CT image shows that these contrast agents can enhance the image significantly and produce a strong contrast image [43].

2.2.2. Iodine (^{131}I)

Iodine-based polymer iodine NP contrast agents were introduced for high vascular contrast and tumour loading. They have low cost and their organic structure provides biodegradation and clearance compared to many metal NPs. They are also very small (~20 nm) in size, which provides better tumour penetration compared to larger NPs. The contrast agents have long blood half-life (40 h) that provides better tumour uptake and clearance from the liver when compared to Au NPs. The agents also efficiently accumulate in tumours and provide high contrast vascular tumour imaging [44]. In the imaging of thyroid diseases and radionuclide therapy, iodine has been routinely used due to its high affinity for thyroid and relatively long half-life (8.01 days). It also has other adventitious properties, such as gamma emission that can be used for SPECT imaging and beta minus decay, which can be used for therapeutic purposes. Iodine-labelled glioma targeting ligands such as chlorotoxin have high potential in targeted SPECT imaging and radionuclide therapy of glioma. A study was carried out to functionalize polyethylenimine (PEI)-entrapped Au NPs, which were PEGylated and combined with targeting peptide BmK, and used in CT for targeted CT/SPECT imaging and radionuclide therapy of glioma [45]. The regional lymph node is one of the most frequent sites of early carcinoma metastasis. There was a study to develop a sentinel lymph node tracer consisting of iodine and docetaxel. The results of the study showed that it can simultaneously perform sentinel lymph node CT and locoregional chemotherapy of the draining lymphatic system [46]. In functional imaging of tumours, simultaneous imaging of multiple contrast agents is useful due to simultaneous visualization of multiple targets that allow observation of cancer progression and its development. Iodine and Gd have a previous record of clinical use as image enhancing agents. A study was carried out to see the viability of them to be used as contrast agents in both dual-energy micro CT with energy integrating detectors and photon-counting detector-based spectral micro CT. The experimental results showed that the contrast agents provided enhanced images. The photon-counting detector provided a lower background signal, a better simultaneous visualization of tumour vasculature, and an intratumoural distribution pattern of NPs compared to dual-energy micro CT with energy integrating detectors [47].

2.2.3. Bismuth

In a study, a hybrid cluster was synthesized using PEG 2000-DSPE. It contained hydrophobic bismuth (Bi_2S_3) NPs and quantum dots, and could be used as a contrast enhancer for combined CT/fluorescence imaging. The cluster produced contrast enhancement in CT imaging of the liver and spleen after 30 min and lasted for more than 4 h. The experimental results showed that the probe had good biocompatibility and did not disrupt normal organ function [48].

2.3. Positron Emission Tomography

Positron emission tomography (PET) is a nuclear medicine imaging technique. It uses radiotracers to produce images of radionuclide distribution. These tracers can provide information on biological pathways via a noninvasive method [49].

2.3.1. Gold Nanoparticles

Gold nanoparticles are commonly used in PET. Visualization of dendritic cell migration is possible with the recent development in highly sensitive, biocompatible, and stable imaging agents. Tracking dendritic cell migration is important in dendritic-based immunotherapy. Novel radioiodine-124-labelled tannic acid gold core–shell NPs were introduced for dendritic cell labelling and tracking using PET imaging. This nanoplatform had good labelling efficiency, high radiosensitivity, and excellent chemical stability. It also had a negligible effect on cell biological function, including phenotype marker expression and proliferation. The experimental results showed they were successful at tracking dendritic cell migration [50]. For early evaluation of photothermal therapy (PTT), a study combined ^{18}F—FDG PET with CT, and diffusion weighted images in tumour-bearing mice using silica gold nanoshells. The NP-treated mice exhibited inhibited tumour growth compared to control mice. Changes in ^{18}F—FDG uptake and apparent diffusion coefficient correlates with tumour survival and it can be used for early evaluation of PTT [51]. For brain tumours, a new ^{124}I-labelled gold nanostar probe using PET was introduced. The experimental results showed that it can potentially reach sub-mm intracranial brain tumour detection, which is superior to any available noninvasive imaging modality [52]. Another study focused on the PEGylated crushed gold shell- radioactive ^{124}I-labelled gold core nanoballs for in vivo imaging application with PET. It has high stability and sensitivity in various pH solutions. Positron emission tomography in combination with Cerenkov luminescent imaging showed tumour lesions at 1 h after an injection of NPs and signals remained visible in tumour lesions up to 24 h [53].

2.3.2. Copper (^{64}Cu)

Copper sulfide (CuS) NPs have noncomplex chemistry, low toxicity, and small particle size, which makes them an ideal imaging agent. Radioactive [^{64}Cu]CuS NPs can be used as a radiotracer for PET and photothermal ablation therapy using near infra-red NIR laser irradiation. When [^{64}Cu]CuS

NPs are conjugated to RGDfK peptide through PEG linkers, they have targeting ability and significantly higher tumour uptake (8.4 ± 1.4% injected dose/tissue). They can be used as an enhancing PET imaging contrast agent and also be used for theranostic application [54]. A study conjugated natriuretic peptide receptor-binding peptide (targeting entity) with a C-type atrial natriuretic factor was conducted to produce comb ^{64}Cu-CANF NPs. The study showed improved biodistribution profiles and significantly reduced accumulation in both the liver and spleen compared to the control. The study results also demonstrated the potential for it to be a PET imaging agent to detect atherosclerosis progression [55]. For quantitative PET imaging macrophages in tumours, pharmacokinetically optimized ^{64}Cu-labelled polyglucose NPs (Macrin) were developed [56]. Single chain antibodies have high antigen specificity and affinity, modular structure, and fast urinary clearance, which makes them ideal to be used as targeting ligands. An antiprostate membrane antigen, scFv, has site-specific cysteine and was evaluated in the prostate cancer xenograft model by Cu-64 PET imaging. scFv-cys was conjugated to copolymer distearoyl phosphatidyl ethanolamine monomethoxy polyethylene glycol-maleimide that spontaneously assemble into homogeneous multivalent lipid NPs, which enhances tumour accumulation. It exhibited a 2-fold increase in tumour uptake compared to scFv alone. The antiprostate membrane antigen scFv lipid NPs exhibited a 1.6-fold increase in tumour targeting over the nontargeted lipid NPs. This shows its potential to be used in PET as an image enhancer [57].

2.3.3. Other Nanoparticles

Abundant inflammatory macrophages destructing tissue leads to atherosclerosis, myocardial infarction, and heart failure. Monitoring macrophages in patients can be useful for avoiding or early treating many of these diseases. ^{18}F-Macroflor modified polyglucose NPs have high avidity for macrophages. They have a small size and can excrete renally. Macroflor enriches cardiac and plaque macrophages and they increase the PET signal [58]. A nanoplatform of farnesylthiosalicylate-based copolymer consisting of a poly (oligo (ethylene glycol) methacrylate) hydrophilic block, a poly hydrophobic block, and a poly (4-vinyl benzyl azide) middle block was introduced. The in vivo and vitro nanoplatform inhibits tumour growth and can also serve as a carrier for paclitaxel. It also provides an active azide group for incorporating a PET imaging modality via a facile strategy based on metal-free click chemistry. Its compatible properties allow it to be used for PET image-guided drug delivery [59]. The pH-sensitive pharmaceutical-grade carboxymethylcellulose-based NPs were introduced for white blood cells to be used in PET imaging. $^{68}Ga^{3+}$ was used for labelling, which provides greater spatial resolution and patient convenience for PET over SPECT [60]. Polyphenol and poloxamer self-assembled supramolecular NPs have multiple hydrogen bonding between tannic acid and Pluronic F-127 in combination with hydrophobic reactions of poly (propylene oxide) chains, which can be applied in NIRF and PET imaging. Their excess phenolic hydroxyl groups chelating positron-emitting radionuclide ^{89}Zr function as PET contrast agents. They have good biocompatibility in various cell lines, and in vitro, they do not induce hemolysis [61]. Cerium oxide NPs have unique surface chemistry. Cerium oxide NPs coated with ^{89}Zr, a clinical PET isotope, for PET imaging and in vivo biodistribution were synthesized and showed great potential to be used in PET imaging [62].

2.4. Single Photon Emission Computerized Tomography

Single photon emission computerized tomography is a nuclear imaging technique that uses gamma rays to assess biochemical changes and the level of the molecular target within a living subject. For the past few decades, SPECT has been the nuclear imaging technique thanks to $^{99m}T_c$ [63].

2.4.1. Gold Nanoparticles

Gold nanoparticles have high potential in SPECT imaging and can be used as a contrast agent [64]. A study showed an alternative method for functionalizing Au NPs with mannose. Technetium ($^{99m}T_c$)-radiolabelled Au NPs functionalized with mannose can track and accumulate in lymph nodes. It can be used as a SPECT contrast agent for lymphatic mapping [65].

2.4.2. Technetium ($^{99m}T_c$)

For the diagnosis of metastases in early-stage cervical cancer patients, a study was carried out to evaluate the accuracy of $^{99m}T_c$ SPECT/MRI fusion for selective assessment of nonenlarged sentinel lymph nodes (SLN). The fused datasets of the SPECT and MR images can be used to identify SLN on the MRI with an accurate correlation to the histologic result of each SLN. The results of the study showed that the size and absence of sharp demarcation can be used to noninvasively assess the presence of metastasis in cervical cancer patients without enlarged lymph nodes [66]. $^{99m}T_c$ can be used as a targeting agent in SPECT for mapping SLN. $^{99m}T_c$ in conjunction with SPECT-MRI has been used for SLN mapping in preoperative assessment of SLN metastases in the early-stage cervical cancer in women [67]. Single photon emission computerized tomography following 2D planer lymphoscintigraphy in conjunction with $^{99m}T_c$ NP can be used for dynamic sentinel lymph node biopsy in penile cancer patients. Single photon emission computerized tomography and $^{99m}T_c$ improved the rate of detection of true tracer acid lymph nodes and delineated their precise anatomic localization in drainage basins [68]. With the help of $^{99m}T_c$ nanocolloid tracer, lymph drainage mapping with SPECT/CT can be used to select patients with minimal risk of contralateral nodal failure for unilateral elective nodal irradiation in head-and-neck squamous cell carcinoma patients [69]. Sentinel lymph node biopsy after intertumoural injection of $^{99m}T_c$-labelled nanocolloid with imaging of scintigraphy and SPECT/CT in renal tumours is feasible. However, the nondetection rate is high [70].

2.5. Optical Imaging

Noninvasive optical imaging can visualize various classes of structures involved in autophagy at macroscopic and microscopic dynamic levels. Optical imaging is involved in fluorescence, chemiluminescence, and Raman imaging, which can obtain noninvasive 2D or multidimensional image data at both the macro and micro scale. Fluorescence imaging provides intuitive results, is less time consuming, and can more easily be interpreted than other methods. That is why it is widely preferred by researchers and is used in biomedical imaging application [71].

2.5.1. Fluorescence

In biological study, fluorescent NPs are generally used to localize molecule or highlight processes in living organisms or cell culture. For fluorescence imaging, the excitation and absorption wavelengths should be in the NIR optical window to allow good signal detection. In general, 700–750 nm excitation and 750–800 nm emission wavelengths are found to be the optimal range [72]. Although fluorescence has been used for a long time in biomarker analysis, immunoassays, and diagnostic imaging, it has several shortcomings such as wavelength range, photobleaching, and fluorescence self-quenching. Fluorescent NPs can mitigate some of the shortcomings as they often contain multiple fluorophore entities, which leads to increased photoluminescent emission. Their encapsulation into the particle provides improved stability, reduced photobleaching, and reduced toxicity [73]. Fluorescence imaging in the NIR II window using organic fluorophores has great advantages, but has a few shortcomings, such as relatively low fluorescence quantum yield (less than 2%). There was a study to develop a system with organic NPs (L1013 NPs) with a high fluorescence quantum yield of 9.9%. This was able to noninvasively visualize real-time mouse hindlimb and vessels under a very low power density and short exposure time. It was also able to localize tumour pathology with a tumour to normal tissue ratio of 11.7 ± 1.3. The study results showed its great potential to be used in optical imaging application [74]. The NIR IIb (1500–1700 nm) window is ideal for deep tissue optical imaging, but it faces the same general NIR issues such as lack of bright and biocompatible probes. Cubic phase (α-phase) erbium-based rare earth NPs were introduced to be used in the NIR IIb window. It was functionalized with a cross-linked hydrophilic polymer layer that was attached to the anti-PF-L1 antibody for molecular imaging of PD-L1 in a mouse model of colon cancer. It achieved a tumour to normal tissue signal ratio of ~40%. It had a luminescence lifetime of ~4.6 ms that enabled simultaneous imaging of the nanocomplex. Its cross-linked functionalized layer facilitated 90% of the nanocomplex excretion within two weeks and showed negligible toxicity in mice [75]. Indocyanine green (ICG) is an FDA-approved dye that has been shown to exhibit NIRII fluorescence. It was used to perform imaging tests of real-time visualization of vascular structures in hindlimb and intracranial regions in vivo. Fluorescence spectra show strong NIR II fluorescence of liposomal ICG. In vivo results show the enhanced performance of liposomal ICG over control for imaging of deep (>4 mm) vascular mimicking structures. It also provided a significantly higher contrast to signal ratio for an extended period which allows visualization of the hindlimb and intracranial vasculature for up to 4 h post injection [76]. In current clinical practices, the recent development of fluorescent probes is very important for cancer diagnosis and surgery. Functionalized fluorescent probes can be used as contrast agents. This allows for real-time visualization of the molecular edge between cancer and adjacent normal tissue. Fluorescence-guided surgery helps the operator decide the tissue spearing margin and generally results in a good surgical outcome. It also reduces costs. Fluorescent Au NPs conjugated with diatriozoic acid and nucleolin targeted AS_{1411}; the aptamer can be used as a molecular contrast agent to reveal tumour location in the CL_{1-5} tumour. It can also be used as an enhancer for CT due to its high attenuation. The conjugate has good biocompatibility, high water solubility, strong x-ray attenuation, and visible fluorescence [77]. For triple-negative breast cancer and ovarian cancer, a fluorinated tracer, which enables MRI (^{19}F MRI), shows potential for repeated imaging sessions due to the use of nonionizing radiation. A fluorous particle is derived from the low molecular weight amphiphilic copolymer. It self-assembles into micelles with a hydrodynamic diameter of 260 nm, and it shows negligible toxicity. Fluorine MRI detects molecular signatures by imaging a fluorinated tracer. In vitro and vivo, it was capable of tracking and monitoring immune cells and cancer cells. Their systemic administration exhibited significant uptake into triple negative breast cancer and ovarian cancer with minimum accumulation in off-target tissue [78]. Unravelling complex neural interactions at multiple scales in the brain is complex and often very difficult. However, optical imaging offers a solution. A fluorescent NPs-based probe, particularly calcium-based NPs, correlate with neuronal activity and can be used to monitor a full array of chemicals in the brain with improved spatial temporal and chemical resolution. This enables mapping of the neurochemical circuit with finer precision [79]. Treatment of inflammatory disorders with glucocorticoids is possible with NPs delivery, but their delivery needs to be controlled and monitored to minimize adverse side effects. In vivo glucocorticoid betamethasone phosphate, in conjunction with NPs and fluorescent dye DY-647, can improve the treatment of inflammation with simultaneous monitoring of the delivery [80].

2.5.2. Quantum Dots

Fluorescence imaging allows for visualization of real-time details at a cellular level. However, long-term imaging is difficult due to the poor light stability of organic fluorescent dyes. Graphene quantum dots are a good alternative solution. They have outstanding optical properties and unique structural features. Graphene quantum dots are loaded on the surface of NPs for example optical magneto ferrofleric oxide@polypyrrole core–shell NPs. They have longer metabolic processes in blood. In vivo results show they are capable of monitoring the distribution and metabolism of NPs [81]. Mesoporous silica NPs with graphene quantum dots can simultaneously monitor real-time localization of the doxorubicin (DOX) carrier for proper drug targeting as a fluorescent imaging agent. The nanoplatform shows stable suspension and excitation-dependent photoluminescence. They also show pH and temperature-dependent release behaviour that can be utilized in theranostic applications. Their fluorescence properties make them suitable for optical imaging with minimal cytotoxicity [82]. Quantum dots offer superior optical characteristics compared to organic dyes. Their potential toxicity, however, limits their application. Topical administration can reduce toxicity. In vivo endoscopic imaging of human bladder cancer by topical administration of quantum dots conjugated to anti-CD47 was successful and showed no indication of acute toxicity up to 7 days after installation [83]. The molecular profile of most cancer varies greatly between patients as well as spatially and temporally within a single tumour mass. To account for such variance, multiplexed molecular imaging has high potential. Multiplexed molecular imaging enables multiplexed imaging of large panels of cancer biomarkers. Polymer dots can be used in multiplexed molecular imaging and utilizes semiconducting polymers with strong fluorescence. Studies show a 10-fold enhanced brightness of polymer dots over commercial fluorescent dyes. Quantum dots are fluorescent semiconductor NPs that typically contain group II-VI (e.g., CdSe and CdTe), III-V (e.g., InP and InAs), IV-VI (e.g., PbTe, PbSe), or I-III-VI (e.g., $CuInS_2$) elements. They have a narrow and symmetric emission band (~30 nm) that can be tuned precisely by changing the NP sizes and compositions. The broad absorption spectra and large stokes shifts of quantum dots allow simultaneous imaging of multiple types of quantum dots with single wavelength excitation. Quantum dots are also often coupled to a biomolecule for targeted imaging [84]. Lead sulfide quantum dots with 1100 nm emission peaks can be used in NIR fluorescence imaging of cerebral venous thrombosis. This was tested in septic mice and the results showed it to be a useful tool for the evaluation of the pathological state of cerebral blood vessels in septic mice [85]. A study introduced short wavelength infrared region emissive indium arsenide quantum dots. They have high-resolution multicolour imaging, are readily modifiable, provide deep penetration, and have fast acquisition speed in small-animal model. It was capable of quantifying metabolic turnover rates of lipoproteins in several organs simultaneously. It was also able to generate detailed 3D quantitative flow maps of the mouse brain vasculature [86]. Carbon quantum dot (CDs) have excitation dependent emission, high fluorescence quantum yields, photostability, and long photoluminescence decay lifetime. These properties make them ideal to be used in imaging modalities [87]. A versatile imaging probe with highly luminescent cadmium free $CuInSe_2$/ZnS core/shell quantum dots conjugated to CGKRK (cys-Gly-Lys-Arg-Lys) tumour-targeting peptide was developed. It had strong tumour-specific homing property, long circulation time, excellent photostability, and minimal toxicity. It was tested on the glioblastoma mouse model and the targeted probe distinguished tumour boundaries and positively labels a population of diffusely infiltrating tumour cells. This shows their potential to be used in optical imaging [88].

2.5.3. Gold Nanoparticles

The identification and characterization of disease-related mRNA in cells are of great significance for early diagnosis and treatment of numerous diseases. Oligonucleotide functionalized Au NPs have high stability, high intracellular delivery efficiency by endocytosis and high signal-to-background ratio for mRNA detection. Spherical nucleic acid Au NPs conjugates consisting of densely packed recognition oligonucleotides with complementary sequences to the target mRNA was studied. It was able to detect intracellular mRNA level [89]. Ultrasmall polyaminocarboxylate-coated Au NPs, a dithiolated derivative of diethylenetriaminepentaacetic acid, and 1,4,7,10-tetraazacyclododecan-1-glutaric acid-4,7,10-triacetic acid functionalized by thioctic acid show potential for image-guided radiotherapy. The immobilization of organic Cy5-NH_2 dyes onto the Au NPs adds radiosensitizer fluorescence properties that can be used for monitoring their internalization in cancer cells for determining their localization in cells by fluorescence microscopy. This allows for following up their accumulation in tumour after intravenous injection [90].

2.5.4. Persistent Luminescence NPs

Recently, optical imaging nanoprobes are studied as contrast agents for biomedical imaging. These nanoprobes are used to provide early detection, accurate diagnosis, and treatment monitoring at the cellular and molecular level. One type of nanoprobes, called PLNPs, are developed as biomedical imaging agents (bioluminescence and fluorescence imaging), because their optical property can be varied by chemical and physical variables such as composition, size, and surface nature [2]. The PL mechanism is that when the PL materials are irradiated by light and the materials are charged until the excitation is stopped. Then, the PL materials emit light [91]. Preclinical studies on bioimaging were carried out to show that PLNPs have advantages of high signal-to-noise ratio, high sensitivity, deep penetration, and no interference from tissue autofluorescence [92,93]. For biocompatibility of PLNPs, a study was conducted on small animals using the zinc gallate (ZGO) in vivo. Mice were injected various amounts of ZGO from 1 to 8 mg. Toxicity was investigated after one day, one month, and half a year after injection. It is found that only the elevated amount of ZGO (i.e., 8 mg per mouse) would cause significant weight change in the mice, and this amount is about 5 times larger than the amount typically used for in vivo imaging [94].

2.6. Ultrasound

Ultrasound is a noninvasive imaging technique that can assess morphology, internal structure, orientation, and margins of the lesion from multiple planes with a high resolution both in predominantly fatty breast and dense glandular structures [95]. Ultrasound-guided drug delivery using nanobubbles (NBs) has become a promising strategy in recent years. Nanobubbles are usually composed of gas cores and stabilized shells. They can cross the capillary wall easily and have been used in many targeted therapies for cancer treatment, such as 5-fluorouracil loaded NBs for hepatocellular carcinoma. Chitosan is the N-deacetylated derivative of chitin and is one of the most abundant biological materials on earth. Chitosan NBs have gained considerable attention in cancer therapy due to their biosafety and drug transportability. A study was conducted to synthesize DOX-loaded biocompatible chitosan NBs. Nanobubbles-mediated DOX uptake and apoptosis on Michigan cancer foundation-7 cells were measured with flow cytometry and the results showed it to have excellent drug loading capability and ultrasound enhancement [96]. A new ultrasound imaging contrast agent was introduced, where the NBs were conjugated to poly (lactic-co-glycolic acid) and carried DOX as a cancer drug. The diameter of the NBs was 500 nm and the potential was −23 mV. Their multifunctionality allow it to be a great theranostic agent as well. The enhanced ultrasonic and antitumour functions were observed in in vivo results. The DOX-NBs had a drug loading efficiency of 78.6% and an encapsulation efficiency of 7.4% [97]. Bypassing the brain blood–brain barrier opening is possible with focused ultrasound. A study examined the stimulated acoustic emission of NBs at a different concentration to evaluate the blood–brain barrier opening under real-time acoustic feedback control across concentration. The study results showed that the successful opening of the blood–brain barrier was reliably achievable under real-time feedback [98]. An ultrasound-responsive phosphatidylserine-based paclitaxel liposomes NBs conjugate that has a proapoptotic effect toward enhanced anticancer efficacy and image guidance was studied. In vitro results showed the conjugate had a 10-fold increase in cellular internalization as compared to the control. The synergy between phosphatidylserine and paclitaxel (combination index, CI < 0.1) provides significantly high tumour efficacy both in vitro and in vivo (98.3 ± 0.8% tumour grown inhibition). The results also showed a significant reduction in tumour proliferation index [99]. Enhancement of macromolecular permeation through layers of retina is possible with ultrasound-responsive NBs. In one study, intracellular delivery of the antibody in the cell was quantified using Cy3-streptavidin with negligible toxicity. The results showed that macromolecular internalization was achieved to a significant amount [100]. Fluorescence upconversion NPs are highly sensitive and can function as nanocarriers. They can also label the tumour in a specific organ under NIR light. NIR has a few drawbacks to it, such as having a penetration depth of approximately 15 mm. Fluorescence in combination with ultrasound can overcome that shortcoming and provide a high-resolution signal-to-noise ratio. A system in combination with Nd^{3+}-sensitized upconversion NPs, graphic carbon nanodots, and NBs were used for a dual modality imaging and treatment on a mouse model [101]. Apatinib is an oral molecular antiangiogenetic medicine used to treat patients with advanced hepatocellular carcinoma. It has significant systemic toxic side effects. Ultrasound-targeted NBs destruction technology can minimize systemic drug exposure and maximize therapeutic efficacy. A study was carried out to develop novel GPC3-targeted and drug-loaded NBs for this purpose and to be used on hepatocellular carcinoma cells. The results showed ultrasound-targeted and drug-loaded NBs successfully achieved the desired destruction, selective growth inhibition, and apoptosis in HepG3 cells in vitro [102]. There was a study done to investigate the possibility of cancer therapy using a combination of NB-liposomes and ultrasound. NB-liposome was injected intratumourally, then, exposed to ultrasound (1 MHz, 0–4 W/cm^2, 2 min) in BALB/c mice that were inoculated with colon-6 cells. Tumour temperature was significantly higher when treated with NB-liposome compared to just ultrasound. It caused extensive tissue necrosis at 3–4 W/cm^2 of ultrasound exposure [103]. An oxygen encapsulated cellulosic NB agent for imaging and ultrasound-guided drug delivery was introduced. It was tested on a urothelial carcinoma model. It was propelled (max 40 mm/s) and guided oxygen NBs to the tumour using an ultrasound beam. This can localize 500 μm inside the tumour using beam guidance. It enhanced the efficacy of mitomycin-C, which yielded significantly lower tumour progression rate, while using 50% lower concentration of chemotherapeutic drug [104]. An antitumour-targeted FoxM1 siRNA-loaded cationic NBs conjugated to A10-3.2 aptamer was introduced for prostate cancer. It has high specificity to the binding of prostate-specific membrane antigen positive LNCaP cells. In vitro results showed it significantly improved transfection efficiency, cell cycle arrest, and cell apoptosis, while reducing FoxM1 expression [105].

2.7. Photoacoustic Imaging

Photoacoustic imaging (PAI) is based on the photoacoustic effect. It reconstructs images from captured ultrasound signals generated from the materials that thermally expand by laser pulse [106]. Photoacoustic imaging is often referred to as optoacoustic imaging. It is a low-cost modality that can provide regional imaging of blood vessels. It has high spatial and temporal resolution with clinically approved imaging depth [107].

2.7.1. Gold Nanoparticles

In cancer patients, metastases rather than the primary tumour often determine tumour mortality. A new noninvasive immune functional imaging method was proposed, where ultrasound-guided PAI can be used to detect sentinel lymph node metastases with the aid of chitosan-coated Au NPs (GC-Au NPs). This was tested on tumour-bearing mice. Volumetric analysis was used to quantify GC-Au NP accumulation in the sentinel lymph node after cellular uptake and transport by immune cells. The analysis results showed that the spatial-temporal distribution of GC-Au NPs in the sentinel lymph node was affected by the presence of metastases. This imaging method can successfully detect metastatic from nonmetastatic lymph nodes using Au NPs [108]. There was a study to visualize murine lymph vessels using PAI and Au NPs as a contrast agent, and the study showed great potential for it to be used to detect sentinel lymph nodes [109]. Another study found that ultrasound-guided PAI and anti-epidermal growth factor (EGFR) antibody conjugated to gold nanorods can effectively detect EGF-expressing primary tumour and regional lymph node metastases. The nanoconjugation was tested on tumour-bearing mice. Anti-EGFR gold nanorods provided significant enhancement in PAI signal in MDA-MB-231 tumour and axillary lymph node metastases relative to MCF-7 tumour and non-lymph node metastases [110]. Moreover, a new nanorod was synthesized through seed-mediated synthesis with an aspect ratio ranging from 8.5 to 15.6. It could tune a longitudinal surface plasmon resonance absorption band that covered a broad NIR range (~680–1100nm). The gold nanorods showed good biocompatibility and stability. The nanorods provided great contrast enhancement in PAI (3.1 times to the control group) and excellent signal-to-noise ratio (5.6 times to the control group) [111]. When administering Au NPs as a contrast agent in PAI, it is important to note that the Au NPs are below the renal clearance (10 nm). A study showed that biodegradable Au NPs assembled from 5 nm primary gold particles had strong NIR absorbance. Ultra-small 5 nm Au NPs can be used to develop molecular-activated plasmonic nanosensors for molecular-specific PAI [112]. In NIR-II tissue generating the least background signal in PAI, large contrast agents in the spectral range delay their pharmacokinetics and reduce their thermal stability that yields unreliable PAI. Miniaturized Au NPs can help to solve that problem. They are 5–11 times smaller than regular gold nanorods with a similar aspect ratio in NIR-II. They are 3 times more thermally stable and can generate 3.5 times stronger PA signal under nanosecond pulsed laser illumination. These results were verified with thermotical and numerical analysis [113]. Gold nanoparticles coated with glycol chitosan (GC) can be used as a contrast agent in PAI. In breast cancer cells, GC-Au NPs have strong cellular uptake and yield a strong PA signal in a tissue phantom. After just 3 h of incubation, the phantom displayed a strong signal and did not require any additional antibodies or complex surface modification. The endocytosis of GC-Au NPs was also confirmed with dark microscopy, which is beneficial for minimizing toxicity [114]. Photoacoustic tomography (PAT) is an emerging technology that can image cells or tissue using contrast agents such as NPs and pigments. An interesting UV–vis absorption peak in NIR was observed when Au NPs were synthesized with astaxanthin. Studies showed that this astaxanthin-based Au NPs had the potential to be used in PAI and therapy [115].

In brain tumours, getting past the blood–brain barrier (BBB) is a major obstacle. The majority of contrast agents cannot get past the BBB; thus, a study was done to use gas microbubble-assisted focused ultrasound to transiently open the blood–brain barrier and locally deliver silica-coated gold nanorods across the BBB. This contrast agent had strong optical absorption, which allowed for visualization of the agent using ultrasound-guided PAI [116]. The enhancement of the amplitude of the PA signal with microbubbles conjugated to gold nanorods (Au MBs) was studied. Fluence below 5 mJ cm^{-2} provided negligible microbubble wall motion and weak PA signal. However, fluence above 5 mJ cm^{-2} produced significantly higher thermal expansion and emitted 10-fold greater amplitude PA signal compared to the control. This phenomenon can be explained by the idea that explosive boiling may occur at the nanorod surface, which produces vapor NBs and contributes to Au MBs expansion. In vivo imaging of Au MBs in a murine kidney model shows that it is an effective alternative to the existing contrast agents for PAI [117].

2.7.2. Carbon Nanotube (CNT)

Carbon-based NPs have gained considerable attention due to their unique physicochemical properties in nanotechnology [118]. In one study, a single-wall CNT complex with long circulation was fabricated. It was capable of self-assembly loading of an albumin-coupled fluorescent photosensitizer and Chlorin e6 via high affinity between albumin and Evans blue, which provided them with fluorescent imaging and photodynamic ability. It was capable of providing fluorescence and PAI of tumours for optimizing therapeutic time window [119].

2.7.3. Fluorescent

A metabolically digestible imaging probe was developed from nanoprecipitation of biliverdin. These NPs are composed of a biliverdin network and are cross-linked with a bifunctional amine linker. Their excitation at NIR wavelengths provides a strong photoacoustic signal. In vivo, they accumulated in a lymph node in mice and have the potential to be used as a photoacoustic agent for sentinel lymph node detection [120]. The nanocomplex consists of split fluorescent protein fragment used as a molecular glue and switchable Raman reporters to assemble Au NPs into photonic clusters. The fluorescent protein-driven assembly of metal colloids yields an enhanced PA signal that can be used as PAI agent [121]. A photoacoustic contrast agent, formulated from an FDA-approved antimycobacterial agent, clofazimine hydrochloride NPs, for a different purpose, was introduced to be used for prostate cancer. It had macrophage targeting ability and high contrast absorbance at 495 nm. The experimental results on transgenic adenocarcinoma of the mouse prostate model showed a preferential accumulation of the NPs in a cancerous prostate cell over the control. This allows PAI and analysis of prostate cancer [122]. Photoacoustic imaging has a penetration depth of a few cm and can generate useful endogenous contrast from melanin and oxy-/deoxyhemoglobin. ICG is a small molecule dye with fast clearance, bleaching effects, and rapid protein binding, and it can be used for PAI. A study was done to entrap ICG in poly (lactic-co-glycolic acid) NPs together with perfluorocarbon using a single emulsion method. The encapsulation of ICG within NPs decreases its photobleaching and increases the retention of signals within the cells. It can detect as little as 0.1×10^6 cells in PAI and the nanocomplex [123]. Core–shell silica PEG NPs were developed with photothermal, photoacoustic, and NIR optical imaging properties. They were doped with triethoxysilane-derivatized cyanine 5.5 and cyanine 7 dyes, which give them photoacoustic properties. The study results showed they have outstanding stability and enhanced photoacoustic signal [124]. Photoswitchable hybrid probes with thermochromic dye and absorbing NPs were introduced where temperature-sensitive light–dark states and spectral shifts in absorption can be switched through controllable photothermal heating of doped NPs. It provided high contrast in PEI [125]. Hypoxia is often correlated with tumour aggressiveness and poor treatment outcome. Early diagnosis of hypoxic tumour cells has a high potential in tumour control. Hypoxia-activated NPs can be used to enhance the efficiency of photoacoustic intensity, fluorescence, and chemotherapy. Hypoxia-activated NPs are inactive during blood circulation and normal physiological conditions. They activate in the hypoxic condition when they extravasate into the hypoxic tumour microenvironment. Azobenzene hypoxia-activated fluorescence nanoparticles have high potential to be used in PAI [126].

3. Cancer Therapy

Cancer therapy is the technique of inhibition or irradiation of cancer cells. There are several techniques available and each one is more beneficial to one type of cancer treatment than others. Nanomaterials offer significant enhancement to many of the cancer therapies and they are discussed below:

3.1. Photothermal Therapy

Photothermal therapy is a hyperthermia-based cancer therapy. The goal of this therapy is to destroy tumour tissue while avoiding excessive heating of normal tissues. Biological tissue lacks NIR-absorbing chromophores. The use of laser wavelength in the 'tissue optical window' (700–1000 nm) minimizes tissue heating, while Au NPs have strong and tunable absorption in the NIR region. Therefore, Au NPs and NIR can be used to facilitate selective heating of tumours with NPs [127]. Gold nanoparticles with thiol and amine groups can be functionalized with targeted antibodies or drug products. Colloidal gold exhibits localized plasmon surface resonance. It can absorb light at specific wavelengths, which makes them useful for hyperthermic cancer treatment application. A gold nanoparticle's localized plasmon surface resonance can be changed with the modification of the particle's shape and size, which alters its photothermal and photoacoustic properties, allowing utilization of different wavelengths of light. Its nanosize allows the particle to localize in the tumour through passive distribution and excrete through the urinary system [128]. One of the major problems with PTT is that heat distribution is often heterogeneous throughout the tumour, which leaves part of the tumour untreated. A new idea was proposed which uses silica gold nanoshells to deliver fractionated PTT [129]. Gold-based NPs are the main mediator of PTT because they offer biocompatibility, efficient light to hear conversion, ability to be tuned to absorb NIR light which penetrates tissue more deeply, a small diameter that enables tumour penetration, and simple gold thiol bioconjugation chemistry for the attachment of the desired molecule. Nanoshells, nanocages, nanorods, and nanostars are the most common nanomaterials as photothermal transducers. The majority of Au NPs have been designed to maximally absorb within the first NIR window, which can safely penetrate 2–3 cm of tissue [130]. A PET-based nanoplatform was introduced to quantitatively correlate to the heat generation of plasmonic NPs with their potential as a cancer-killing agent. Heat generation was evaluated in human tumour xenografts in mice using 2-deoxy-2-[F-18]-fluoro-D-glucose (^{18}F—FDG) PET imaging. The platform was validated by quantifying the photothermal efficiency of the NIR silica gold nanosphere and benchmarked it against the solid Au NPs. The results showed the heat generation of the resonant gold nanospheres (in vitro and in vivo) performed better compared to the control. It also showed PET could reliably be used to monitor early treatment response in PTT [131].

In PTT, the temperature of the tumour is raised above 42 degrees Celsius to destroy the cancer cells. A light-absorbing material or photothermal agent must be introduced into the tumour to improve the efficacy and selectivity of the energy to heat transduction. Even though gold is the most employed agent in PTT, magnetic NPs are a good alternative. Magnetic NPs formed by iron oxide can be used in combination with other substances or used by themselves as photothermal agents. They can be directed to the tumour site magnetically and their distribution in tumours and other organs can be imaged. Their molar absorption coefficient in NIR is low when they are used alone. However, this can be mitigated by clustering of the NPs. They can also be designed to release a drug upon heat generation, which can be beneficial for combination therapy of PTT and chemotherapy [132].

Polymer-based NP systems have been investigated to overcome some of the limitations associated with traditional inorganic NPs. Some of the materials that have been investigated for this purpose include polyaniline, polypyrrole, polydopamine, and poly-(3,4-ethylene dioxythiophene): poly(4-styrene sulfonate). They are often conjugated with ligands for targeting ability. A specific set of requirements should be met for NPs to be an ideal candidate for PTT, such as suitable size and uniform shape, good dispersibility in aqueous solution, respond to light in NIR range 650–950 nm to prevent damage to surrounding healthy tissue, sufficiently photostable to ensure adequate diffusion time to reach tumour before losing their photosensitivity, and exhibit low or no cytotoxicity in a living system. Current available PTT enabling agents mainly comprise metal NPs such as gold, palladium, silver, germanium, and carbon-based NPs. Some of the polymer-based NPs systems are listed in Table 1 below [133].

Table 1. Polymer-based nanoparticle system for PTT [133].

Polymer	Configuration	Testing Stage
Polyaniline	NPs	In vitro and in vivo
	F-127 Conjugated NPs	
	Silver core, Polyaniline shell (ICG-Ag@PANI)	
	NPs with lanreotide and methotrexate (LT-MTX/PANI NPs)	
	WS core, polyaniline shell with hyaluronic acid and chlorin e6 (Ce6)	
	Polyaniline and cisplastin within folate-poly (ethylene glycol)-distearoylphosphatidylcholine (FA-PEG-DSPE), cRGD[cyclic (Arg-GLY-Asp-D-Phe-Lys)]-PEG-DSPE, and lecithin conjugates dubbed FA/cRGD-PNPs	
Polydopamine	Dopamine-melanin colloidal nanospheres	In vitro and in vivo
	PEGylated polydopamine NPs conjugated with ICG (PDA-ICG-PEF) loaded with DOX	In vitro
	Pegylated NPs loaded with 7-ethyl-10-hydroxycamptjotheticin (SN38)	In vivo
	DOX encapsulated with DSPE-PEG micelles coated with polydopamine	In vitro and in vivo
	Fe(3)O(4) core polydopamine coated nanoshell	In vitro
	Polydopamine coated gold nanorods	In vitro
	Polydopamine coated gold/silver NPs	In vitro
Polypyrrole	Base NPs	In vitro and in vivo
	Base NPs	In vitro
	Spindle-like hollow polypyrrole nanocapsules (PPy HNCs) loaded with DOX	In vivo
	Ppy and rapamycin loaded into liposomes conjugated with trastuzumab (LRPmAB)	In vitro
TBDOPV-DT	D-A conjugated polymer (TBDOPV-DT), with 2,2-bithiophene serving as a donor and thiophene-fused benzo-difuran dione-based oligo (p-phenylenevinylene) as an acceptor (TBDOPV-DT NPs)	In vitro and in vivo
PEDOT:PSS	PEGylated PEDOT:PSS NPs (PDOT:PSS-PEG)	In vivo
	PEDOT: PSS-PEG loaded with DOX, SN38, and Ce6	In vitro
	Magnetic NPs with PEDOT: PSS Cyanine7 (Cy7), and 2-deoxyglucose (2-DG)-polyethylene glcol (MNP@PES-Cy7/2-DG)	In vitro and in vivo
	Magnetic NPs with PEDOT: PSS coating	In vivo

In PTT, red blood cell-coated NPs show improved efficacy with a faster decrease in tumour volumes and a higher survival rate than bare NPs. It is speculated that red blood cell NPs inherit the photothermal conversion effect from inner cores and the long blood retention from the red blood cell coating. One study showed that the combination of biodegradable, natural, and nontoxic melanin NPs extracted from living cuttlefish and red blood cell membrane have significantly higher PTT efficacy. Au NPs encapsulated with the antitumour drug paclitaxel-coated by anti-EpCam antibodies-modified red blood cell membranes show increased cancer-targeting ability due to anti-EpCam antibodies. Paclitaxel can be released when the membrane is destroyed by the heat generated from the Au NPs under laser irradiation to yield the anticancer effect [134].

3.2. Photodynamic Therapy (PDT)

Photodynamic therapy is a form of light therapy that uses molecular oxygen, visible light, and photosensitizers (PS) to destroy cancer cells and pathogenic bacteria. Photodynamic therapy is noninvasive and selectively cytotoxic to malignant cells. It causes direct tumour cell damage by apoptosis necrosis and autophagy. The photosensitizer is distributed directly into the tumour site or systematically via the vascular system. In the presence of molecular oxygen, light at a specific wavelength is applied in PDT, followed by the production of reactive oxygen species (ROS), which results in oxidative damage of the intracellular elements within the cell. This leads to cancer cell death. When PS targets the vascular system of the tumour, it results in hemostasis, vessel constriction, and breakdown. This ultimately leads to a decrease in oxygen and nutrient supply to the tumour, which eventually results in tumour cell death. Gold nanoparticles are primarily used in PDT [135]. Porphyrins have been approved for the treatment of cancer in PDT. They have low physiological solubility and lack of selectivity toward tumours, which is not efficient. Nanoparticles can be used to transport porphyrins. Silica NPs (80 nm) coated with xylan–TPPOH conjugate was studied for such purpose and showed significant phototoxic effects from post-PDT ROS generation, and stronger cellular uptake in the human colorectal cancer cell line. They showed high anticancer efficacy [136]. The dual specificity of PDT relies on the accumulation of PS in tumour tissue and localized light delivery. Tetrapyrrole structures such as bacteriochlorins, porphyrins, chlorins, and phthalocyanines with functionalization have been widely investigated in PDT. Several compounds have already received clinical approval. Photosensitizers conjugated to antibody, proteins, peptide, and other ligands with specific cellular receptors are used in targeted PDT. Nanotechnology has also been widely used for targeted delivery. Fullerene-based PS, titania photocatalysis, and the use of upconverting NPs to increase light penetration into tissue have been studied [137]. Table 2 is a list of several nanoplatforms for PDT and their advantages [138].

Table 2. Nanoplatforms for PDT and their advantages [138].

Nanoparticle Platform	Advantages
Passive PDT PS tumour drug micelles and Liposomes	Enhanced tumour uptake and improved phototoxicity
Dendrimer encapsulated NPs	High loading drug
Metal oxide NPs	High loading capability, biocompatibility, easy surface modification
Immuno NPs	The highly specific molecule, improved drug release within the desired cell
Quantum dots	Large absorbance cross-section and size-tunable optical properties

To achieve synergistic chemiexcited photodynamic starvation therapy against tumour metastasis, a biomimetic nanoreactor was developed. Photosensitizers on the hollow mesoporous silica NPs were excited by chemical energy in deep metastatic tumour tissue to generate singlet oxygen, and then, glucose oxidase catalyzed glucose into hydrogen peroxide in PDT. This blocked nutrient supply for starvation therapy and provided hydrogen peroxide to synergistically enhance PDT [139].

Photosensitizer chlorin e6 (Ce6) and the ferroptosis inducer erastin were self-assembled into a novel supramolecular Ce6-erastin nanodrug though bonding and π–π stacking. Ferroptosis with nanodrug enhances anticancer actions by relieving hypoxia and promoting ROS production [140].

3.3. Chemotherapy

Chemotherapeutic agent DOX is a member of the anthracycline class. It is heavily used in many clinical cancer therapies. It is also one of the most used chemotherapeutic drugs for the treatment of breast cancer. Paclitaxel is another popular chemotherapeutic agent used in breast cancer. Other commonly used chemotherapy regimens are cisplatin, tamoxifen, trastuzumab, and docetaxel. The efficiency of the drug increases significantly with targeted drug delivery. Nanoparticle-based carriers are often conjugated to them for targeted delivery. Some of the NPs that are used in chemotherapy for breast cancer are polymer-based NPs, liposomal NPs, metal-based NPs (Au NPs, SPIONP), carbon-based NPs, mesoporous silica NPs, and protein-based NPs [141]. Nanoparticle vehicles are currently in clinical use and some are undergoing clinical investigation for anticancer therapies, including dendrimers, liposomes, polymeric micelles, and protein drug NPs. There are many new NPs drug formulations in development and undergoing early and late phase clinical trials, including several that utilize active targeting or triggered release based on environmental stimuli. A variety of NP formulations have been approved by the FDA and EMA for the treatment of a wide range of cancers. Some examples are pegylated liposomal doxorubicin and liposomal daunorubicin, which are available in the United States. Nonpegylated liposomal doxorubicin is approved in Europe. Nab-paclitaxel is an FDA- and EMA-approved therapy using NP albumin-bound particles [142]. Various types of proteins and small peptides are often conjugated to the surface of NPs to improve the selectivity of chemotherapeutic drugs. Serum glycoprotein is one of the targeting ligands used with NPs in chemotherapy drug delivery [143]. The antimalarial agent chloroquine can reduce the immunological clearance of NPs by resident macrophages in the liver, leading to increased tumour accumulation of the nanodrug [144].

Gold nanoparticles have high stability, surface area-to-volume ratio, surface plasmon resonance, and multifunctionalities. The nontoxic, nonimmunogenic nature, high permeability, and retention effect of Au NPs provide additional benefits by enabling penetration and accumulation of the drug at tumour sites. DOX-BLM-PEG-Au NPs and EpCAM-RPAnN are two Au NP carriers that have high potential to be used in chemotherapy [145]. Cisplatin is a genotoxic agent that can be used alone or in combination with radiation or other chemotherapeutic agents. It is used in chemotherapy for a broad range of cancers. However, the agent is limited by the intrinsic and acquired resistance, and the dose to normal tissue. It shows little selectivity for tumour vs. normal tissue, which leads to toxicity. Nanoparticles can be used to deliver cisplatin to reduce toxicity. Some organic NPs that can be used to transport cisplatin are liposomes, polymeric NPs, polymeric micelles, and dendrimers. Some inorganic NPs are Au NPs, ferromagnetic NPs, and mesoporous silica NPs. Some hybrid NPs are CNT, nanoscale coordination polymers, and polysilsesquioxane NPs [146].

Organic NPs are a popular choice for chemotherapeutic drug delivery. They can increase the circulation half-life and tumour accumulation of a drug. Combination chemotherapy is used in the treatment of a broad range of cancers. Nanoparticles are essential to delivering many of these drugs to the target site and also provide a theranostic platform for multifunction [147]. Multidrug-loaded NPs formulation consists of different classes of therapeutic agents. It has been studied for breast cancer therapy in preclinical breast cancer models. One example would be polymer lipid hybrid NPs for coencapsulated DOX and mitomycin C. It has demonstrated its efficacy in the human breast cancer model, including multidrug resistance cells. Multidrug-loaded NPs micellar formulation was also developed for the delivery of three drugs: paclitaxel, 17-AAG (Triolimus), and rapamycin. They were evaluated on MDA-MB-231 tumour-bearing mice [148]. Hypoxia promotes the invasiveness of tumour cells and chemoresistance. Tumour-associated macrophages (TAMs) reside in the hypoxic region to promote proliferation and chemoresistance. Nanoparticles MnO_2 with high reactivity toward hydrogen peroxide for the simultaneous production of O_2 and regulation of pH can affectively alleviate tumour hypoxia by targeted delivery of MnO_2 to the hypoxic area. It was conjugated to DOX and significantly increased the apparent diffusion coefficient value of breast cancer and inhibited tumour growth [149]. A novel carrier, targeting nanomicelles for synchronous delivery of curcumin and baicalin, was introduced, which could effectively overcome tumour resistance. Mannose binds to CD206 receptors on the surface of tumour-associated macrophages, subsequently increasing the number of nanodandelions engulfed by tumour-associated macrophages. To increase tumour cellular uptake, oligomeric hyaluronic acid can also be used as a targeting material. Nanodandelions can easily enter tumour tissue through the vascular barrier due to their small size. Effective antitumour activity and reduced side effects were confirmed in antitumour experiments in A549 tumour-bearing mice [150]. Sustained-release characteristics of NPs may aid the effectiveness of chemotherapy by maintaining drug concentrations at the tumour site for longer durations. Nanoparticles can increase penetration and accumulation of the inhaled drug in tumour tissue and cells. This yield improved antitumour activity compared to the free drug. These characteristics make them suitable for chemotherapy for lung cancer [151].

3.4. Immunotherapy

During recent decades, cancer immune therapy has made significant progress with the improvement in nanotechnology. Immunotherapy is a therapy based on stimulation or activation of the patient's immune system to recognize and destroy cancer cells [152]. Understanding how to increase the response rate to various classes of immunotherapy is to improving cancer treatment efficacy and minimizing adverse side effects. There are five classes of cancer immunotherapy: lymphocyte-promoting cytokines, agonistic antibodies against co-stimulatory receptors, checkpoint inhibitors, engineered T cells such as CAR T and T cell receptor (TCR) T cells, and cancer vaccines. Nanoparticles can be used to target T cells in the blood or transport mRNA to the cancer cell, or transport other vaccines in immunotherapy [153]. Nanoparticle systems have shown to be a promising tool for effective antigen delivery. The antigen is generally in peptide form that can stimulate an adaptive immune response. For conditioning a robust and long-lasting adaptive immune response, stimulation of the innate immune system through natural killer cells is necessary. Therefore, an adjuvant that works to recruit natural killer cell response is vital for effective vaccination. Table 3 summarizes the different antigens being studied for different cancer treatments and their delivery NP conjugate [154].

Table 3. Nanoparticle vaccine delivery for various cancer [154].

Cancer Type	Nanoparticles	Antigen
Melanoma	Poly(lactic-co-glycolic acid) (PLGA) NPs	Ag, Poly(I:C)
	Liposome	TRP2, α GalCer
	CNT	α CD40, CpG
	Cowpea mosaic virus (CPMV) NPs	Empty Cowpea mosaic virus (eCPMV)
Non-small cell lung cancer	L-BLP25 liposome	MUC1
Breast cancer	PLGA-PEG	Ovalbumin (OVA), Monophosphoryl lipid A (MPLA), CpG
Prostate cancer	Virus-like particle	Polyethylenimine-stearic acid (PSA)
Cervical cancer	Tumour virus vaccine	HPV

An adjuvant is a molecule that increases immunogenicity. They sometimes are lacking in tumour antigens when presented alone. Commonly used adjuvant in cancer treatment are 3-O-desacyk-4'-monophosphoryl lipid A (MPLA), CpG oligodeoxynucleotides (ODNs), lipopolysaccharide (LPS), polyinosinic:polycytidylic acid (poly I:C), and agonists of the stimulator of IFN genes (STING).

When they are internalized in antigen-presenting cells with tumour antigens, they promote anticancer immune response [155]. Nanoparticles have a multifaceted role in modern immunotherapy. They can reduce tumour-associated macrophages and act as a tumour suppressor agent, selectively knockdown Kras oncogene addiction by the nano-Crisper-Cas9 delivery system, and serve as an efficient alternative to the chimeric antigen receptor [(CAR)-T] [156]. Immunotherapy is one of the effective modalities for cancer treatment. Targeting the tumour environment along with the immune system is a viable strategy to use for cancer treatment. Systematic delivery of immunotherapeutic agents to the body using NP delivery is of great importance. Liposomes, Au NPs, polylactic-co-glycolic acid (PLGA) NPs, micelles, iron oxide NPs, and dendrimers are widely used for immunotherapy. Polymeric NPs are the most commonly used ones in immunotherapy where PLGA is an FDA-approved polymeric carrier. Table 4 below lists the commonly used NPs used in immunotherapy, their therapeutic agent conjugate, target, function, and studied tumour model [157].

Table 4. Nanoparticle used in immunotherapy [157].

NP Materials	Therapeutic Agents	Target	Function	Tumour Model
PLGA-based NPs	AUNP12 anti-PD-1 peptide	Tumour cells	Blockage of PD-1/PDL-1 pathway	4T1 Subcutaneous tumour
	Trastuzumab	Human epidermal growth factor 2 (HER2)	GER2 degradation and antibody-dependent cell-mediated cytotoxicity	In vitro HER2 Positive breast model
	Pam3CSK4 and α-CD40-mAb	CD40	T cell response	B16-OVA Subcutaneous tumour
Liposomes	SB505124 TGF-β 1 inhibitor	Tumour specific cytotoxic T-lymphocyte CTLs	Block TGF-β Signal and promote CD8 + T cell infiltration	E.g7-OVA Subcutaneous tumour
	Curdlan and mannan	Cytosol of DCs	Activation of DCs via Th1 cytokine production	DC2.4 in vitro model
	Stimulator of interferon genes (STING) agonists and c GAMP	Tumour microenvironment (TME)	Proinflammatory gene induction and production of immunological memory	B16-F10 Lung metastatic tumour
Micelles	Pyranine antigen	Cytoplasm of DCs	Antigen-specific cellular immunity	C57BL/6 intradermal immunized mice
	NLG919/IR780	Lymph node	Suppression of growth of tumour margin in primary tumours	4T1 subcutaneous tumour
	ROS inducing ZnPP PM/PIC	Tumour-associated macrophages (TAMs)	Activation of NK cells and T lymphocytes	B16-F10 Subcutaneous tumour
AuNPs	OVA peptide antigen/CpG adjuvant	Dendritic cells	Induce systemic antigen-specific immune response	B-16 OVA Subcutaneous tumour
	α-PDL1	Tumour cells	Imaging and tumour reduction	Colon cancer Subcutaneous tumour
Iron Oxide NPs	Superparamagnetic Fe_3O_4	DCs and macrophages	Immune cell activation and cytokine production	CT2 Subcutaneous tumour
	Ferumoxytol	Macrophages	Increased caspase-3 activity and proinflammatory Th1 response	MMTV-PyMT Mammary tumour
Dendrimers	mAbK1/PTX	Tumour cells—mesothelin receptor	Specific binding and antitumour activity	OVCAR3 Subcutaneous tumour
Artificial exosomes	DEC205 monoclonal antibody	Dendritic cells	Targeting to DCs	In vitro studies-DCs

Cyclic dinucleotides (CDNs) is a potent stimulator of the interferon receptor (STING) agonist. Its efficacy is limited to micromolar concentration due to the cytosolic residence of STING in the ER membrane. Biodegradable poly (beta-amino ester) NPs were introduced to deliver CDNs to the cytosol, which leads to robust immune response > 100-fold lower extracellular CDN concentration in vitro. This NP-mediated cytosolic delivery for STING agonists synergizes with checkpoint inhibitors and has the potential for enhanced immunotherapy [158]. A new strategy of cancer immunotherapy using plant virus-based NPs was proposed. In vaccine development, plant virus has already been utilized extensively. Successful employment of plant viruses in cancer treatment has been observed using hibiscus chlorotic ringspot virus, tomato bushy stunt virus, and red clover necrotic mosaic virus. Plant viruses offer the advantage of uniformity concerning shape and size and ability to self assemble into highly repeating nanostructures. They also exhibit structurally defined chemical attachment sites, cargo capacity, and tolerance against high temperature and pH [159]. Metallic NPs also have high potential in immunotherapy. Several metallic NPs such as Au NPs have been studied to be used with several immunotherapeutic agents such as ovalbumin (OVA). Metallic NPs have also shown to improve antitumour cytotoxic T cell response. Metallic NPs have advantages which can be utilized with combination therapy of immunotherapy and PTT [160]. Elimination or reprogramming of the immune-suppressive tumour microenvironment is a major challenge in immunotherapy. Immune checkpoint inhibition targets regulatory pathways in T cells to enhance tumour response and has been the most successful method in immunotherapy. Some FDA-approved immune checkpoint agents are ipilimumab against CTLA-4, and pembrolizumab and nivolumab against PD-1. Lipid-based NPs are generally used to transport these materials to the target site [161]. A study showed that R848-loaded β—cyclodextrin NPs can efficiently be delivered to tumour-associated macrophages in vivo to macrophages to acquire an antitumourigenic M1-like phenotype. The functional orientation of the tumour immune microenvironment toward an M1 phenotype was achieved through the administration of CDNP-R848 in multiple mouse models. An improved immune response rate was observed when combined with immune checkpoint inhibitor anti-PD-1 [162]. Exosomes are nanosized particles secreted from most cells. This allows crosstalk between cells and their surrounding environment through cargo transfer. Tumour cells also secrete exosomes, known as tumour-derived exosomes. They have tumour modulation activity and can affect the tumour microenvironment and antitumour response. Their immunological activity influences both innate and adaptive immune systems, including regulatory T-cell maturation, natural killer cell activity, and anti-inflammatory response. Their characteristics allow them to be used for metastasis lung cancer treatment [163].

4. Theranostics

Theranostics involves the administration of a diagnosis agent. They are referred to as a combination of diagnosis and therapy using the same agent [164].

4.1. Multimodality Imaging

SPIONs, (Feraheme, FH) and [^{89}Zr]Zr was used as a nanoplatform for PET and MRI. PET-MRI integrates the excellent sensitivity of PET with the spatial resolution and contrast of soft tissue by MRI. Feraheme can shorten the transverse relaxation time, T_2, and is generally used for dark contrast enhancement. However, dark contrast is often difficult to implement in clinical settings for applications such as detection and diagnosis of metastases in the lymph nodes. FH radiolabelled with OET tracer can take advantage of highly sensitive bright signals from PET. It can detect the presence of FH in regions, where the MRI contrast is too low or noisy. Experimental results showed that FH is a very suitable SPION for chelate-free labelling of PET tracers, and can be used in hybrid PET-MRI [165]. For combined magnetomotive ultrasound PET/CT and MRI for sentinel lymph nodes, ^{68}Ga-labelled SPIONs were proposed. The results showed that the SPIONs provided viable contrast enhancement [166]. TAM is significantly associated with poor prognosis of tumours. Using super magnetic iron oxide and perfluorocarbon nanoemulsions, quantitative monitoring of TAM is possible with MRI-based TAM imaging. A study was conducted using MRI-based measurements of TAMs as a prognostic marker and PET to observe tumour behaviour with ^{18}F-2-fluroro-2-deoxy-D-glucose as a radioactive tracer [167]. Ultra-small AGuIX NPs are made of polysiloxane and are surrounded by gadolinium chelates. They are generally obtained via the top-down process. They are the first multifunctional silica-based NPs that are small enough to escape hepatic clearance. Their hydrodynamic diameter is under 5 nm, and they have excellent radiosensitizing properties for radiotherapy. They can be used in four different types of imaging modalities: MRI, SPECT, fluorescence imaging, and CT. A recent study showed that they can be used in MRI-guided radiotherapy. The study found that ^{68}Ga-AGuIX@NODAGA has great potential in PET/MRI-guided radiotherapy. They can be used as a dual modality PET/MRI imaging agent with passive accumulation in the diseased area [168].

Image-guided radiotherapy can improve cancer outcomes significantly [169–171]. A theranostic platform and a combination of bismuth and gadolinium were proposed for onsite radiosensitization and image contrast enhancement. A study showed that NPs provided image enhancement in both CT and MRI, and tumour suppression with prolonged survival in non-small cell lung carcinoma models with minimal off-target toxicity [172]. Mesoporous silica NPs for CT and optical imaging were introduced. The high density of platinum NPs in the surface of mesoporous silica NPs greatly enhances CT contrast. NIR fluorescent dye Dy800 was conjugated to the platform to enhance optical imaging contrast. It was tested on a breast tumour mouse model. In vivo imaging showed significant enhancement in images after 24 h injection [173]. A multimodal imaging probe for PET/SPECT and MRI (T_2) was developed using SPIONs and deblock copolymer with either methoxy polyethylene glycol or primary amine NH_2 end groups. $^{57}Co^{2+}$ ions were used as a radioactive tracer and the study results found the probe to be nontoxic [174]. Another biomedical probe with an Au NP platform was introduced that is capable of coordinating Gd^{3+} for MRI and $^{67}Gd^{3+}$ for SPECT imaging. The Au NPs had high affinity toward the gastrin-releasing peptide receptor. These receptors are overexpressed in various human cancer cells, mainly in PC3 prostate cancer cells [175]. A multifunctional targeting NP probe for pancreatic cancer was introduced that consists of 1,2 Distearoyl-sn-glycero-3-phosphoethanolamine-N-amino (polyethylene glycol)-modified SPIONs, which were conjugated with the plectin-1 antibody. In vivo optical imaging and MRI show that they highly accumulate in MIAPaCa2 and XPA-1 carcinoma cells. They can be used as a theranostic tool in fluorescence and MRI to visualize pancreatic cancer [176]. Myocardial infection (MI) is a common disease and has a high mortality rate. MnO-based NPs in conjunction with MRI and NIR fluorescence imaging can help to combat against MI. MnO possess high r_1 relaxivity and has none or minimal toxicity. They can be used as an MRI contrast agent and as a drug carrier due to their preference to accumulate in the infarcted myocardium, as shown in fluorescence imaging [177]. Dendrimers with size range between 7–12 nm have advantages over other NPs due to their improved tumour penetration ability and inclusion of a tumour-specific drug release mechanism. G5 PAMAM dendrimer can be used with a paramagnetic chemical exchange saturation transfer (PARACEST) MRI contrast agent in MRI-optical imaging as dual mode MRI-optical glioma imaging NPs. Experimental results showed they were able to identify glioma tumours at a mm scale due to the perseverance of the MRI contrast throughout the glioma [178].

Nanoparticles that have high absorption in the NIR region are valuable in biomedical applications. Photoacoustic imaging (PAI) is an imaging modality that makes use of optical excitation. The imaging provides deep tissue penetration and high spatial resolution. In PAI, the photoacoustic signal is primarily determined by the pulsed laser. Therefore, the contrast agents used in PAI generally can also be used in PTT. Mesoporous carbon nanospheres (Meso-CNS), as a stable suspension with broadband and intense absorption in the UV–vis–NIR region, were studied. The analysis of photothermal conversion and photoacoustic generation show Meso-CNS possess absorption coefficients that are 1.5–2 times higher than those of CNT and graphene in the broad wavelength region, and comparable to gold nanorod in both NIR-I and NIR-II region. They can efficiently (35 wt%) load DOX due to their large surface area, appropriate pore volume, and size. All of these characteristics make them an excellent theranostic platform [179]. A dual-mode imaging system of photoacoustic microscopy and fluorescence optical microscopy with Au NPs was also proposed. Gold nanoparticles have a large absorption coefficient and enough fluoresce emission with a wavelength of 512 nm. They can be used to label certain drugs in tobacco cells, and also can be used to carry the labelled drug in the target position [180].

4.2. Image-Guided Therapy

A semiconducting plasmonic nanovesicle was proposed that consisted of semiconducting poly (perylene diimide) (PPDI) and poly(ethylene glycol) (PEG) tethered to Au NPs (Au@PPDI/PEG). The complex was highly localized and had a strong electromagnetic field between adjacent Au NPs in the vesicular shell. The electromagnetic field enhanced the light absorption efficiency of PPDI. It generates a great photothermal effect. It also provides a strong photoacoustic signal that can be used in PAI. Overall, the complex has high potential as a theranostic agent [181]. Gold nanorods in PAI and plasmonic PTT have been studied. The advantageous properties of Au NPs such as biocompatibility, tuneable surface plasmonic resonance, and controlled synthesis make them a great choice for theranostic applications. PAI-guided PTT is possible when the pulse is used to destroy the cancer cells. This application has great potential to be used for lung cancer [182]. A hybrid reduced graphene oxide (rGO)-loaded ultra-small plasmonic gold nanorod vesicle (rGO-AuNRVe) had excellent photoacoustic signal amplification ability, and the photothermal effect was proposed as a theranostic tool to be used in PIA, PTT, and chemotherapy. It had high DOX loading capability and efficiency, and it can unload upon light NIR photothermal heating. This ability makes them ideal for a combination of photochemotherapy. When rGO-AuNRVe was labelled with ^{64}Cu, it showed high accumulation in U87MG tumours via passive accumulation in PET imaging [183]. Pure bismuth NPs have ultrahigh x-ray attenuation coefficient and light to heat conversion capabilities. These characteristics make them suitable to be used in PAI and PTT. In one study, bismuth NPs were able to increase the temperature by 70 degrees Celsius within 4 min under infrared irradiation in PTT [184]. Carbon nanotubes have advantageous optical, thermal, mechanical, electrical, and magnetic properties. Some of the applications of CNT in biology are as a heating agent, contrast agent, and drug delivery agent. Carbon nanotubes can increase the temperature in the tissue during laser irradiation in PTT, and at the same time, enhance photoacoustic signals. The nanotubes can potentially be used as a theranostic agent in PTT and PAI [185]. A theranostic agent was developed that consists of perfluorohexane liquid and Au NPs that make up the core and is stabilized by a polymer shell (poly (lactide-co-glycolic acid)(PLGA)). When PLGA-Au NPs localize in tumour cells and are exposed to laser pulses, cell viability decreases, leading to cell death. The study results showed they have viable potential to be used as a PAI and therapeutic agent for future clinical cancer therapy [186].

Gold nanoparticles have a high atomic number and they strongly absorb low and medium energy x-rays by the photoelectric effect [187–189]. During the photoelectric effect, characteristic x-rays and Auger electrons released in the surroundings are in a short-range. They can cause additional local damage [190]. Gold nanoparticles can be conjugated to targeting ligands or they can selectively be accumulated into the tumour via passive permeability and retention effects. Due to these abilities, they have high potential to be very effective in tumour radiotherapy augmentation without increasing the dose to the surrounding normal tissues, and can also be used as a contrast agent in CT, making it an excellent theranostic tool [191,192]. A hyaluronic acid-functionalized bismuth oxide NP was synthesized using a one-pot hydrothermal method used in targeting specific CT imaging and radiosensitizing of tumour. The integration of hyaluronic acid Bi_2O_3 NPs provides solubility in water and excellent biocompatibility. Targeting mechanism allows them to be taken up specifically by CD44 receptors overexpressed in cancer cells. HA-Bi_2O_3 NPs have high x-ray attenuation efficiency. They also have ideal radiosensitivity through synergizing x-rays to induce cell apoptosis and arrest cell cycle in a dose-dependent manner. A study showed that these active targeting NPs provide excellent CT imaging enhancement and can be used as a theranostic tool [193].

A liposome-coencapsulated DOX, hollow Au NPs, and perfluorocarbon were synthesized into a theranostic agent. It had an efficient light-to-heat conversion effect under 808 nm NIR laser irradiation and small size that enabled high accumulation in the tumour sites. It also had an efficient DOX release and enhanced ultrasound signal. All of these properties make it an excellent theranostic agent in PTT and ultrasound imaging [194]. Another ultrasonic photothermal agent was introduced that consists of NBs, graphene oxide, and hairpin sulfate proteoglycan glypican-3 (target molecule). It can work as a molecularly targeted contrast agent and contrast enhancer for ultrasound imaging. It can also be used in combination with ultrasound and PTT [195]. A new NBs–paclitaxel liposome complex for ultrasound imaging and ultrasound responsive drug delivery was introduced. The complex was 528.7 ± 31.7 nm in size with paclitaxel entrapment efficiency of 85.4 ± 4.39%, and conjugation efficiency of ~98.7 ± 0.14% with 200 nm-sized liposomes. When treated with the NBs–paclitaxel liposome, the sonoporation of MiaPaCa-2 cells had 2.5-fold higher uptake of liposomes compared to the control. It also had more than 300-fold higher anticancer activity compared to the commercial formulation ABRAZANE. The conjugate exhibits echogenicity comparable to the commercial ultrasound contrast agent SonoVue, where the echogenic stability of NBs–paclitaxel was more than one week. These properties and the image enhancing properties make it an excellent theranostic agent [196].

Silica NPs have been intensively studied in drug delivery and can be integrated with other materials for theranostic capabilities. The MnO/SiO_2 core–shell can be used for multimodal imaging. Its localization can be monitored with MRI and poly (propylene fumarate) scaffolds. The anticancer drug DOX can be loaded into it. Its porous silica shell enhances the water dispersibility of the core and minimizes leakage of the core iron [197]. Carbon dots are widely used in optical imaging nanoprobes. They are generally used for labelling cells in cancer treatment. A study proposed a gadolinium complex that consists of carbon nanodots. They have high fluorescent properties, excellent water solubility, and biocompatibility. They can also be conjugated to apoferritin nanocages for drug loading capabilities such as DOX. Folic acid can be used as a targeting molecule for MCF-7 cells and the results showed it is a viable theranostic tool with negligible toxicity [198]. A new iron (III)–tannic complex-based NP (Fe–TA NP) was introduced. It had good physicochemical properties with the capability of inducing autophagy in both hepatocellular carcinoma cells (HePG2.2.15) and normal rat hepatocytes (AML12). Experimental results showed the Fe–TA NP was capable of inducing HepG2.2.15 cell death via autography and did not affect cell viability in AML12 cells due to much higher uptake of the Fe-TA NPs by the HepG2.2.15 cells. Enhancement of the T_1 MRI contrast was achieved in HepG2.2.15 cells due to these circumstances. These results also suggest that the Fe–TA NP can provide new strategies for combining diagnostic and therapeutic functions for hepatocellular carcinoma [199].

A synergistic platform for synergistic therapy and real-time imaging was studied. It is very advantageous when treating cancer patients. However, it also faces many challenges for clinical use. Novel theranostic agent, bismuth sulfide@mesoporous silica ($Bi_2S_3@mPs$) core–shell NPs were introduced to be used in targeted image-guided therapy for EGFR-2 positive breast cancer. The agent was obtained by decorating polyvinylpyrrolidone with Bi_2S_3 NR. It was chemically encapsulated with a mesoporous silica layer loaded with DOX, an anticancer drug. Trastuzumab was used as a targeting molecule that targets EGFR-2. They overexpressed in breast cancer cells. Experimental results showed the agent has good drug loading capabilities, biocompatibility, strong x-ray attenuation of the bismuth element, and precise tumour targeting and accumulation. These characteristics allow it to simultaneously act as a contrast enhancer for CT in deep tissue and as a therapeutic agent in synergistic photothermal chemotherapy [200]. Another synergistic treatment platform was developed for PAI, targeted PTT, and chemotherapy. Its use was studied in triple-negative breast cancer. The nanoplatform was composed of magnetic hybrid NP (lipid, doxorubicin), gold nanorods, and an iron oxide nanocluster (LDGI) loaded with mesenchymal stem cells. LDGIs have efficient cellular uptake by stem cells and are still be able to maintain their cellular function. LDGI can simultaneously release drugs and achieve photothermal properties upon light irradiation. The drug can then enter the cell and activate cell apoptosis. Mesenchymal stem cells have the highest enhanced migration and penetration abilities in tumours. It also showed the best antitumour efficacy in chemophotothermal therapy compared to other treatment groups in triple-negative breast cancer [201]. Another study showed a new strategy to use gold nanorod conjugated with polyacrylic acid/calcium phosphate (AuNR@PAA/CaP) yolk-shell NPs for dual-mode x-ray CT/PAI and PTT. It possesses extremely high DOX loading capabilities, pH and NIR dual responsive drug delivery ability, and high photothermal conversion properties. At low pH, the CaP shell takes damage and releases DOX. When the conjugate is exposed to NIR irradiation, burst-like drug release occurs [202]. A human cytokine-induced killer cell (CIK) was loaded with gold nanorods that were used for targeted PAI, enhanced immunotherapy, and PTT for gastric cancer. The study results showed that CIK-labelled gold nanorods actively target gastric cancer MGC803 cells and activate cell apoptosis under NIR laser irradiation. The results also showed CIKAuNR can actively target and image subcutaneous gastric cancer vessels via PIA after 4 h of injection. It can also enhance immunotherapy by regulating cytokines and kill gastric cancer cells by PTT [203]. SPIONs have high r_1 and r_2 relativities and they can be completely eliminated from the body. They can accumulate in cancer through passive targeting permeability, and retention effects or active targeting. The magnetite and maghemite cores of SPIONs can easily be detected with MRI. Polymer coating SPIONs can be loaded with therapeutic agents to facilitate MRI-guided drug delivery, PTT, PDT, gene therapy, or magnetic hyperthermia. SPIONs-delivered chemotherapy has high potential, and a variety of small chemotherapeutic agents have been incorporated into SPIONs-based nanocarriers through a cleavable linker or π–π stacking. They can increase blood circulation half-life, promote tumour retention, and enable real-time drug tracking. Accumulation of SPIONs in the spleen or other reticuloendothelial systems can exert toxic effects after multiple-dose administration. Smart or responsive SPIONs have been developed to mediate that problem. SPIONs can also be used as a carrier for small interfering RNA (siRNA) or microRNA (miRNA), which can protect the ribonucleic acid and prevent enzyme degradation [204].

4.3. Combination Therapy

Combination therapy provides treatment of several malignancies to improve clinical outcomes. They generally induce synergistic drug action and try to work around drug resistance. There are several NPs used in combination therapy such as liposomes. Various liposomal formulation of DOX include DaunoXome, Doxil, DepoCyt, and ONCO-TCS. Liposomes are one of the most established drug delivery vehicles, with many clinical products. Some other NPs that are used in combination therapy are polymeric NPs. They have high thermodynamic and kinetic properties used in site-specific delivery of the anticancer drug to tumours. Metallic NPs, dendrimers, nanodiamonds, carbon NPs, and CNT are some other ones used in combination therapy [205]. A mesoporous NP-based drug delivery system was introduced to be used for real-time imaging in photothermal/photodynamic therapy and nanozyme oxidative therapy. In one study on synthesized mesoporous carbon–gold hybrid nanozyme nanoprobes, carbon nanospheres were doped with small Au NPs, and stabilized with a complex of reduced serum albumin and folic acid. They were then loaded with IR780 iodide. Their large surface area and numerous -COOH groups allowed for chemical modification for numerous targeting molecules, load abundant NIR dye, and photothermal agents. Small Au NPs were utilized as nanozymes to catalyze H_2O_2 located in the tumour cells to generate OH for intracellular oxidative damage to the tumour. In vivo and vitro results showed the nanoprobe had excellent tumour targeting efficacy, long tumour retention, and favorable therapeutic effect [206]. For combined PDT/PTT with photodecomposable, photothermal, and photodynamic properties, SP^3NPs were prepared from self-assembled PEGylated cypate that consists of PEG and ICG derivate. It can generate singlet oxygen for PDT and photothermal effect for PTT. It has high accumulation in tumour due to PEGylated surface and small size (~60 nm). All of these properties make it a potential candidate to be used in image-guided PDT/PTT [207].

Chemotherapy is one of the most common cancer treatment options, but it has showed off-target toxicity issues. Theranostic NPs integrates diagnostic and therapeutic functions within one platform, increases tumour selectivity for more effective therapy, and assists in diagnosis and monitoring of therapeutic response. Core–shell NPs were synthesized by nanoprecipitation of blends of the biodegradable and biocompatible amphiphilic copolymers poly (lactic-co-glycolic acid)-b-ply-L-lysine and poly (lactic acid)-b-ply (ethylene glycol). The NPs were spherical and had an average size of 60–90 nm. DOX was encapsulated in the core of the NPs. The results showed a 33-fold increase in NIR fluorescence in the mouse model and found it to be suitable for a controlled drug delivery system and a contrast agent for imaging cancer cells [208]. PTT in combination with chemotherapy can trigger powerful antitumour immunity against tumours. Polydopamine-coated spiky Au NPs with high photothermal stability were introduced for PTT and chemotherapy. A single round of PTT combined with a subtherapeutic dose of DOX can yield good antitumour immune response and eliminate primary and untreated distant metastasis in 85% of animals bearing CT26 colon carcinoma. Their efficacy was studied against TC-1 submucosa-lung metastasis, a highly aggressive model for advanced head-and-neck squamous cell carcinoma [209]. Monotherapy of cancer is usually subjected to some sacrifice and as such, limits therapeutic benefits. Generally, in the form of systemic toxicity, a combination of chemo and PTT elevates the therapeutic benefits and is generally considered a maximal cooperation effect achieved in combination therapy. Silica NPs with Cetuximab to target the epidermal growth factor receptor were developed. They had a high drug loading capacity of Cet-SLN that can be used to encapsulate photothermal agent ICG. It can simultaneously codeliver ICG and Cet for combinational chemophotothermal therapy of breast cancer [210]. Approximately 90% of the cancer therapeutic failure in patients is due to chemoresistance. Some cancer cells such as progenitor cells or cancer stem cells develop radioresistance from a variety of chemotherapy agents. Chemo agents generally aim to destroy rapidly dividing cells and do not have much effect on undifferentiated cancer stem cells. Hepatocellular carcinoma is responsible for the third leading cause of cancer-related death and the fifth most common type of cancer. Gold nanorods have been studied to provide a solution. Gold nanoparticles in conjunction with PTT can destroy these cells and gold nanorods can provide suitable contrast agents for PAI. Gold nanoparticles can also act as a carrier. They can carry therapeutic agents such as Adr when in conjunction with EpCAM antibody on the surface of the nanosystem. Adr/AuNPs@Pms-antiEpCAM can specifically target cancer stem cells and enhance the concentration of drugs in the tumour. This complex can be useful as a future theranostic tool [211]. Modification of NPs allows administration of the drug across the brain and provide a theranostic platform for Alzheimer's, Parkinson's, Huntington's, and epilepsy disease. NPs can be used as a carrier to get past the blood–brain barrier and deliver the drug to the brain [212].

Photoacoustic and fluorescence imaging in NIR-II hold great potential due to their noninvasive nature and excellent spatial resolution properties. NIR-II is superior in biological imaging due to its higher signal-to-noise ratio and deeper tissue penetration. Photoacoustic imaging in NIR-II allows direct and wide visualization of dynamic biological tissues with high spatiotemporal resolution and sensitivity. It cannot provide comprehensive and accurate diagnosis information, so fluoroscopic imaging in NIR-II can make up the missing information in this dual imaging system. It can be used to facilitate image-guided synergistic chemophotodynamic therapy using gold nanorods. It can also be used as a carrier and allow precise controlled $^1O_2$ drug release [213]. Nanoscale coordination polymer core–shell NPs carry oxaliplatin in the core and photosensitize the pyropheophorbide–lipid conjugate in the shell for effective chemotherapy and PDT. The synergy between oxaliplatin and pyrolipid-induced PDT kills tumour cells and provokes an immune response. This results in calreticulin exposure on the cell surface, antitumour vaccination, and an abscopal effect [214].

Photothermal therapy can be an effective antitumour therapy but it may not eliminate tumour cells. This can lead to the risk of recurrence or metastasis. Photothermal therapy in combination with immunotherapy can minimize that risk. Polydopamine-coated Al_2O_3 NPs were introduced for this type of combination therapy. NIR laser irradiation can kill the majority of the tumour tissue via PTT. It also releases tumour-associated antigens. The Al_2O_3 within the NPs, together with CpG that acts as an adjuvant to trigger robust cell-mediated immune responses, can help eliminate the residual tumour cells. Fifty percent of mice, after going through combined therapy, achieved goal tumour eradication and survived for 120 days, which was the end goal of the experiment [215]. Photothermal therapy can be combined with blockage checkpoints to achieve an even more enhanced antitumour effect. Table 5 below summarizes different NPs that can be used in photothermal immunotherapy [216].

Table 5. Nanoparticles used in photothermal therapy (PTT) immunotherapy [216].

Photothermal NPs	Checkpoint Blockade	Effector Cells	Tumours
Prussian blue NPs	Anti-CTLA-4	$CD4^+/CD8^+$ T cells	Neuroblastoma
PEGylated single-walled nanotubes	Anti-CTLA-4	DCs, $CD4^+/CD8^+$ T cells, $CD20^+$ TILs	4T1 murine breast tumour, murine B16 musculus skin melanoma
PLGA-ICG-R837 NPs	Anti-CTLA-4	DCs, $CD4^+/CD8^+$, memory T cells	4T1 murine breast tumour, CT26 colorectal cancer
Gold nanostars	Anti-PD-L1	$CD4^+/CD8^+$ T cells, $CD19^+$ B cells	MB49 bladder tumour

ICG is a photothermal agent and imiquimod (R837) is a toll-like receptor-7 agonist. In one study, they were coencapsulated by poly (lactic-co-glycolic) acid (PLGA). The formed NPs were composed purely by three clinically approved components that can be used for NIR laser-triggered photothermal elimination of primary tumours. This generates tumour-associated antigens, which in the presence of adjuvant R837-containing NPs, show vaccine-like functions. In combination with the checkpoint blockade using anticytotoxic T-lymphocyte antigen-4 (CTTLA4), the generated immunological responses will be able to eliminate remaining tumour cells and will be very useful in metastasis inhibition [217]. Metastatic breast cancer is one of the most devastating cancers and has very limited therapeutic options. Nanoparticle-based platforms can offer some therapeutic options for it with different combinations of therapy. The chemotherapeutic drug DOX can be delivered using NPs. PTX formulated with albumin to form NPs is currently used in the clinic for breast cancer therapy. siRNA can also be delivered using NPs for gene therapy. Nanoparticles offer an option for photothermal therapy and magnetothermal therapy. They can also be used as a contrast enhancement agent for image-guided radiotherapy [218]. Gastric cancer is the second most malignant tumour in the world. HER-2 is one of the key targets for gastric cancer therapy. A gold nanoshell drug carrier was developed for delivery of immunotherapeutic agent and selective photothermal release of genes that targets HER-2 and the immunologic adjuvant CPG sequence in gastric tumour cells. This allows multidimensional treatment strategies such as gene, immune, and PTT. The study results showed good gene transduction ability and combined treatment effect [219]. A nanosystem consisting of ER targeting pardaxin peptides modified ICG conjugated to hollow gold nanospheres, together with oxygen delivering hemoglobin liposome was studied in PDT, PTT, and immunotherapy. It induces robust ER stress and calreticulin exposure on the cell surface under NIR light irradiation. CRT, a marker for ICD, acts as an eat-me signal to stimulate the antigen-presenting function of dendritic cells. It triggers a series of immunological responses including cytotoxic cytokine secretion and $CD8^+$ T cell proliferation [220]. A theranostic nanoplatform that was capable of PAI, as well as a combination of gene and photothermal therapy, were studied. A gold nanorod was coated with dipicolyl amine, which forms stable complexes with Zn^{2+} cations and yields a Zn (II) dipicolyl amine gold nanorod. It has a strong complexation with anti-polo like kinase 1 siRNA used for gene silencing. The Au NPs can act as a photothermal agent as well as an enhancer for photoacoustic imaging upon laser irradiation. Experimental results showed that they yield significant antitumour activity in the PC-3 tumour mouse model [221].

5. Conclusions

Recent advances in nanotechnology have resulted in great progress of synthetic techniques, which benefit from the design of many nanomaterials, such as nanoparticles, nanocages, nanodiamonds, nanoshells, and nanotubes. These nanomaterials can act as very effective contrast agents in various medical imaging modalities and provide a large number of options in modern cancer therapy. The nanomaterials allow delivery of many drugs to target sites that otherwise would not be possible and provide a fundamental basis for some cancer therapy that is showing promising clinical outcomes. It is expected that continuous discovery in nanotechnology will significantly influence future cancer therapy and medical imaging. However, some of the limitations of nanomaterials as drug carriers, contrast agents, and sensitizers, such as cytotoxicity and nonbiodegradability, should be studied further in order to minimize the side effects on humans.

For the transition of nanomaterial applications in biomedical imaging and cancer therapy into commercial clinical practice, it can be seen that many in vitro and in vivo studies have shown promising results. However, numerous challenges, such as physicochemical properties, drug metabolism, cytotoxicity and biocompatibility, pharmacokinetic screening, surface engineering, in vivo efficacy, nanomaterial uptake, immunogenic issues, and preparation costs, still remain. The mechanisms of action such as the potential impact on the cellular communication, which would limit its clinical transformation, are still unclear. Based on the above challenges, possible future directions include further optimizing various nanomaterials and elucidating the precise mechanisms between the cell and nanomaterials, to achieve better imaging and therapeutic effects, and accelerate the translation of nanomaterials into clinical practice.

Author Contributions: Methodology, J.C.L.C. and S.S.; writing-original draft preparation, S.S.; writing—review and editing, J.C.L.C.; supervision, J.C.L.C. All authors have read and agreed to the published version of the manuscript.

Funding: This research received no external funding.

Conflicts of Interest: The authors declare no conflict of interest.

References

1. Rosado-De-Castro, P.H.; Morales, M.D.P.; Pimentel-Coelho, P.M.; Mendez-Otero, R.; Herranz, F. Development and application of nanoparticles in biomedical imaging. *Contrast Media Mol. Imaging* **2018**. [CrossRef] [PubMed]
2. Lecuyer, T.; Teston, E.; Ramirez-Garcia, G.; Maldiney, T.; Viana, B.; Seguin, J.; Mignet, N.; Scherman, D.; Richard, C. Chemically engineered persistent luminescence nanoprobes for bioimaging. *Theranostics* **2016**, *6*, 2488. [CrossRef] [PubMed]
3. Liu, J.; Lécuyer, T.; Seguin, J.; Mignet, N.; Scherman, D.; Viana, B.; Richard, C. Imaging and therapeutic applications of persistent luminescence nanomaterials. *Adv. Drug Deliv. Rev.* **2019**, *138*, 193–210. [CrossRef] [PubMed]
4. Baetke, S.C.; Lammers, T.; Kiessling, F. Applications of nanoparticles for diagnosis and therapy of cancer. *Br. J. Radiol.* **2015**, *88*. [CrossRef] [PubMed]
5. Kim, J.; Lee, N.; Hyeon, T. Recent development of nanoparticles for molecular imaging. *Philos. Trans. R. Soc. A Math. Phys. Eng. Sci.* **2017**, *375*. [CrossRef] [PubMed]
6. Burke, B.P.; Cawthorne, C.; Archibald, S.J. Multimodal nanoparticle imaging agents: Design and applications. *Philos. Trans. R. Soc. A Math. Phys. Eng. Sci.* **2017**, *375*. [CrossRef]
7. Yousaf, T.; Dervenoulas, G.; Politis, M. Advances in MRI Methodology. *Int. Rev. Neurobiol.* **2018**, *141*, 31–76. [CrossRef]
8. Hemond, C.C.; Bakshi, R. Magnetic resonance imaging in multiple sclerosis. *Cold Spring Harb. Perspect. Med.* **2018**, *8*, 1–21. [CrossRef]
9. Behzadi, A.H.; Farooq, Z.; Newhouse, J.H.; Prince, M.R. MRI and CT contrast media extravasation. *Medcine* **2018**, *97*. [CrossRef]
10. Esqueda, A.C.; López, J.A.; Andreu-de-Riquer, G.; Alvarado-Monzón, J.C.; Ratnakar, J.; Lubag, A.J.; Sherry, A.D.; De León-Rodríguez, L.M. A new gadolinium-based MRI zinc sensor. *J. Am. Chem. Soc.* **2009**, *131*, 11387–11391. [CrossRef]

11. Lux, J.; Sherry, A.D. Advances in gadolinium-based MRI contrast agent designs for monitoring biological processes in vivo. *Curr. Opin. Chem. Biol.* **2018**, *45*, 121–130. [CrossRef] [PubMed]
12. Liu, X.; Madhankumar, A.B.; Miller, P.A.; Duck, K.A.; Hafenstein, S.; Rizk, E.; Slagle-Webb, B.; Sheehan, J.M.; Connor, J.R.; Yang, Q.X. MRI contrast agent for targeting glioma: Interleukin-13 labeled liposome encapsulating gadolinium-DTPA. *Neuro. Oncol.* **2016**, *18*, 691–699. [CrossRef] [PubMed]
13. McMahon, M.T.; Bulte, J.W.M. Two decades of dendrimers as versatile MRI agents: A tale with and without metals. *Wiley Interdiscip. Rev. Nanomed. Nanobiotechnol.* **2018**, *10*, e1496. [CrossRef] [PubMed]
14. Moghimi, H.; Zohdiaghdam, R.; Riahialam, N.; Behrouzkia, Z. The assessment of toxicity characteristics of cellular uptake of paramagnetic nanoparticles as a new magnetic resonance imaging contrast agent. *Iran. J. Pharm. Res.* **2019**, *18*, 2083–2092. [CrossRef]
15. Rogosnitzky, M.; Branch, S. Gadolinium-based contrast agent toxicity: A review of known and proposed mechanisms. *BioMetals* **2016**, *29*, 365–376. [CrossRef]
16. Layne, K.A.; Dargan, P.I.; Archer, J.R.H.; Wood, D.M. Gadolinium deposition and the potential for toxicological sequelae – A literature review of issues surrounding gadolinium-based contrast agents. *Br. J. Clin. Pharmacol.* **2018**, *84*, 2522–2534. [CrossRef]
17. Ramalho, J.; Semelka, R.C.; Ramalho, M.; Nunes, R.H.; AlObaidy, M.; Castillo, M. Gadolinium-based contrast agent accumulation and toxicity: An update. *Am. J. Neuroradiol.* **2016**, *37*, 1192–1198. [CrossRef]
18. Wei, H.; Bruns, O.T.; Kaul, M.G.; Hansen, E.C.; Barch, M.; Wiśniowska, A.; Chen, O.; Chen, Y.; Li, N.; Okada, S.; et al. Exceedingly small iron oxide nanoparticles as positive MRI contrast agents. *Proc. Natl. Acad. Sci. USA* **2017**, *114*, 2325–2330. [CrossRef]
19. Dulińska-Litewka, J.; Łazarczyk, A.; Hałubiec, P.; Szafrański, O.; Karnas, K.; Karewicz, A. Superparamagnetic iron oxide nanoparticles-current and prospective medical applications. *Materials* **2019**. [CrossRef]
20. Kim, S.J.; Lewis, B.; Steiner, M.S.; Bissa, U.V.; Dose, C.; Frank, J.A. Superparamagnetic iron oxide nanoparticles for direct labelling of stem cells and in vivo MRI tracking. *Contrast Media Mol. Imaging* **2016**, *11*, 55–64. [CrossRef]
21. Iyer, S.R.; Xu, S.; Stains, J.P.; Bennett, C.H.; Lovering, R.M. Superparamagnetic iron oxide nanoparticles in musculoskeletal biology. *Tissue Eng. Part. B Rev.* **2017**, *23*, 373–385. [CrossRef] [PubMed]
22. Kumar, S.; Kumar, B.S.H.; Khushu, S. Increased transverse relaxivity in ultrasmall superparamagnetic iron oxide nanoparticles used as MRI contrast agent for biomedical imaging. *Contrast Media Mol. Imaging* **2016**. [CrossRef]
23. Hobson, N.J.; Weng, X.; Siow, B.; Veiga, C.; Ashford, M.; Thanh, N.T.K.; Schätzlein, A.G.; Uchegbu, I.F. Clustering superparamagnetic iron oxide nanoparticles produces organ-Targeted high-contrast magnetic resonance images. *Nanomedicine* **2019**, *14*, 1135–1152. [CrossRef] [PubMed]
24. Shari, S.; Seyednejad, H.; Laurent, S.; Atyabi, F. Superparamagnetic iron oxide nanoparticles for in vivo molecular and cellular imaging. *Contrast Media Mol. Imaging* **2015**. [CrossRef]
25. Wang, Z.J.; Ohliger, M.A.; Larson, P.E.Z.; Gordon, J.W.; Bok, R.A.; Slater, J.; Villanueva-Meyer, J.E.; Hess, C.P.; Kurhanewicz, J.; Vigneron, D.B. Hyperpolarized 13C MRI: State of the art and future directions. *Radiology* **2019**, *291*, 273–284. [CrossRef]
26. Kurhanewicz, J.; Vigneron, D.B.; Ardenkjaer-Larsen, J.H.; Bankson, J.A.; Brindle, K.; Cunningham, C.H.; Gallagher, F.A.; Keshari, K.R.; Kjaer, A.; Laustsen, C.; et al. Hyperpolarized 13C MRI: Path to Clinical Translation in Oncology. *Neoplasia* **2019**, *21*, 1–16. [CrossRef]
27. Cho, A.; Lau, J.Y.C.; Geraghty, B.J.; Cunningham, C.H.; Keshari, K.R. Noninvasive interrogation of cancer metabolism with hyperpolarized 13C MRI. *J. Nucl. Med.* **2017**, *58*, 1201–1206. [CrossRef]
28. Malik, M.; Chaudhary, R.; Pundir, C.S. An improved enzyme nanoparticles based amperometric pyruvate biosensor for detection of pyruvate in serum. *Enzym. Microb. Technol.* **2019**, *123*, 30–38. [CrossRef]
29. Waddington, D.E.J.; Sarracanie, M.; Zhang, H.; Salameh, N.; Glenn, D.R.; Rej, E.; Gaebel, T.; Boele, T.; Walsworth, R.L.; Reilly, D.J.; et al. Nanodiamond-enhanced MRI via in situ hyperpolarization. *Nat. Commun.* **2017**, *8*, 1–8. [CrossRef]
30. Kostarelos, K.; Bianco, A.; Prato, M. Promises, facts and challenges for carbon nanotubes in imaging and therapeutics. *Nat. Nanotechnol.* **2009**, *4*, 627–633. [CrossRef]
31. De La Zerda, A.; Zavaleta, C.; Keren, S.; Vaithilingam, S.; Bodapati, S.; Liu, Z.; Levi, J.; Smith, B.R.; Ma, T.J.; Oralkan, O.; et al. Carbon nanotubes as photoacoustic molecular imaging agents in living mice. *Nat. Nanotechnol.* **2008**, *3*, 557–562. [CrossRef] [PubMed]

32. Welsher, K.; Liu, Z.; Sherlock, S.P.; Robinson, J.T.; Chen, Z.; Daranciang, D.; Dai, H. A route to brightly fluorescent carbon nanotubes for near-infrared imaging in mice. *Nat. Nanotechnol.* **2009**, *4*, 773–780. [CrossRef] [PubMed]
33. Garg, B.; Sung, C.H.; Ling, Y.C. Graphene-based nanomaterials as molecular imaging agents. *Wiley Interdiscip. Rev. Nanomed. Nanobiotechnol.* **2015**, *7*, 737–758. [CrossRef] [PubMed]
34. Nurunnabi, M.; Khatun, Z.; Reeck, G.R.; Lee, D.Y.; Lee, Y.K. Photoluminescent graphene nanoparticles for cancer phototherapy and imaging. *ACS Appl. Mat. Interf.* **2014**, *6*, 12413–12421. [CrossRef]
35. Cai, X.; Zhu, Q.; Zeng, Y.; Zeng, Q.; Chen, X.; Zhan, Y. Manganese oxide nanoparticles as mri contrast agents in tumor multimodal imaging and therapy. *Int. J. Nanomed.* **2019**, *14*, 8321–8344. [CrossRef]
36. Kwiatkowski, G.; Jähnig, F.; Steinhauser, J.; Wespi, P.; Ernst, M.; Kozerke, S. Nanometer size silicon particles for hyperpolarized MRI. *Sci. Rep.* **2017**, *7*, 1–6. [CrossRef]
37. Yoo, S.P.; Pineda, F.; Barrett, J.C.; Poon, C.; Tirrell, M.; Chung, E.J. Gadolinium-functionalized peptide amphiphile micelles for multimodal imaging of atherosclerotic lesions. *ACS Omega* **2016**, *1*, 996–1003. [CrossRef]
38. Dong, Y.C.; Hajfathalian, M.; Maidment, P.S.N.; Hsu, J.C.; Naha, P.C.; Si-Mohamed, S.; Breuilly, M.; Kim, J.; Chhour, P.; Douek, P.; et al. Effect of gold nanoparticle size on their properties as contrast agents for computed tomography. *Sci. Rep.* **2019**, *9*, 1–13. [CrossRef]
39. Silvestri, A.; Zambelli, V.; Ferretti, A.M.; Salerno, D.; Bellani, G.; Polito, L. Design of functionalized gold nanoparticle probes for computed tomography imaging. *Contrast Media Mol. Imaging* **2016**, *11*, 405–414. [CrossRef]
40. Nakagawa, T.; Gonda, K.; Kamei, T.; Cong, L.; Hamada, Y.; Kitamura, N.; Tada, H.; Ishida, T.; Aimiya, T.; Furusawa, N.; et al. X-ray computed tomography imaging of a tumor with high sensitivity using gold nanoparticles conjugated to a cancer-specific antibody via polyethylene glycol chains on their surface. *Sci. Technol. Adv. Mater.* **2016**, *17*, 387–397. [CrossRef]
41. Mok, P.L.; Leow, S.N.; Koh, A.E.H.; Mohd Nizam, H.H.; Ding, S.L.S.; Luu, C.; Ruhaslizan, R.; Wong, H.S.; Halim, W.H.W.A.; Ng, M.H.; et al. Micro-computed tomography detection of gold nanoparticle-labelled mesenchymal stem cells in the rat subretinal layer. *Int. J. Mol. Sci.* **2017**, *18*, 345. [CrossRef] [PubMed]
42. Farooq Aziz, A.I.; Nazir, A.; Ahmad, I.; Bajwa, S.Z.; Rehman, A.; Diallo, A.; Khan, W.S. Novel route synthesis of porous and solid gold nanoparticles for investigating their comparative performance as contrast agent in computed tomography scan and effect on liver and kidney function. *Int. J. Nanomed.* **2017**, *12*, 1555. [CrossRef] [PubMed]
43. Cheheltani, R.; Ezzibdeh, R.M.; Chhour, P.; Pulaparthi, K.; Kim, J.; Jurcova, M.; Hsu, J.C.; Blundell, C.; Litt, H.I.; Ferrari, V.A.; et al. Tunable, biodegradable gold nanoparticles as contrast agents for computed tomography and photoacoustic imaging. *Biomaterials* **2016**, *102*, 87–97. [CrossRef] [PubMed]
44. Hainfeld, J.F.; Ridwan, S.M.; Stanishevskiy, Y.; Smilowitz, N.R.; Davis, J.; Smilowitz, H.M. Small, long blood half-life iodine nanoparticle for vascular and tumor imaging. *Sci. Rep.* **2018**, *8*, 2–11. [CrossRef]
45. Sun, N.; Zhao, L.; Zhu, J.; Li, Y.; Song, N.; Xing, Y.; Qiao, W.; Huang, H.; Zhao, J. 131I-labeled polyethylenimine-entrapped gold nanoparticles for targeted tumor Spect/Ct imaging and radionuclide therapy. *Int. J. Nanomed.* **2019**, *14*, 4367–4381. [CrossRef]
46. Kim, H.; Jang, E.J.; Kim, S.K.; Hyung, W.J.; Choi, D.K.; Lim, S.J.; Lim, J.S. Simultaneous sentinel lymph node computed tomography and locoregional chemotherapy for lymph node metastasis in rabbit using an iodine-docetaxel emulsion. *Oncotarget* **2017**, *8*, 27177–27188. [CrossRef]
47. Badea, C.T.; Clark, D.P.; Holbrook, M.; Srivastava, M.; Mowery, Y.; Ghaghada, K.B. Functional imaging of tumor vasculature using iodine and gadolinium-based nanoparticle contrast agents: A comparison of spectral micro-CT using energy integrating and photon counting detectors. *Phys. Med. Biol.* **2019**, *64*, 65007. [CrossRef]
48. Chen, J.; Yang, X.Q.; Qin, M.Y.; Zhang, X.S.; Xuan, Y.; Zhao, Y.D. Hybrid nanoprobes of bismuth sulfide nanoparticles and CdSe/ZnS quantum dots for mouse computed tomography/fluorescence dual mode imaging. *J. Nanobiotechnol.* **2015**, *13*, 1–10. [CrossRef]
49. Santos, B.S.; Ferreira, M.J. Positron emission tomography in ischemic heart disease. *Rev. Port. Cardiol.* **2019**, *38*, 599–608. [CrossRef]

50. Lee, S.B.; Lee, S.W.; Jeong, S.Y.; Yoon, G.; Cho, S.J.; Kim, S.K.; Lee, I.K.; Ahn, B.C.; Lee, J.; Jeon, Y.H. Engineering of radioiodine-labeled gold core-shell nanoparticles as efficient nuclear medicine imaging agents for trafficking of dendritic cells. *ACS Appl. Mater. Interfaces* **2017**, *9*, 8480–8489. [CrossRef]
51. Simón, M.; Jørgensen, J.T.; Norregaard, K.; Kjaer, A. 18F-FDG positron emission tomography and diffusion-weighted magnetic resonance imaging for response evaluation of nanoparticle-mediated photothermal therapy. *Sci. Rep.* **2020**, *10*, 1–9. [CrossRef]
52. Liu, Y.; Carpenter, A.B.; Pirozzi, C.J.; Yuan, H.; Waitkus, M.S.; Zhou, Z.; Hansen, L.; Seywald, M.; Odion, R.; Greer, P.K.; et al. Non-invasive sensitive brain tumor detection using dual-modality bioimaging nanoprobe. *Nanotechnology* **2019**, *30*, 275101. [CrossRef] [PubMed]
53. Lee, S.B.; Kumar, D.; Li, Y.; Lee, I.K.; Cho, S.J.; Kim, S.K.; Lee, S.W.; Jeong, S.Y.; Lee, J.; Jeon, Y.H. PEGylated crushed gold shell-radiolabeled core nanoballs for in vivo tumor imaging with dual positron emission tomography and Cerenkov luminescent imaging. *J. Nanobiotechnol.* **2018**, *16*, 1–12. [CrossRef] [PubMed]
54. Cui, L.; Xiong, C.; Zhou, M.; Shi, S.; Chow, D.S.L.; Li, C. Integrin αvβ3-targeted [64 Cu]CuS nanoparticles for PET/CT imaging and photothermal ablation therapy. *Bioconjug. Chem.* **2018**, *29*, 4062–4071. [CrossRef]
55. Woodard, P.K.; Liu, Y.; Pressly, E.D.; Luehmann, H.P.; Detering, L.; Sultan, D.E.; Laforest, R.; McGrath, A.J.; Gropler, R.J.; Hawker, C.J. Design and modular construction of a polymeric nanoparticle for targeted atherosclerosis positron emission tomography imaging: A Story of 25% (64)Cu-CANF-Comb. *Pharm. Res.* **2016**, *33*, 2400–2410. [CrossRef] [PubMed]
56. Kim, H.Y.; Li, R.; Ng, T.; Courties, G.; Rodell, C.B.; Prytyskach, M.; Kohler, R.H.; Pittet, M.J.; Nahrendorf, M.; Weissleder, R.; et al. Quantitative imaging of tumor-associated macrophages and their response to therapy using (64)Cu-labeled macrin. *ACS Nano* **2018**, *12*, 12015–12029. [CrossRef]
57. Wong, P.; Li, L.; Chea, J.; Delgado, M.K.; Crow, D.; Poku, E.; Szpikowska, B.; Bowles, N.; Channappa, D.; Colcher, D.; et al. PET imaging of (64)Cu-DOTA-scFv-anti-PSMA lipid nanoparticles (LNPs): Enhanced tumor targeting over anti-PSMA scFv or untargeted LNPs. *Nucl. Med. Biol.* **2017**, *47*, 62–68. [CrossRef]
58. Keliher, E.J.; Ye, Y.X.; Wojtkiewicz, G.R.; Aguirre, A.D.; Tricot, B.; Senders, M.L.; Groenen, H.; Fay, F.; Perez-Medina, C.; Calcagno, C.; et al. Polyglucose nanoparticles with renal elimination and macrophage avidity facilitate PET imaging in ischaemic heart disease. *Nat. Commun.* **2017**, *8*, 1–12. [CrossRef]
59. Sun, J.; Sun, L.; Li, J.; Xu, J.; Wan, Z.; Ouyang, Z.; Liang, L.; Li, S.; Zeng, D. A multi-functional polymeric carrier for simultaneous positron emission tomography imaging and combination therapy. *Acta Biomater.* **2018**, *75*, 312–322. [CrossRef]
60. Piras, A.M.; Fabiano, A.; Sartini, S.; Zambito, Y.; Braccini, S.; Chiellini, F.; Cataldi, A.G.; Bartoli, F.; de la Fuente, A.; Erba, P.A. pH-responsive carboxymethylcellulose nanoparticles for 68Ga-WBC labelling in PET imaging. *Polymers* **2019**, *11*. [CrossRef]
61. Wang, X.; Yan, J.; Pan, D.; Yang, R.; Wang, L.; Xu, Y.; Sheng, J.; Yue, Y.; Huang, Q.; Wang, Y.; et al. Polyphenol–poloxamer self-assembled supramolecular nanoparticles for tumor NIRF/PET imaging. *Adv. Healthc. Mater.* **2018**, *7*, 1–8. [CrossRef] [PubMed]
62. McDonagh, P.R.; Sundaresan, G.; Yang, L.; Sun, M.; Mikkelsen, R.; Zweit, J. Biodistribution and PET imaging of 89-zirconium labeled cerium oxide nanoparticles synthesized with several surface coatings. *Nanomedicine* **2018**, *14*, 1429–1440. [CrossRef] [PubMed]
63. Chakravarty, R.; Hong, H.; Cai, W. Image-guided drug delivery with single-photon emission computed tomography: A review of literature. *Curr. Drug Targets* **2015**, *16*, 592–609. [CrossRef]
64. Si-Mohamed, S.; Cormode, D.P.; Bar-Ness, D.; Sigovan, M.; Naha, P.C.; Langlois, J.B.; Chalabreysse, L.; Coulon, P.; Blevis, I.; Roessl, E.; et al. Evaluation of spectral photon counting computed tomography K-edge imaging for determination of gold nanoparticle biodistribution in vivo. *Nanoscale* **2017**, *9*, 18246–18257. [CrossRef] [PubMed]
65. Estudiante-Mariquez, O.J.; Rodríguez-Galván, A.; Ramírez-Hernández, D.; Contreras-Torres, F.F.; Medina, L.A. Technetium-radiolabeled mannose-functionalized gold nanoparticles as nanoprobes for sentinel lymph node detection. *Molecules* **2020**, *25*, 1982. [CrossRef] [PubMed]
66. Hoogendam, J.P.; Zweemer, R.P.; Hobbelink, M.G.G.; Van Den Bosch, M.A.A.J.; Verheijen, R.H.M.; Veldhuis, W.B. 99mTc-nanocolloid SPECT/MRI fusion for the selective assessment of nonenlarged sentinel lymph nodes in patients with early-stage cervical cancer. *J. Nucl. Med.* **2016**, *57*, 551–556. [CrossRef] [PubMed]

67. Collarino, A.; Vidal-Sicart, S.; Perotti, G.; Valdés Olmos, R.A. The sentinel node approach in gynaecological malignancies. *Clin. Transl. Imaging* **2016**, *4*, 411–420. [CrossRef]
68. Saad, Z.Z.; Omorphos, S.; Michopoulou, S.; Gacinovic, S.; Malone, P.; Nigam, R.; Muneer, A.; Bomanji, J. Investigating the role of SPECT/CT in dynamic sentinel lymph node biopsy for penile cancers. *Eur. J. Nucl. Med. Mol. Imaging* **2017**, *44*, 1176–1184. [CrossRef]
69. De Veij Mestdagh, P.D.; Schreuder, W.H.; Vogel, W.V.; Donswijk, M.L.; Van Werkhoven, E.; Van Der Wal, J.E.; Dirven, R.; Karakullukcu, B.; Sonke, J.J.; Van Den Brekel, M.W.M.; et al. Mapping of sentinel lymph node drainage using SPECT/CT to tailor elective nodal irradiation in head and neck cancer patients (SUSPECT-2): A single-center prospective trial. *BMC Cancer* **2019**, *19*, 1–9. [CrossRef]
70. De Veij Mestdagh, P.D.; Schreuder, W.H.; Vogel, W.V.; Donswijk, M.L.; Van Werkhoven, E.; Van Der Wal, J.E.; Dirven, R.; Karakullukcu, B.; Sonke, J.J.; Van Den Brekel, M.W.M.; et al. An analysis of SPECT/CT non-visualization of sentinel lymph nodes in renal tumors. *EJNMMI Res.* **2018**. [CrossRef]
71. Wang, Y.; Li, Y.; Wei, F.; Duan, Y. Optical imaging paves the way for autophagy research. *Trends Biotechnol.* **2017**, *35*, 1181–1193. [CrossRef] [PubMed]
72. Boschi, F.; de Sanctis, F. Overview of the optical properties of fluorescent nanoparticles for optical imaging. *Eur. J. Histochem.* **2017**, *61*, 245–248. [CrossRef]
73. De-La-Cuesta, J.; González, E.; Pomposo, J.A. Advances in fluorescent single-chain nanoparticles. *Molecules* **2017**, *22*, 1–14. [CrossRef] [PubMed]
74. Wu, W.; Yang, Y.Q.; Yang, Y.; Yang, Y.M.; Wang, H.; Zhang, K.Y.; Guo, L.; Ge, H.F.; Liu, J.; Feng, H. An organic NIR-II nanofluorophore with aggregation-induced emission characteristics for in vivo fluorescence imaging. *Int. J. Nanomed.* **2019**, *14*, 3571–3582. [CrossRef] [PubMed]
75. Zhong, Y.; Ma, Z.; Wang, F.; Wang, X.; Yang, Y.; Liu, Y.; Zhao, X.; Li, J.; Du, H.; Zhang, M.; et al. In vivo molecular imaging for immunotherapy using ultra-bright near-infrared-IIb rare-earth nanoparticles. *Nat. Biotechnol.* **2019**, *37*, 1322–1331. [CrossRef] [PubMed]
76. Bhavane R, Starosolski Z, Stupin I, Ghaghada KB, Annapragada, A. NIR-II fluorescence imaging using indocyanine green nanoparticles. *Sci. Rep.* **2018**, *8*, 1–10. [CrossRef]
77. Li, C.H.; Kuo, T.R.; Su, H.J.; Lai, W.Y.; Yang, P.C.; Chen, J.S.; Wang, D.Y.; Wu, Y.C.; Chen, C.C. Fluorescence-guided probes of aptamer-targeted gold nanoparticles with computed tomography imaging accesses for in vivo tumor resection. *Sci. Rep.* **2015**, *5*, 1–11. [CrossRef] [PubMed]
78. Wallat, J.D.; Czapar, A.E.; Wang, C.; Wen, A.M.; Wek, K.S.; Yu, X.; Steinmetz, N.F.; Pokorski, J.K. Optical and magnetic resonance imaging using fluorous colloidal nanoparticles. *Biomacromolecules* **2017**, *18*, 103–112. [CrossRef]
79. Kim, E.H.; Chin, G.; Rong, G.; Poskanzer, K.E.; Clark, H.A. Optical probes for neurobiological sensing and imaging. *Acc. Chem. Res.* **2018**, *51*, 1023–1032. [CrossRef]
80. Napp, J.; Andrea Markus, M.; Heck, J.G.; Dullin, C.; Möbius, W.; Gorpas, D.; Feldmann, C.; Alves, F. Therapeutic fluorescent hybrid nanoparticles for traceable delivery of glucocorticoids to inflammatory sites. *Theranostics* **2018**, *8*, 6367–6383. [CrossRef]
81. Wang, Y.; Xu, N.; He, Y.; Wang, J.; Wang, D.; Gao, Q.; Xie, S.; Li, Y.; Zhang, R.; Cai, Q. Loading graphene quantum dots into optical-magneto nanoparticles for real-time tracking in vivo. *Materials* **2019**, *12*, 2191. [CrossRef] [PubMed]
82. Flak, D.; Przysiecka, Ł.; Nowaczyk, G.; Scheibe, B.; Kościński, M.; Jesionowski, T.; Jurga, S. GQDs-MSNs nanocomposite nanoparticles for simultaneous intracellular drug delivery and fluorescent imaging. *J. Nanopart. Res.* **2018**, *20*. [CrossRef] [PubMed]
83. Pan, Y.; Chang, T.; Marcq, G.; Liu, C.; Kiss, B.; Rouse, R.; Mach, K.E.; Cheng, Z.; Liao, J.C. In vivo biodistribution and toxicity of intravesical administration of quantum dots for optical molecular imaging of bladder cancer. *Sci. Rep.* **2017**, *7*, 1–9. [CrossRef]
84. Wang, Y.W.; Reder, N.P.; Kang, S.; Glaser, A.K.; Liu, J.T.C. Multiplexed optical imaging of tumor-directed nanoparticles: A review of imaging systems and approaches. *Nanotheranostics* **2017**, *1*, 369–388. [CrossRef] [PubMed]
85. Imamura, Y.; Yamada, S.; Tsuboi, S.; Nakane, Y.; Tsukasaki, Y.; Komatsuzaki, A.; Jin, T. Near-infrared emitting PbS quantum dots for in vivo fluorescence imaging of the thrombotic state in septic mouse brain. *Molecules* **2016**, *21*, 80. [CrossRef] [PubMed]

86. Bruns, O.T.; Bischof, T.S.; Harris, D.K.; Franke, D.; Shi, Y.; Riedemann, L.; Bartelt, A.; Jaworski, F.B.; Carr, J.A.; Rowlands, C.J.; et al. Next-generation in vivo optical imaging with short-wave infrared quantum dots. *Nat. Biomed. Eng.* **2017**. [CrossRef]
87. Mintz, K.J.; Zhou, Y.; Leblanc, R.M. Recent development of carbon quantum dots regarding their optical properties, photoluminescence mechanism, and core structure. *Nanoscale* **2019**, *11*, 4634–4652. [CrossRef]
88. Liu, X.; Braun, G.B.; Zhong, H.; Hall, D.J.; Han, W.; Qin, M.; Zhao, C.; Wang, M.; She, Z.-G.; Cao, C.; et al. Tumor-targeted multimodal optical imaging with versatile cadmium-free quantum dots. *Adv. Funct. Mater.* **2016**, *26*, 267–276. [CrossRef]
89. Ou, J.; Zhou, Z.; Chen, Z.; Tan, H. Optical diagnostic based on functionalized gold nanoparticles. *Int. J. Mol. Sci.* **2019**, *20*, 4346. [CrossRef]
90. Sánchez, G.J.; Maury, P.; Stefancikova, L.; Campion, O.; Laurent, G.; Chateau, A.; Hoch, F.B.; Boschetti, F.; Denat, F.; Pinel, S.; et al. Fluorescent radiosensitizing gold nanoparticles. *Int. J. Mol. Sci.* **2019**, *20*, 4618. [CrossRef]
91. Brito, H.F.; Hölsä, J.; Laamanen, T.; Lastusaari, M.; Malkamäki, M.; Rodrigues, L.C. Persistent luminescence mechanisms: Human imagination at work. *Opt. Mater. Exp.* **2012**, *2*, 371–381. [CrossRef]
92. Lecuyer, T.; Teston, E.; Maldiney, T.; Scherman, D.; Richard, C. Physico-chemical characterizations of CR doped persistent luminescence nanoparticles. *SPIE Bios.* **2016**, *9722*, 97220X.
93. Sharma, S.K.; Gourier, D.; Viana, B.; Maldiney, T.; Teston, E.; Scherman, D.; Richard, C. Persistent luminescence in nanophosphors for long term in-vivo bio-imaging. *SPIE Bios.* **2015**, *9337*, 93370I.
94. Ramírez-García, G.; Gutiérrez-Granados, S.; Gallegos-Corona, M.A.; Palma-Tirado, L.; d'Orlyé, F.; Varenne, A.; Mignet, N.; Richard, C.; Martínez-Alfaro, M. Long-term toxicological effects of persistent luminescence nanoparticles after intravenous injection in mice. *Int. J. Pharm.* **2017**, *532*, 686–695. [CrossRef]
95. Guo, R.; Lu, G.; Qin, B.; Fei, B. Ultrasound imaging technologies for breast cancer detection and management: A review. *Ultrasound Med. Biol.* **2018**, *44*, 37–70. [CrossRef]
96. Zhou, X.; Guo, L.; Shi, D.; Duan, S.; Li, J. Biocompatible chitosan nanobubbles for ultrasound-mediated targeted delivery of doxorubicin. *Nanoscale Res. Lett.* **2019**. [CrossRef]
97. Meng, M.; Gao, J.; Wu, C.; Zhou, X.; Zang, X.; Lin, X.; Liu, H.; Wang, C.; Su, H.; Liu, K.; et al. Doxorubicin nanobubble for combining ultrasonography and targeted chemotherapy of rabbit with VX2 liver tumor. *Tumor Biol.* **2016**, *37*, 8673–8680. [CrossRef]
98. Cheng, B.; Bing, C.; Xi, Y.; Shah, B.; Exner, A.A.; Chopra, R. Influence of nanobubble concentration on blood–brain barrier opening using focused ultrasound under real-time acoustic feedback control. *Ultrasound Med. Biol.* **2019**, *45*, 2174–2187. [CrossRef]
99. Chandan, R.; Banerjee, R. Pro-apoptotic liposomes-nanobubble conjugate synergistic with paclitaxel: A platform for ultrasound responsive image-guided drug delivery. *Sci. Rep.* **2018**, *8*, 1–15. [CrossRef]
100. Thakur, S.S.; Ward, M.S.; Popat, A.; Flemming, N.B.; Parat, M.; Barnett, N.L.; Parekh, H.S. Stably engineered nanobubblesand ultrasound—An effective platform for enhanced macromolecular delivery to representative cells of the retina. *PLoS ONE* **2017**, *12*, 1–17. [CrossRef]
101. Chan, M.H.; Pan, Y.T.; Chan, Y.C.; Hsiao, M.; Chen, C.H.; Sun, L.; Liu, R.S. Nanobubble-embedded inorganic 808 nm excited upconversion nanocomposites for tumor multiple imaging and treatment. *Chem. Sci.* **2018**, *9*, 3141–3151. [CrossRef] [PubMed]
102. Tian, Y.; Liu, Z.; Zhang, L.; Zhang, J.; Han, X.; Wang, Q.; Cheng, W. Apatinib-loaded lipid nanobubbles combined with ultrasound-targeted nanobubble destruction for synergistic treatment of HepG2 cells in vitro. *OncoTargets Ther.* **2018**, *11*, 4785–4795. [CrossRef] [PubMed]
103. Suzuki, R.; Oda, Y.; Omata, D.; Nishiie, N.; Koshima, R.; Shiono, Y.; Sawaguchi, Y.; Unga, J.; Naoi, T.; Negishi, Y.; et al. Tumor growth suppression by the combination of nanobubbles and ultrasound. *Cancer Sci.* **2016**, *107*, 217–223. [CrossRef] [PubMed]
104. Bhandari, P.; Novikova, G.; Goergen, C.J.; Irudayaraj, J. Ultrasound beam steering of oxygen nanobubbles for enhanced bladder cancer therapy. *Sci. Rep.* **2018**, *8*, 1–10. [CrossRef] [PubMed]
105. Wu, M.; Zhao, H.; Guo, L.; Wang, Y.; Song, J.; Zhao, X.; Li, C.; Hao, L.; Wang, D.; Tang, J. Ultrasound-mediated nanobubble destruction (UMND) facilitates the delivery of A10-3.2 aptamer targeted and siRNA-loaded cationic nanobubbles for therapy of prostate cancer. *Drug Deliv.* **2018**, *25*, 226–240. [CrossRef]
106. Choi, W.; Park, E.-Y.; Jeon, S.; Kim, C. Clinical photoacoustic imaging platforms. *Biomed. Eng. Lett.* **2018**, *8*, 139–155. [CrossRef]

107. Steinberg, I.; Huland, D.M.; Vermesh, O.; Frostig, H.E.; Tummers, W.S.; Gambhir, S.S. Photoacoustic clinical imaging. *Photoacoustics* **2019**. [CrossRef]
108. Dumani, D.S.; Sun, I.-C.; Emelianov, S.Y. Ultrasound-guided immunofunctional photoacoustic imaging for diagnosis of lymph node metastases. *Nanoscale* **2019**, *11*, 11649–11659. [CrossRef]
109. Nagaoka, R.; Tabata, T.; Yoshizawa, S.; Umemura, S. Photoacoustics visualization of murine lymph vessels using photoacoustic imaging with contrast agents. *Biochem. Pharmacol.* **2018**, *9*, 39–48. [CrossRef]
110. Zhang, M.; Kim, H.S.; Jin, T.; Yi, A.; Moon, W.K. Ultrasound-guided photoacoustic imaging for the selective detection of EGFR-expressing breast cancer and lymph node metastases. *Biomed. Opt. Express* **2016**, *7*, 1920–1931. [CrossRef]
111. Li, P.; Wu, Y.; Li, D.; Su, X.; Luo, C.; Wang, Y.; Hu, J.; Li, G.; Jiang, H.; Zhang, W. Seed-mediated synthesis of tunable-aspect-ratio gold nanorods for near-infrared photoacoustic imaging. *Nanoscale Res. Lett.* **2018**. [CrossRef] [PubMed]
112. Han, S.; Bouchard, R.; Sokolov, K.V. Molecular photoacoustic imaging with ultra-small gold nanoparticles. *Biomed. Opt. Express* **2019**, *10*, 3472. [CrossRef] [PubMed]
113. Chen, Y.-S.; Zhao, Y.; Yoon, S.J.; Gambhir, S.S.; Emelianov, S. Miniature gold nanorods for photoacoustic molecular imaging in the second near-infrared optical window. *Nat. Nanotechnol.* **2019**, *14*, 465–472. [CrossRef]
114. Sun, I.-C.; Ahn, C.-H.; Kim, K.; Emelianov, S. Photoacoustic imaging of cancer cells with glycol-chitosan-coated gold nanoparticles as contrast agents. *J. Biomed. Opt.* **2019**, *24*, 1. [CrossRef] [PubMed]
115. Bharathiraja, S.; Manivasagan, P.; Bui, N.Q.; Oh, Y.O.; Lim, I.G.; Park, S.; Oh, J. Cytotoxic induction and photoacoustic imaging of breast cancer cells using astaxanthin-reduced gold nanoparticles. *Nanomaterials* **2016**, *6*, 78. [CrossRef] [PubMed]
116. Hartman, R.K.; Hallam, K.A.; Donnelly, E.M.; Emelianov, S.Y. Photoacoustic imaging of gold nanorods in the brain delivered via microbubble-assisted focused ultrasound: A tool for in vivo molecular neuroimaging. *Laser Phys. Lett.* **2019**. [CrossRef]
117. Dixon, A.J.; Hu, S.; Klibanov, A.L.; Hossack, J.A. Oscillatory dynamics and in vivo photoacoustic imaging performance of plasmonic nanoparticle-coated microbubbles. *Small* **2015**, *11*, 3066–3077. [CrossRef]
118. Augustine, S.; Singh, J.; Srivastava, M.; Sharma, M.; Das, A.; Malhotra, B.D. Recent advances in carbon based nanosystems for cancer theranostics. *Biomater. Sci.* **2017**, *5*, 901–952. [CrossRef]
119. Xie, L.; Wang, G.; Zhou, H.; Zhang, F.; Guo, Z.; Liu, C.; Zhang, X.; Zhu, L. Functional long circulating single walled carbon nanotubes for fluorescent/photoacoustic imaging-guided enhanced phototherapy. *Biomaterials* **2016**, *103*, 219–228. [CrossRef]
120. Fathi, P.; Knox, H.J.; Sar, D.; Tripathi, I.; Ostadhossein, F.; Misra, S.K.; Esc, M.B.; Chan, J.; Pan, D. Biodegradable biliverdin nanoparticles for efficient photoacoustic imaging. *ACS Nano* **2019**, *13*, 7690–7704. [CrossRef]
121. Köker, T.; Tang, N.; Tian, C.; Tian, C.; Zhang, W.; Wang, X.; Martel, R.; Pinaud, F. Cellular imaging by targeted assembly of hot-spot SERS and photoacoustic nanoprobes using split-fluorescent protein scaffolds. *Nat. Commun.* **2018**. [CrossRef] [PubMed]
122. Tan, J.W.Y.; Murashov, M.D.; Rosania, G.R.; Wang, X. Photoacoustic imaging of clofazimine hydrochloride nanoparticle accumulation in cancerous vs normal prostates. *PLoS ONE* **2019**. [CrossRef] [PubMed]
123. Swider, E.; Daoudi, K.; Staal, A.H.J.; Koshkina, O.; Koen van Riessen, N.; van Dinther, E.; de Vries, I.J.M.; de Korte, C.L.; Srinivas, M. Clinically-applicable perfluorocarbon-loaded nanoparticles for in vivo photoacoustic,19f magnetic resonance and fluorescent imaging. *Nanotheranostics* **2018**, *2*, 258–268. [CrossRef]
124. Biffi, S.; Petrizza, L.; Garrovo, C.; Rampazzo, E.; Andolfi, L.; Giustetto, P.; Nikolov, I.; Kurdi, G.; Danailov, M.B.; Zauli, G.; et al. Multimodal near-infrared-emitting PluS Silica nanoparticles with fluorescent, photoacoustic, and photothermal capabilities. *Int. J. Nanomed.* **2016**, *11*, 4865–4874. [CrossRef]
125. Harrington, W.N.; Haji, M.R.; Galanzha, E.I.; Nedosekin, D.A.; Nima, Z.A.; Watanabe, F.; Ghosh, A.; Biris, A.S.; Zharov, V.P. Photoswitchable non-fluorescent thermochromic dye-nanoparticle hybrid probes. *Sci. Rep.* **2016**, *6*, 1–11. [CrossRef]
126. Wang, Y.; Shang, W.; Niu, M.; Tian, J.; Xu, K. Hypoxia-active nanoparticles used in tumor theranostic. *Int. J. Nanomed.* **2019**, *14*, 3705–3722. [CrossRef]
127. Hirschberg, H.; Madsen, S.J. Cell mediated photothermal therapy of brain tumors. *J. Neuroimmune Pharmacol. Off. J. Soc. Neuroimmune Pharmacol.* **2017**, *12*, 99–106. [CrossRef]

128. Vines, J.B.; Yoon, J.H.; Ryu, N.E.; Lim, D.J.; Park, H. Gold nanoparticles for photothermal cancer therapy. *Front. Chem.* **2019**. [CrossRef]
129. Simón, M.; Norregaard, K.; Jørgensen, J.T.; Oddershede, L.B.; Kjaer, A. Fractionated photothermal therapy in a murine tumor model: Comparison with single dose. *Int. J. Nanomed.* **2019**, *14*, 5369–5379. [CrossRef]
130. Riley, R.S.; Day, E.S. Gold nanoparticle-mediated photothermal therapy: Applications and opportunities for multimodal cancer treatment. *Wiley Interdiscip. Rev. Nanomed. Nanobiotechnol.* **2017**. [CrossRef]
131. Jørgensen, J.T.; Norregaard, K.; Tian, P.; Bendix, P.M.; Kjaer, A.; Oddershede, L.B. Single particle and PET-based platform for identifying optimal plasmonic nano-heaters for photothermal cancer therapy. *Sci. Rep.* **2016**. [CrossRef]
132. Estelrich, J.; Antònia Busquets, M. Iron oxide nanoparticles in photothermal therapy. *Molecules* **2018**, *23*, 1567. [CrossRef] [PubMed]
133. Vines, J.B.; Lim, D.J.; Park, H. Contemporary polymer-based nanoparticle systems for photothermal therapy. *Polymers* **2018**, *10*, 1357. [CrossRef]
134. Wu, M.; Le, W.; Mei, T.; Wang, Y.; Chen, B.; Liu, Z.; Xue, C. Cell membrane camouflaged nanoparticles: A new biomimetic platform for cancer photothermal therapy. *Int. J. Nanomed.* **2019**, *14*, 4431–4448. [CrossRef] [PubMed]
135. Mokoena, D.R.; George, B.P.; Abrahamse, H. Enhancing breast cancer treatment using a combination of cannabidiol and gold nanoparticles for photodynamic therapy. *Int. J. Mol. Sci.* **2019**, *20*, 4771. [CrossRef] [PubMed]
136. Bretin, L.; Pinon, A.; Bouramtane, S.; Ouk, C.; Richard, L.; Perrin, M.; Chaunavel, A.; Carrion, C. Photodynamic therapy activity of new human colorectal cancer. *Cancers* **2019**, *11*, 1474. [CrossRef]
137. Abrahamse, H.; Hamblin, M.R. New photosensitizers for photodynamic therapy. *Biochem. J.* **2016**, *473*, 347–364. [CrossRef]
138. Honors, C.N.; Kruger, C.A.; Abrahamse, H. Photodynamic therapy for metastatic melanoma treatment: A review. *Technol. Cancer Res. Treat.* **2018**, *17*, 1–15. [CrossRef]
139. Yu, Z.; Zhou, P.; Pan, W.; Li, N.; Tang, B. A biomimetic nanoreactor for synergistic chemiexcited photodynamic therapy and starvation therapy against tumor metastasis. *Nat. Commun.* **2018**, *9*, 1–9. [CrossRef]
140. Zhu, T.; Shi, L.; Yu, C.; Dong, Y.; Qiu, F.; Shen, L.; Qian, Q.; Zhou, G.; Zhu, X. Ferroptosis promotes photodynamic therapy: Supramolecular photosensitizer-inducer nanodrug for enhanced cancer treatment. *Theranostics* **2019**, *9*, 3293–3307. [CrossRef]
141. Liyanage, P.Y.; Hettiarachchi, S.D.; Zhou, Y.; Ouhtit, A.; Seven, E.S.; Oztan, C.Y.; Celik, E.; Leblanc, R.M. Nanoparticle-mediated targeted drug delivery for breast cancer treatment. *Biochim. Biophys. Acta Rev. Cancer* **2019**, *1871*, 419–433. [CrossRef] [PubMed]
142. Lee, M.S.; Dees, E.C.; Wang, A.Z. Nanoparticle-delivered chemotherapy: Old drugs in new packages. *Oncology* **2017**, *31*, 198–208. [PubMed]
143. Press, D. Application of active targeting nanoparticle delivery system for chemotherapeutic drugs and traditional/herbal medicines in cancer therapy: A systematic review. *Int. J. Nanomed.* **2018**, *13*, 3921.
144. Pelt, J.; Busatto, S.; Ferrari, M.; Thompson, E.A.; Mody, K.; Wolfram, J. Chloroquine and nanoparticle drug delivery: A promising combination. *Pharmacol. Ther.* **2018**, *191*, 43–49. [CrossRef] [PubMed]
145. Singh, P.; Pandit, S.; Mokkapati, V.R.S.S.; Garg, A.; Ravikumar, V.; Mijakovic, I. Gold nanoparticles in diagnostics and therapeutics for human cancer. *Int. J. Mol. Sci.* **2018**, *19*, 1979. [CrossRef] [PubMed]
146. Duan, X.; He, C.; Kron, S.J.; Lin, W. Nanoparticle formulations of cisplatin for cancer therapy. *Wiley Interdiscip. Rev. Nanomed. Nanobiotechnol.* **2016**, *8*, 776–791. [CrossRef]
147. Meng, F.; Han, N.; Yeo, Y. Organic nanoparticle systems for spatiotemporal control of multimodal chemotherapy. *Expert Opin. Drug Deliv.* **2017**, *14*, 427–446. [CrossRef]
148. Fisusi, F.A.; Akala, E.O. Drug combinations in breast cancer therapy. *Pharm. Nanotechnol.* **2019**, *7*, 3–23. [CrossRef]
149. Song, M.; Liu, T.; Shi, C.; Zhang, X.; Chen, X. Bioconjugated manganese dioxide nanoparticles enhance chemotherapy response by priming tumor-associated macrophages toward M1-like phenotype and attenuating tumor hypoxia. *ACS Nano* **2016**, *10*, 633–647. [CrossRef]
150. Wang, B.; Zhang, W.; Zhou, X.; Liu, M.; Hou, X.; Cheng, Z.; Chen, D. Development of dual-targeted nano-dandelion based on an oligomeric hyaluronic acid polymer targeting tumor-associated macrophages for combination therapy of non-small cell lung cancer. *Drug Deliv.* **2019**, *26*, 1265–1279. [CrossRef]

151. Mangal, S.; Gao, W.; Li, T.; Zhou, Q.T. Pulmonary delivery of nanoparticle chemotherapy for the treatment of lung cancers: Challenges and opportunities. *Acta Pharmacol. Sin.* **2017**, *38*, 782–797. [CrossRef] [PubMed]
152. Saleh, T.; Shojaosadati, S.A. Multifunctional nanoparticles for cancer immunotherapy. *Hum. Vaccines Immunother.* **2016**, *12*, 1863–1875. [CrossRef] [PubMed]
153. Riley, R.S.; June, C.H.; Langer, R.; Mitchell, M.J. Delivery technologies for cancer immunotherapy. *Nat. Rev. Drug Discov.* **2019**, *18*, 175–196. [CrossRef] [PubMed]
154. Wen, R.; Umeano, A.C.; Kou, Y.; Xu, J.; Farooqi, A.A. Nanoparticle systems for cancer vaccine. *Nanomedicine* **2019**, *8*, 627–648. [CrossRef]
155. Park, W.; Heo, Y.-J.; Han, D.K. New opportunities for nanoparticles in cancer immunotherapy. *Biomater. Res.* **2018**, *22*, 1–10. [CrossRef]
156. Sau, S.; Alsaab, H.O.; Bhise, K.; Alzhrani, R.; Nabil, G.; Iyer, A.K. Multifunctional nanoparticles for cancer immunotherapy: A groundbreaking approach for reprogramming malfunctioned tumor environment. *J. Control. Release* **2018**, *274*, 24–34. [CrossRef]
157. Surendran, S.P.; Moon, M.J.; Park, R.; Jeong, Y.Y. Bioactive nanoparticles for cancer immunotherapy. *Int. J. Mol. Sci.* **2018**, *19*, 3877. [CrossRef]
158. Wilson, D.R.; Sen, R.; Sunshine, J.C.; Pardoll, D.M.; Green, J.J.; Kim, Y.J. Biodegradable STING agonist nanoparticles for enhanced cancer immunotherapy. *Nanomedicine* **2018**, *14*, 237–246. [CrossRef]
159. Shoeb, E.; Hefferon, K. Future of cancer immunotherapy using plant virus-based nanoparticles. *Future Sci. OA* **2019**. [CrossRef]
160. Evans, E.R.; Bugga, P.; Asthana, V.; Drezek, R. Metallic nanoparticles for cancer immunotherapy. *Mater. Today* **2018**, *21*, 673–685. [CrossRef]
161. Jia, Y.; Omri, A.; Krishnan, L.; McCluskie, M.J. Potential applications of nanoparticles in cancer immunotherapy. *Hum. Vaccines Immunother.* **2017**, *13*, 63–74. [CrossRef] [PubMed]
162. Rodell, C.B.; Arlauckas, S.P.; Cuccarese, M.F.; Garris, C.S.; Li, R.; Ahmed, M.S.; Kohler, R.H.; Pittet, M.J.; Weissleder, R. TLR7/8-agonist-loaded nanoparticles promote the polarization of tumour-associated macrophages to enhance cancer immunotherapy. *Nat. Biomed. Eng.* **2018**, *2*, 578–588. [CrossRef] [PubMed]
163. Alipoor, S.D.; Mortaz, E.; Varahram, M.; Movassaghi, M.; Kraneveld, A.D.; Garssen, J.; Adcock, I.M. The potential biomarkers and immunological effects of tumor-derived exosomes in lung cancer. *Front. Immunol.* **2018**. [CrossRef] [PubMed]
164. Ballinger, J.R. Theranostics and precision medicine special feature: Review Article Theranostic radiopharmaceuticals: Established agents in current use. *Br. J. Radiol.* **2018**. [CrossRef]
165. Yuan, H.; Wilks, M.Q.; Maschmeyer, R.; Normandin, M.D.; Josephson, L.; Fakhri, G.E. Original research a radio-nano-platform for T1/T2 dual-mode PET-MR imaging. *Int. J. Nanomed.* **2020**, *15*, 1253.
166. Evertsson, M.; Kjellman, P.; Cinthio, M.; Andersson, R.; Tran, T.A.; In't Zandt, R.; Grafström, G.; Toftevall, H.; Fredriksson, S.; Ingvar, C.; et al. Combined magnetomotive ultrasound, PET/CT, and MR imaging of 68Ga-labelled superparamagnetic iron oxide nanoparticles in rat sentinel lymph nodes in vivo. *Sci. Rep.* **2017**, *7*, 1–9. [CrossRef]
167. Shin, S.H.; Park, S.H.; Kang, S.H.; Kim, S.W.; Kim, M.; Kim, D. Fluorine-19 magnetic resonance imaging and positron emission tomography of tumor-associated macrophages and tumor metabolism. *Contrast Media Mol. Imaging* **2017**. [CrossRef]
168. Thomas, E. Ga-radiolabeled AGuIX nanoparticles as dual-modality imaging agents for PET/MRI-guided radiotherapy. *Nanomedicine* **2017**, *12*, 1561–1574.
169. Martelli, S.; Chow, J.C.L. Dose enhancement for the flattening-filter-free and flattening-filter photon beams in nanoparticle-enhanced radiotherapy: A monte carlo phantom study. *Nanomaterials* **2020**, *10*, 637. [CrossRef]
170. Mututantri-Bastiyange, D.; Chow, J.C.L. Imaging dose of cone-beam computed tomography in nanoparticle-enhanced image-guided radiotherapy: A Monte Carlo phantom study. *AIMS Bioeng.* **2020**, *7*, 1–11. [CrossRef]
171. Chow, J.C.L. Monte carlo nanodosimetry in gold nanoparticle-enhanced radiotherapy. In *Recent Advancements and Applications Applications in Dosimetry*; Chan, M.F., Ed.; Nova Science Publishers: New York, NY, USA, 2018; Chapter 2.

172. Detappe, A.; Thomas, E.; Tibbitt, M.W.; Kunjachan, S.; Zavidij, O.; Parnandi, N.; Reznichenko, E.; Lux, F.; Tillement, O.; Berbeco, R. Ultrasmall silica-based bismuth gadolinium nanoparticles for dual magnetic resonance-computed tomography image guided radiotherapy. *Nano Lett.* **2017**, *17*, 1733–1740. [CrossRef] [PubMed]
173. Chu, C.H.; Cheng, S.H.; Chen, N.T.; Liao, W.N.; Lo, L.W. Microwave-synthesized platinum-embedded mesoporous silica nanoparticles as dual-modality contrast agents: Computed tomography and optical imaging. *Int. J. Mol. Sci.* **2019**, *20*, 1560. [CrossRef] [PubMed]
174. Nguyen Pham, T.H.; Lengkeek, N.A.; Greguric, I.; Kim, B.J.; Pellegrini, P.A.; Bickley, S.A.; Tanudji, M.R.; Jones, S.K.; Hawkett, B.S.; Pham, B.T.T. Tunable and noncytotoxic PET/SPECT-MRI multimodality imaging probes using colloidally stable ligand-free superparamagnetic iron oxide nanoparticles. *Int. J. Nanomed.* **2017**, *12*, 899–909. [CrossRef] [PubMed]
175. Silva, F.; Paulo, A.; Pallier, A.; Même, S.; Tóth, É.; Gano, L.; Marques, F.; Geraldes, C.F.G.C.; Castro, M.M.C.A.; Cardoso, A.M.; et al. Dual imaging gold nanoplatforms for targeted radiotheranostics. *Materials* **2020**, *13*, 513. [CrossRef] [PubMed]
176. Chen, X.; Zhou, H.; Li, X.; Duan, N.; Hu, S.; Liu, Y.; Yue, Y.; Song, L.; Zhang, Y.; Li, D.; et al. Plectin-1 targeted dual-modality nanoparticles for pancreatic cancer imaging. *EBioMedicine* **2018**, *30*, 129–137. [CrossRef]
177. Zheng, Y.; Zhang, H.; Hu, Y.; Bai, L.; Xue, J. MnO nanoparticles with potential application in magnetic resonance imaging and drug delivery for myocardial infarction. *Int. J. Nanomed.* **2018**, *13*, 6177–6188. [CrossRef]
178. Gonawala, S.; Ali, M.M. Application of dendrimer-based nanoparticles in glioma imaging. *J. Nanomed. Nanotechnol.* **2017**. [CrossRef]
179. Zhou, L.; Jing, Y.; Liu, Y.; Liu, Z.; Gao, D.; Chen, H.; Song, W.; Wang, T.; Fang, X.; Qin, W.; et al. Mesoporous carbon nanospheres as a multifunctional carrier for cancer theranostics. *Theranostics* **2018**, *8*, 663–675. [CrossRef]
180. Zhang, Y.; Tang, Z.; Wu, Y. The dual-mode imaging of nanogold-labeled cells by photoacoustic microscopy and fluorescence optical microscopy. *Technol. Cancer Res. Treat.* **2018**, *17*, 1–4. [CrossRef]
181. Yang, Z.; Song, J.; Dai, Y.; Chen, J.; Wang, F.; Lin, L.; Liu, Y.; Zhang, F.; Yu, G.; Zhou, Z.; et al. Theranostics self-assembly of semiconducting-plasmonic gold nanoparticles with enhanced optical property for photoacoustic imaging and photothermal therapy. *Theranostics* **2017**. [CrossRef]
182. Knights, O.B.; McLaughlan, J.R. Gold nanorods for light-based lung cancer theranostics. *Int. J. Mol. Sci.* **2018**, *19*, 3318. [CrossRef] [PubMed]
183. Song, J.; Yang, X.; Jacobson, O.; Lin, L.; Huang, P.; Niu, G.; Ma, Q.; Chen, X. Sequential drug release and enhanced photothermal and photoacoustic effect of hybrid reduced graphene oxide-loaded ultrasmall gold nanorod vesicles for cancer therapy. *ACS Nano* **2015**, *9*, 9199–9209. [CrossRef] [PubMed]
184. Lu, S.T.; Xu, D.; Liao, R.F.; Luo, J.Z.; Liu, Y.H.; Qi, Z.H.; Zhang, C.J.; Ye, N.L.; Wu, B.; Xu, H.B. Single-component bismuth nanoparticles as a theranostic agent for multimodal imaging-guided glioma therapy. *Comput. Struct. Biotechnol. J.* **2019**, *17*, 619–627. [CrossRef] [PubMed]
185. Siregar, S.; Oktamuliani, S.; Saijo, Y. A theoretical model of laser heating carbon nanotubes. *Nanomaterials* **2018**, *8*, 580. [CrossRef]
186. Chow, J.C.L. Application of nanoparticle materials in radiation therapy. In *Handbook of Ecomaterials*; Martinez, L.M.T., Kharissova, O.V., Kharisov, B.I., Eds.; Springer Nature: Basel, Switzerland, 2017; Chapter 150, pp. 3661–3681.
187. Chow, J.C.L. Photon and electron interactions with gold nanoparticles: A Monte Carlo study on gold nanoparticle-enhanced radiotherapy. In *Nanobiomaterials in Medical Imaging: Applications of Nanobiomaterials*; Grumezescu, A.M., Ed.; Elsevier: Amsterdam, The Netherlands, 2016; Chapter 2, pp. 45–70.
188. Chow, J.C.L. Recent progress of gold nanomaterials in cancer therapy. In *Handbook of Nanomaterials and Nanocomposites for Energy and Environmental Applications*; Kharissova, O.V., Torres-Martínez, L.M., Kharisov, B.I., Eds.; Springer Nature: Cham, Switzerland, 2020; pp. 1–30.
189. He, C.; Chow, J.C. Gold nanoparticle DNA damage in radiotherapy: A Monte Carlo study. *AIMS Bioeng.* **2016**, *3*, 352. [CrossRef]
190. Wang, Yanjie; Strohm, E.M.; Sun, Y.; Wang, Z.; Zheng, Y.; Wang, Z.; Kolios, M.C. Biodegradable polymeric nanoparticles containing gold nanoparticles and Paclitaxel for cancer imaging and drug delivery using photoacoustic methods. *Biomed. Opt. Express* **2016**, *7*, 4125. [CrossRef] [PubMed]

191. Ashton, J.R.; Castle, K.D.; Qi, Y.; Kirsch, D.G.; West, J.L.; Badea, C.T. Dual-energy CT imaging of tumor liposome delivery after gold nanoparticle-augmented radiotherapy. *Theranostics* **2018**, *8*, 1782–1797. [CrossRef]
192. Siddique, S.; Chow, J.C. Gold nanoparticles for drug delivery and cancer therapy. *Appl. Sci.* **2020**, *10*, 3824. [CrossRef]
193. Du, F.; Lou, J.; Jiang, R.; Fang, Z.; Zhao, X.; Niu, Y.; Zou, S.; Zhang, M.; Gong, A.; Wu, C. Hyaluronic acid-functionalized bismuth oxide nanoparticles for computed tomography imaging-guided radiotherapy of tumor. *Int. J. Nanomed.* **2017**, *12*, 5973–5992. [CrossRef]
194. Li, W.; Hou, W.; Guo, X.; Luo, L.; Li, Q.; Zhu, C.; Yang, J.; Zhu, J.; Du, Y.; You, J. Temperature-controlled, phase-transition ultrasound imaging-guided photothermal-chemotherapy triggered by NIR light. *Theranostics* **2018**, *8*, 3059–3073. [CrossRef]
195. Liu, Z.; Zhang, J.; Tian, Y.; Zhang, L.; Han, X.; Wang, Q.; Cheng, W. Targeted delivery of reduced graphene oxide nanosheets using multifunctional ultrasound nanobubbles for visualization and enhanced photothermal therapy. *Int. J. Nanomed.* **2018**, *13*, 7859–7872. [CrossRef] [PubMed]
196. Prabhakar, A.; Banerjee, R. Nanobubble liposome complexes for diagnostic imaging and ultrasound-triggered drug delivery in cancers: A theranostic approach. *ACS Omega* **2019**, *4*, 15567–15580. [CrossRef]
197. Chen, F.; Hableel, G.; Zhao, E.R.; Jokerst, J.V. Multifunctional nanomedicine with silica: Role of silica in nanoparticles for theranostic, imaging, and drug monitoring. *J. Colloid Interface Sci.* **2018**, *521*, 261–279. [CrossRef] [PubMed]
198. Yao, H.C.; Su, L.; Zeng, M.; Cao, L.; Zhao, W.W.; Chen, C.Q.; Du, B.; Zhou, J. Construction of magnetic-carbon-quantum-dots-probe-labeled apoferritin nanocages for bioimaging and targeted therapy. *Int. J. Nanomed.* **2016**, *11*, 4423–4438. [CrossRef] [PubMed]
199. Saowalak, K.; Titipun, T.; Somchai, T.; Chalermchai, P. Iron(III)-tannic molecular nanoparticles enhance autophagy effect and T1 MRI contrast in liver cell lines. *Sci. Rep.* **2018**, *8*, 1–13. [CrossRef] [PubMed]
200. Li, L.H.; Lu, Y.; Jiang, C.Y.; Zhu, Y.; Yang, X.F.; Hu, X.M.; Lin, Z.F.; Zhang, Y.; Peng, M.Y.; Xia, H.; et al. Actively targeted deep tissue imaging and photothermal-chemo therapy of breast cancer by antibody-functionalized drug-loaded X-ray-responsive bismuth Sulfide@Mesoporous silica core-shell nanoparticles. *Adv. Funct. Mater.* **2018**. [CrossRef]
201. Xu, C.; Feng, Q.; Yang, H.; Wang, G.; Huang, L.; Bai, Q.; Zhang, C.; Wang, Y.; Chen, Y.; Cheng, Q.; et al. A light-triggered mesenchymal stem cell delivery system for photoacoustic imaging and chemo-photothermal therapy of triple negative breast cancer. *Adv. Sci.* **2018**. [CrossRef]
202. Li, G.; Chen, Y.; Zhang, L.; Zhang, M.; Li, S.; Li, L.; Wang, T.; Wang, C. Facile approach to synthesize gold Nanorod@Polyacrylic acid/calcium phosphate yolk–shell nanoparticles for dual-mode imaging and pH/NIR-responsive drug delivery. *Nano-Micro Lett* **2018**. [CrossRef]
203. Yang, Y.; Zhang, J.; Xia, F.; Zhang, C.; Qian, Q.; Zhi, X.; Yue, C.; Sun, R.; Cheng, S.; Fang, S.; et al. Human CIK cells loaded with Au nanorods as a theranostic platform for targeted photoacoustic imaging and enhanced immunotherapy and photothermal therapy. *Nanoscale Res. Lett.* **2016**. [CrossRef]
204. Li, K.; Nejadnik, H. Daldrup-Link HE. Next-generation superparamagnetic iron oxide nanoparticles for cancer theranostics. *Drug Discov. Today* **2017**, *22*, 1421–1429. [CrossRef]
205. Gurunathan, S.; Kang, M.H.; Qasim, M.; Kim, J.H. Nanoparticle-mediated combination therapy: Two-in-one approach for cancer. *Int. J. Mol. Sci.* **2018**, *19*, 1–37. [CrossRef] [PubMed]
206. Zhang, A.; Pan, S.; Zhang, Y.; Chang, J.; Cheng, J.; Huang, Z.; Li, T.; Zhang, C.; De La Fuentea, J.M.; Zhang, Q.; et al. Carbon-gold hybrid nanoprobes for real-time imaging, photothermal/photodynamic and nanozyme oxidative therapy. *Theranostics* **2019**, *9*, 3443–3458. [CrossRef] [PubMed]
207. Miao, W.; Kim, H.; Gujrati, V.; Kim, J.Y.; Jon, H.; Lee, Y.; Choi, M.; Kim, J.; Lee, S.; Lee, D.Y.; et al. Photo-decomposable organic nanoparticles for combined tumor optical imaging and multiple phototherapies. *Theranostics* **2016**, *6*, 2367–2379. [CrossRef] [PubMed]
208. Yildiz, T.; Gu, R.; Zauscher, S.; Betancourt, T. Doxorubicin-loaded protease-activated near-infrared fluorescent polymeric nanoparticles for imaging and therapy of cancer. *Int. J. Nanomed.* **2018**, *13*, 6961–6986. [CrossRef] [PubMed]
209. Nam, J.; Son, S.; Ochyl, L.J.; Kuai, R.; Schwendeman, A.; Moon, J.J. Chemo-photothermal therapy combination elicits anti-tumor immunity against advanced metastatic cancer. *Nat. Commun.* **2018**. [CrossRef]

210. Zhang, X.; Li, Y.; Wei, M.; Liu, C.; Yang, J. Cetuximab-modified silica nanoparticle loaded with ICG for tumor-targeted combinational therapy of breast cancer. *Drug Deliv.* **2019**, *26*, 129–136. [CrossRef]
211. Locatelli, E.; Li, Y.; Monaco, I.; Guo, W.; Maturi, M.; Menichetti, L.; Armanetti, P.; Martin, R.C.; Franchini, M.C. A novel theranostic gold nanorods- and adriamycin-loaded micelle for EpCA M targeting, laser ablation, and photoacoustic imaging of cancer stem cells in hepatocellular carcinoma. *Int. J. Nanomed.* **2019**, *14*, 1877–1892. [CrossRef]
212. Ramanathan, S.; Archunan, G.; Sivakumar, M.; Selvan, S.T.; Fred, A.L.; Kumar, S.; Gulyás, B.; Padmanabhan, P. Theranostic applications of nanoparticles in neurodegenerative disorders. *Int. J. Nanomed.* **2018**, *13*, 5561–5576. [CrossRef]
213. Ge, X.; Fu, Q.; Su, L.; Li, Z.; Zhang, W.; Chen, T.; Yang, H.; Song, J. Light-activated gold nanorod vesicles with NIR-II fluorescence and photoacoustic imaging performances for cancer theranostics. *Theranostics* **2020**, *10*, 4809–4821. [CrossRef]
214. He, C.; Duan, X.; Guo, N.; Chan, C.; Poon, C.; Weichselbaum, R.R.; Lin, W. Core-shell nanoscale coordination polymers combine chemotherapy and photodynamic therapy to potentiate checkpoint blockade cancer immunotherapy. *Nat. Commun.* **2016**, *7*, 1–12. [CrossRef]
215. Chen, W.; Qin, M.; Chen, X.; Wang, Q.; Zhang, Z.; Sun, X. Combining photothermal therapy and immunotherapy against melanoma by polydopamine-coated Al_2O_3 nanoparticles. *Theranostics* **2018**, *8*, 2229–2241. [CrossRef] [PubMed]
216. Hou, X.; Tao, Y.; Pang, Y.; Li, X.; Jiang, G.; Liu, Y. Nanoparticle-based photothermal and photodynamic immunotherapy for tumor treatment. *Int. J. Cancer* **2018**, *143*, 3050–3060. [CrossRef] [PubMed]
217. Chen, Q.; Xu, L.; Liang, C.; Wang, C.; Peng, R.; Liu, Z. Photothermal therapy with immune-adjuvant nanoparticles together with checkpoint blockade for effective cancer immunotherapy. *Nat. Commun.* **2016**, *7*, 1–13. [CrossRef] [PubMed]
218. Mu, Q.; Wang, H.; Zhang, M. Nanoparticles for imaging and treatment of metastatic breast cancer. *Expert Opin. Drug Deliv.* **2017**, *14*, 123–136. [CrossRef] [PubMed]
219. Zhang, J.; Zhao, T.; Han, F.; Hu, Y.; Li, Y. Photothermal and gene therapy combined with immunotherapy to gastric cancer by the gold nanoshell-based system. *J. Nanobiotechnol.* **2019**, *17*, 1–11. [CrossRef]
220. Li, W.; Yang, J.; Luo, L.; Jiang, M.; Qin, B.; Yin, H.; Zhu, C.; Yuan, X.; Zhang, J.; Luo, Z.; et al. Targeting photodynamic and photothermal therapy to the endoplasmic reticulum enhances immunogenic cancer cell death. *Nat. Commun.* **2019**. [CrossRef]
221. Min, K.H.; Kim, Y.H.; Wang, Z.; Kim, J.; Kim, J.S.; Kim, S.H.; Kim, K.; Kwon, I.C.; Kiesewetter, D.O.; Chen, X. Theranostics engineered Zn(II)-dipicolylamine-gold nanorod provides effective prostate cancer treatment by combining siRNA delivery and photothermal therapy. *Theranostics* **2017**. [CrossRef]

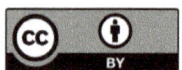

© 2020 by the authors. Licensee MDPI, Basel, Switzerland. This article is an open access article distributed under the terms and conditions of the Creative Commons Attribution (CC BY) license (http://creativecommons.org/licenses/by/4.0/).

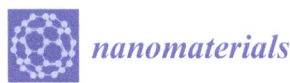

Article

Computational Study Regarding Co$_x$Fe$_{3-x}$O$_4$ Ferrite Nanoparticles with Tunable Magnetic Properties in Superparamagnetic Hyperthermia for Effective Alternative Cancer Therapy

Costica Caizer

Department of Physics, West University of Timisoara, Bv. V. Pârvan No. 4, 300223 Timisoara, Romania; costica.caizer@e-uvt.ro

Abstract: The efficacy in superparamagnetic hyperthermia (SPMHT) and its effectiveness in destroying tumors without affecting healthy tissues depend very much on the nanoparticles used. Considering the results previously obtained in SPMHT using magnetite and cobalt ferrite nanoparticles, in this paper we extend our study on Co$_x$Fe$_{3-x}$O$_4$ nanoparticles for x = 0–1 in order to be used in SPMHT due to the multiple benefits in alternative cancer therapy. Due to the possibility of tuning the basic observables/parameters in SPMHT in a wide range of values by changing the concentration of Co^{2+} ions in the range 0–1, the issue explored by us is a very good strategy for increasing the efficiency and effectiveness of magnetic hyperthermia of tumors and reducing the toxicity levels. In this paper we studied by computational simulation the influence of Co^{2+} ion concentration in a very wide range of values (x = 0–1) on the specific loss power (P_S) in SPMHT and the nanoparticle diameter (D_M) which leads to the maximum specific loss power (P_{sM}). We also determined the maximum specific loss power for the allowable biological limit (P_{sM})$_l$ which doesn't affect healthy tissues, and how it influences the change in the concentration of Co^{2+} ions. Based on the results obtained, we established the values for concentrations (x), nanoparticle diameter (D_M), amplitude (H) and frequency (f) of the magnetic field for which SPMHT with Co$_x$Fe$_{3-x}$O$_4$ nanoparticles can be applied under optimal conditions within the allowable biological range. The obtained results allow the obtaining a maximum efficacy in alternative and non-invasive tumor therapy for the practical implementation of SPMHT with Co$_x$Fe$_{3-x}$O$_4$ nanoparticles.

Keywords: Co-Fe ferrite nanoparticles; magnetic hyperthermia; specific loss power; optimization; alternative therapy; cancer

Citation: Caizer, C. Computational Study Regarding Co$_x$Fe$_{3-x}$O$_4$ Ferrite Nanoparticles with Tunable Magnetic Properties in Superparamagnetic Hyperthermia for Effective Alternative Cancer Therapy. *Nanomaterials* **2021**, *11*, 3294. https://doi.org/10.3390/nano11123294

Academic Editor: James C. L. Chow

Received: 11 October 2021
Accepted: 2 December 2021
Published: 4 December 2021

Publisher's Note: MDPI stays neutral with regard to jurisdictional claims in published maps and institutional affiliations.

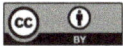

Copyright: © 2021 by the author. Licensee MDPI, Basel, Switzerland. This article is an open access article distributed under the terms and conditions of the Creative Commons Attribution (CC BY) license (https://creativecommons.org/licenses/by/4.0/).

1. Introduction

The magnetic nanoparticles most often used in magnetic hyperthermia therapy in the ferrimagnetic materials class are those of iron oxide due to their good magnetic characteristics and their efficient use at high frequencies. Of these materials, Fe$_3$O$_4$ nanoparticles (magnetite) are still the most used [1–17] due to their great magnetic properties for magnetic hyperthermia [18–20], and also their low toxicity towards cells [21].

However, extensive studies have been conducted on the subject [22–30] with the aim of finding other magnetic nanoparticles and magnetic nanomaterials/nanostructures suitable for use in magnetic hyperthermia, with improved properties. In this regard, of particular interest are cobalt ferrite and cobalt ferrite nanoparticles, Co$_x$Fe$_{3-x}$O$_4$, in order to be applied in magnetic or superparamagnetic hyperthermia due to their magnetic anisotropy which is very different from that of magnetite [18,19], and could lead to substantial improvements in terms of magnetic or superparamagnetic hyperthermia. In terms of magnetic anisotropy, CoFe$_2$O$_4$ ferrite is magnetically hard, having a magnetocrystalline anisotropy constant of 200×10^3 J/m^3, while Fe$_3$O$_4$ ferrite (magnetite) is magnetically soft, having an anisotropy constant of only 11×10^3 J/m^3, although their spontaneous magnetizations (M_s) differ only slightly from each other (M_s = 480 kA/m for Fe$_3$O$_4$ and M_s = 425 kA/m for CoFe$_2$O$_4$) [18].

In superparamagnetic hyperthermia (SPMHT), the very high magnetic anisotropy of CoFe$_3$O$_4$ ferrite nanoparticles compared to that of F$_3$O$_4$ magnetite, radically influences the hyperthermia effect, which is reflected in the specific loss power and, finally, on the heating temperature of the nanoparticles [31,32]. As a result, the maximum effect in SPMHT given by the specific loss power is obtained in the case of soft nanoparticles of Fe$_3$O$_4$ for a diameter (size) of nanoparticles (approximate spherical) of ~16 nm, and in the case of CoFe$_2$O$_4$ hard ferrite nanoparticles for a diameter of only ~6 nm (the exact value depending on the frequency of the alternating magnetic field). These nanoparticle sizes, in terms of SPMHT which uses superparamagnetic nanoparticles would be too large for Fe$_3$O$_4$ nanoparticles and too small for CoFe$_2$O$_4$ nanoparticles, both types of nanoparticles thus having advantages and disadvantages in magnetic hyperthermia for cancer therapy. More detailed results and discussions on these issues were previously presented [31,32].

Considering the above and the sporadic results of the overall research on the matter so far, lacking a systematic approach, we've focused on studying SPMHT on Co$_x$Fe$_{3-x}$O$_4$ nanoparticles for the entire range of values x = 0–1, wherein the bivalent Fe^{2+} ions are replaced by a percentage of Co^{2+} ions (x) in the octahedral lattice of the spinel of Fe^{3+}[Co$_x$$^{2+}Fe_{(1-x)}$$^{2+}$, Fe^{3+}]O$_4$$^{2-}$ ferite (the right bracket comprises the Fe^{3+}, Fe^{2+} ions and Co^{2+} from the octahedral lattice, and outside the parentheses are the Fe^{3+} ions from the tetrahedral lattice within the ferrite structure [18]). Thus, by replacing Fe^{2+} ions with Co^{2+} ions in the entire range of atomic percentage values (0–1), starting from Fe$_3$O$_4$ magnetite (for x = 0) and reaching the CoF$_2$O$_4$ ferrite for x = 1, the magnetic anisotropy will change in a very wide range of values, and thus different Co$_x$Fe$_{3-x}$O$_4$ nanoparticles which have different magnetic characteristics in magnetic hyperthermia depending on the concentration of Co^{2+} ions can be obtained. Therefore, we can modify the parameter x (concentration of Co^{2+} ions in the structure of magnetite) in order to obtain adjustable properties in superparamagnetic hyperthermia, thus, being able to find the optimal values of the parameters which give the best results in magnetic hyperthermia. With this in mind, we focused on a systematic study by using a 3D/2D computational tools and as complete as possible in terms of the specific loss power in magnetic hyperthermia (which is the key value that indicates whether the nanoparticles are good or not to obtain the maximum hyperthermia effect) depending on the concentration of Co^{2+} ions (x), in order to find which nanoparticles would give the best results in SPMHT. At the same time, we studied the maximum specific loss power for the admissible biological limit (without affecting healthy tissues), depending on the concentration of Co^{2+} (x) ions, in order to optimize SPMHT with Co$_x$Fe$_{3-x}$O$_4$ for its practical implementation in vivo and, in the future, in clinical trials with maximum efficacy.

2. Theoretical Considerations on Specific Loss Power in Superparamagnetic Hyperthermia

In superparamagnetic hyperthermia (SPMHT) of tumors with magnetic nanoparticles [14,17,31,33] the basic mechanism that leads to the heating of dispersed and fixed nanoparticles in the tumor are the Néel magnetic relaxation processes [8,9,34]. Thus, under the action of an alternating magnetic field with a frequency in the range of hundreds of kHz [20], superparamagnetic (biocompatible) nanoparticles dispersed in the tumor by different techniques, heat to temperatures of 42–43 °C, thus, leading to the irreversible destruction of tumor cells by apoptosis [35]. However, the efficiency of the method depends very much on the type of magnetic nanoparticles used for this therapy and the magnetic relaxation processes that take place in the alternating magnetic field.

The specific loss power (P_s) in magnetic nanoparticles in the presence of an alternating magnetic field with frequency f and amplitude H is [20,36]:

$$P_s = \frac{\pi \mu_0 \chi''}{\rho} f H^2 \qquad (1)$$

where ρ is the density of the magnetic material, μ_0 is the magnetic permeability of the vacuum and χ'' is the imaginary component of complex magnetic susceptibility, given by the following expression:

$$\chi = \chi' - j\chi'' \tag{2}$$

According to Debye's theory, the components of complex magnetic susceptibility are given by the relations [20,37,38]

$$\chi' = \chi_0 \frac{1}{1 + (\omega\tau)^2} \tag{3}$$

and:

$$\chi'' = \chi_0 \frac{\omega\tau}{1 + (\omega\tau)^2} \tag{4}$$

where χ_0 is the static magnetic susceptibility, τ is the magnetic relaxation time, and ω is the pulsation of the alternating magnetic field ($\omega = 2\pi f$).

Static magnetic susceptibility in the case of magnetization of superparamagnetic nanoparticles [39], according to Langevin's law of magnetization:

$$M = M_{sat}\left(\coth\xi - \frac{1}{\xi}\right) \tag{5}$$

is given by:

$$\chi_0 = \frac{3\chi_i}{\xi}\left(\coth\xi - \frac{1}{\xi}\right) \tag{6}$$

where χ_i is the initial magnetic susceptibility:

$$\chi_i = \frac{\varepsilon\pi\mu_0 M_s^2 D^3}{18k_B T} \tag{7}$$

and the parenthesis from Equation (6) is the Langevin function in the case of magnetic nanoparticles [39,40] having the argument:

$$\xi = \frac{\pi\mu_0 M_s D^3}{6k_B T} H \tag{8}$$

In Equations (5), (7) and (8), M_{sat} is the saturation magnetization, D is the diameter of the nanoparticles (approximate spherical), M_s is the spontaneous magnetization, ε is the packing fraction of nanoparticles k_B is Boltzmann's constant, and T is the temperature. In the case of nanoparticle systems, the magnetic packing fraction expressed by the observable ε in Equation (7) must also be taken into account.

The magnetic relaxation time, according to Néel's theory [34], is:

$$\tau = \tau_0 \exp\left(\frac{\pi K D^3}{6k_B T}\right) \tag{9}$$

where K is the magnetic anisotropy constant, and τ_0 is a time constant which usually has a value of 10^{-9} s [41].

Thus, taking into account all the above formulas, the specific loss power in the magnetic nanoparticles in an alternating magnetic field (harmonic) with frequency f and amplitude H, will have the expression [31]:

$$P_s = \frac{3\pi\mu_0\chi_i}{\rho\xi}\left(\coth\xi - \frac{1}{\xi}\right)\frac{2\pi f\tau}{1 + (2\pi f\tau)^2} f H^2 \; (W/g) \tag{10}$$

This equation and the above will be used in our 3D/2D computational study considering the specific loss power in $Co_xFe_{3-x}O_4$ nanoparticles for $x = 0$–1, as a function of the characteristic observables of the magnetic nanoparticles and the parameters of the alternating magnetic field. The key parameters considered in our study are the size (diameter) of the nanoparticles (D), the concentration of Co^{2+} (x) ions (which determines a certain magnetic anisotropy), and the alternating magnetic field parameters, amplitude (H) and frequency (f), on which will depend to a large extent the specific loss power (P_s) and the efficiency of the SPMHT method. The ultimate goal of the study is to find the optimal observables/parameters that lead to a maximum specific loss power in the biological allowable limit ($P_{sM})_l$, so that the SPMHT method can be applied with maximum effectiveness in tumor therapy in vitro, in vivo and then in the future in clinical trials.

3. Results and Discution

3.1. Characteristic Observables of Nanoparticles Depending on the Concentration of Co^{2+} Ions and Alternating Magnetic Field Parameters, and Input/Output Data Used in SPMHT

3.1.1. Magnetic Anisotropy and Spontaneous Magnetization

In the case of cobalt-iron ferrite (Co-Fe) with the chemical formula $Co_xFe_{3-x}O_4$ for $x = 0$–1, depending on the concentration x of Co^{2+} ions in the structure of $Fe^{3+}[Co_x^{2+}Fe_{(3-x)}^{2+}, Fe^{3+}]O_4^{2-}$ ferrite, where the bivalent Co^{2+} ions occupy the octahedral positions in the spinel structure, the values of the magnetic anisotropy constant and of the saturation magnetization at room temperature were determined by fitting the experimental reference data [18,19] (Figures 1 and 2). These values extracted from the fit curves for different values of concentration x, are given in Table 1.

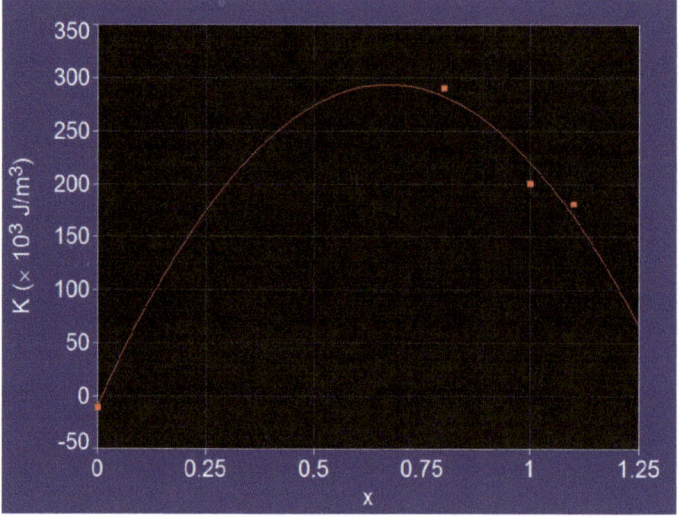

Figure 1. Fit curve on experimental reference values for magnetic anisotropy constant of $Co_xFe_{3-x}O_4$ ferrite.

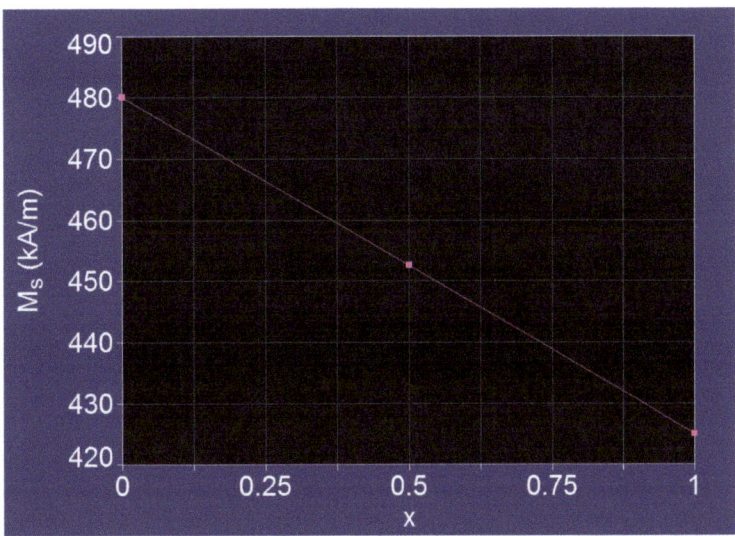

Figure 2. Fit on experimental reference values for spontaneous magnetisation of $Co_xFe_{3-x}O_4$ ferrite.

Table 1. Values of magnetocrystalline anisotropy constant, the spontaneous magnetisation, and the density at room temperature in the case of $Co_xFe_{3-x}O_4$ ferrite for different values of x in the range of 0–1.1 extracted from fit curves.

No.	Observables	x	K ($\times 10^3$ J/m³)	M_s (kA/m)	ρ ($\times 10^3$ kg/m³)
1		0	11 (I)	480 (I)	5.24
2		0.05	38	477	~5.243
3		0.1	82	474	5.245
4		0.2	156	469	5.25
5		0.4	245	458	5.26
6		0.67	294	443	~5.27
7		0.8	290 (I)	436	5.28
8		1	200 (II)	425 (II)	5.29
9		1.1	180 (I)	-	-

(I) [18]; (II) [19].

Thus, a very important result was found for the magnetocrystalline anisotropy constant K of the $Co_xFe_{3-x}O_4$ ferrite, which varies in very wide limits when the concentration of Co^{2+} ions changes from the value 0, corresponding to the spinel Fe_3O_4 (magnetite) with K = 11 × 10³ J/m³, to value 1, corresponding to the cobalt ferrite $CoFe_2O_4$ with K = 200 × 10³ J/m³. Also, it is observed that the variation of the anisotropy constant presents a maximum (294 × 10³ J/m³) at the value x = 0.67, and when the concentration x decreases to 0 the constant K decreases to the value corresponding to the magnetite (11 × 10³ J/m³) (Figure 1).

In order to determine the sponteneous magnetization of the $Co_xFe_{3-x}O_4$ ferrite as a function of the concentration of Co^{2+} ions for the variation of x in the range (0–1), we considered a linear variation of it with the concentration (x) of Co^{2+} ions (Figure 2). Thus, the values for spontaneous magnetization in Table 1 are obtained. However, in the case of nanoparticles the values may sometimes differ depending on the preparation method, nanoparticle size, type of material, etc. Therefore, in order not to cause confusion in our study for determining the values for K and M_s by fitting we used the well known standard values for Co-Fe [18,19] ferrite. For a better accuracy in the applications of magnetic hyperthermia it is beneficial to determine experimentally the effective values of the magnetic anisotropy constant and the saturation magnetisation of nanoparticles that will be used.

3.1.2. Nanoparticles and Alternating Magnetic Field Parameters

Having in view that the values of nanoparticle diameters (D) corresponding to the maximum loss power (P_{sM}) in magnetic hyperthermia are ~16 nm for magnetite and ~6 nm for cobalt ferrite, we considered for this study the range of interest to be 1–20 nm (Table 2) for the nanoparticle size.

Table 2. Characteristic observables for $Co_xFe_{3-x}O_4$ nanoparticles and parameters of magnetic field.

Observables	D (nm)	ε	H (kA/m)	f (kHz)
Value range	1–20	0.1	10–50	100–500

For our study on specific loss power, we considered the nanoparticles to be spherical and the value of the packing volumetric fraction (ε) in Table 2 (which are the most commonly used in magnetic and superparamagnetic hyperthermia). Also, based on our previous results [31,32], we also considered the amplitude (H) and frequency (f) of the alternating magnetic field in the ranges given in Table 2.

3.1.3. Input and Output Data Used in Computational Study of SPMHT

For computational study using $Co_xFe_{3-x}O_4$ ($x = 0-1$) nanoparticles we used a professional software for 3D/2D calculus and representation. The input data are the characteristic observable of nanoparticles and the parameters of magnetic field from Table 2, and the magnetic observables of nanoparticles as a function of Co^{2+} ions concentration (x) from Table 1. The output data is mainly the specific loss power expressed by Equation (10) with Equations (1)–(9). The aim is to determine the specific loss power by $Co_xFe_{3-x}O_4$ nanoparticles for different concentrations of Co^{2+} ions depending on their size and alternating magnetic field parameters. At the same time, the maximum specific loss power for the admissible biological limit was determined.

3.2. The Specific Loss Power in Superparamagnetic Hyperthermia with $Co_xFe_{3-x}O_4$ Ferrite Nanoparticles

Using Equation (10) with the observables given by Equations (7)–(9), we calculated the specific loss power in the case of $Co_xFe_{3-x}O_4$ ferrimagnetic nanoparticles for the values of the concentration of Co^{2+} ions (x) located in the range of $x = 0-1$ (Table 1). The specific loss powers determined are 3D shown in Figure 3, as a function of nanoparticle diameter (D) and magnetic field frequency (f), for a constant magnetic field of 20 kA/m. For each value of the concentration x, the corresponding values for the magnetic anisotropy constant K and the saturation magnetization M_s given in Table 1 were used.

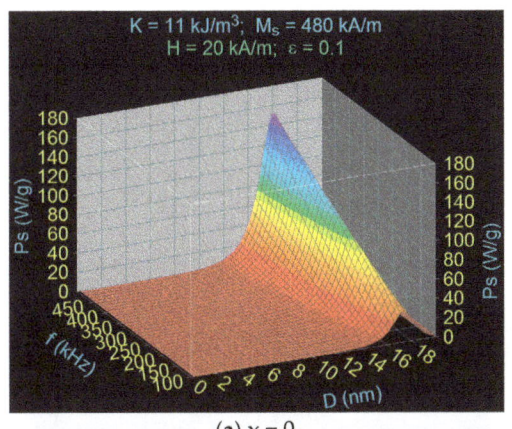

(a) x = 0

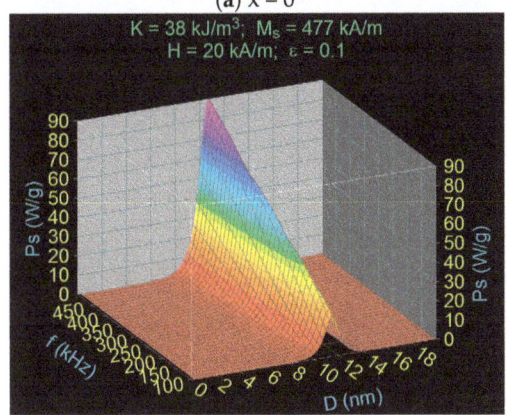

(b) x = 0.05

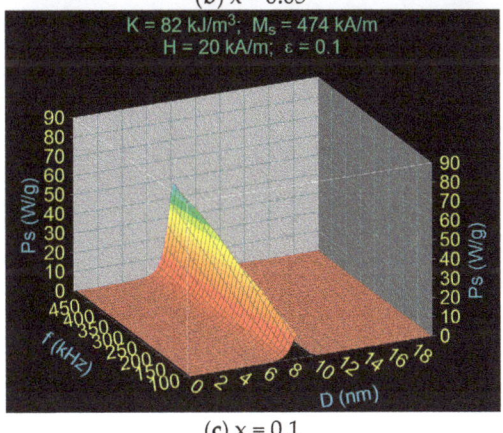

(c) x = 0.1

Figure 3. *Cont.*

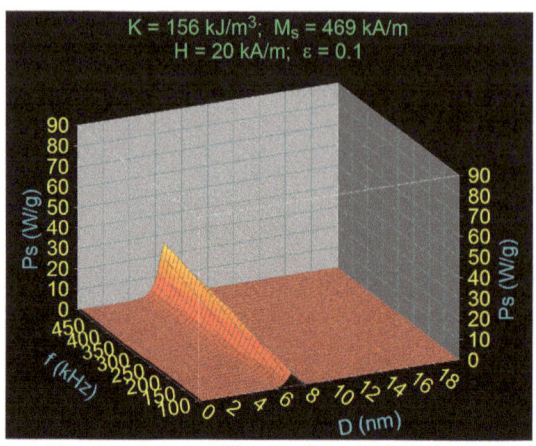

(d) x = 0.2

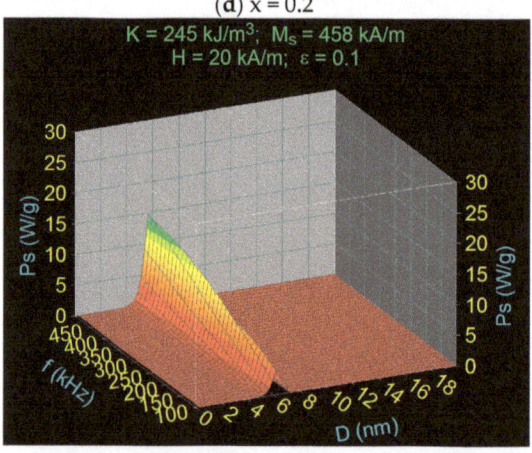

(e) x = 0.4

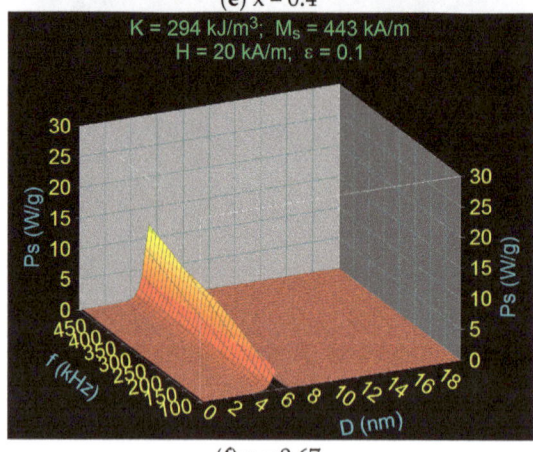

(f) x = 0.67

Figure 3. *Cont.*

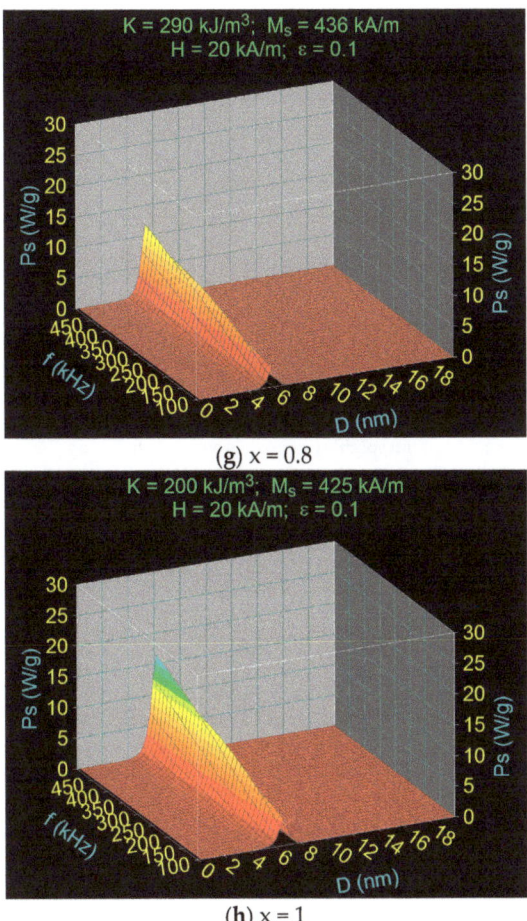

Figure 3. Specific loss power variation in the case of $Co_xFe_{3-x}O_4$ ferrimagnetic nanoparticles as a function of the diameter of nanoparticles and the magnetic field frequency for different Co^{2+} ions concentration: (**a**) 0, (**b**) 0.05, (**c**) 0.1 (**d**) 0.2, (**e**) 0.4, (**f**) 0.67, (**g**) 0.8, and (**h**) 1.

The results obtained and shown in diagrams (a)–(h) of Figure 3 are summarized in Tables 3–5. Figure 3 shows the presence of the maximum specific loss power at a certain values of the nanoparticle diameter (D_M), which is a critical parameter; the maximum specific loss power P_{sM} decrease rapidly to zero for values slightly larger or smaller than the D_M diameter. Also, in all cases, the maximum specific loss power increases with the frequency of the magnetic field (100–500 kHz) as shown in diagrams (a)–(h). These variations of the specific loss power are in agreement with the variations previously observed in the case of nanoparticles of Fe_3O_4 and $CoFe_2O_4$ [31,32]. However, a special result obtained now is that the maximum specific loss power P_{sM} decreases continuously and rapidly at the beginning with the increase of the concentration of Co^{2+} ions (x) from x = 0 to x = 0.8 after which a slow increase is obtained until x = 1 (Figure 4). Thus, the maximum specific loss power P_{sM} has a minimum at the concentration value of x = 0.8.

Table 3. Maximum specific loss powers and corresponding diameter of nanoparticles as a function of the Co^{2+} ions concentration (x) for f = 100 kHz and H = 20 kA/m.

No.	Observables x	P_{sM} (W/g)	D_M (nm)
1	0	31.69	17.4
2	0.05	21.14	11.5
3	0.1	11.85	9
4	0.2	6.45	7.2
5	0.4	3.96	6.2
6	0.67	3.05	5.9
7	0.8	3.03	5.9
8	1	4.11	6.7

Table 4. Maximum specific loss powers and corresponding diameter of nanoparticles as a function of the Co^{2+} ions concentration (x) for f = 250 kHz and H = 20 kA/m.

No.	Observables x	P_{sM} (W/g)	D_M (nm)
1	0	77.6	16.7
2	0.05	48.95	11.1
3	0.1	26.59	8.6
4	0.2	14.23	6.9
5	0.4	8.66	6.
6	0.67	6.81	5.6
7	0.8	6.62	5.6
8	1	9.13	6.4

Table 5. Maximum specific loss powers and corresponding diameter of nanoparticles as a function of the Co^{2+} ions concentration (x) for f = 500 kHz and H = 20 kA/m.

No.	Observables x	P_{sM} (W/g)	D_M (nm)
1	0	152.1	16.1
2	0.05	91.06	10.7
3	0.1	48.13	8.3
4	0.2	25.61	6.7
5	0.4	15.48	5.8
6	0.67	12.2	5.4
7	0.8	11.88	5.4
8	1	16.25	6.2

A similar variation of the concentration x is also obtained for the diameters of nanoparticles D_M corresponding to the maximum specific loss power P_{sM} (Figure 5). The diameter of nanoparticles that give the maximum of the specific loss power decreases very much with the increase of the concentration x; e.g., for the frequency of 500 kHz the diameter of nanoparticles decreases from 16.1 nm for x = 0 to 6.2 nm when x increases to 1, the diameter also having a minimum value, which is 5.4 nm for x = 0.8.

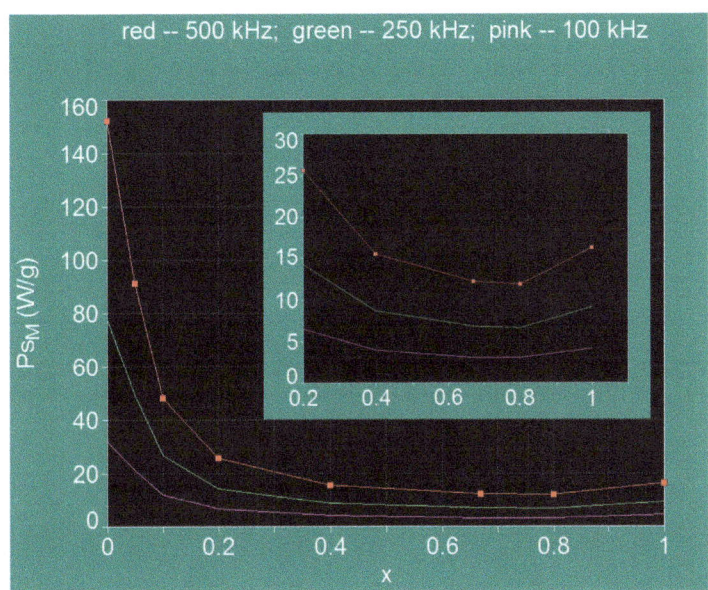

Figure 4. Maximum specific loss power variation in the case of $Co_xFe_{3-x}O_4$ ferrimagnetic nanoparticles as a function of the Co^{2+} ions concentration. Inset: magnified image for the range x = 0.2–1.

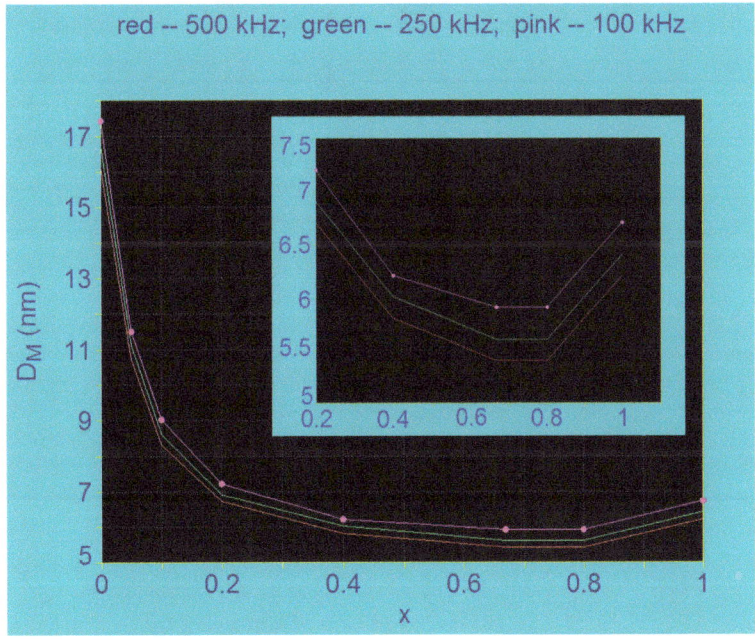

Figure 5. The variation of the nanoparticle diameters corresponding to the maximum specific loss power in the case of $Co_xFe_{3-x}O_4$ ferrimagnetic nanoparticles as a function of the Co^{2+} ions concentration. Inset: magnified image in the range x = 0.2–1.

This result, as well as the one regarding the specific loss power, are very important from the SPMHT point of view, because it suggests that it is possible to tune the observables and parameters of interest in magnetic hyperthermia, such as the specific loss power, nanoparticle size, and implicitly heating temperature and toxicity, magnetic packing fraction, etc., in a very wide range of values, just by simply changing the concentration of Co^{2+} ions. Thus, by changing the x concentration, the most suitable conditions can be obtained for the application of SPMHT in optimal conditions: obtaining maximum efficiency in SPMHT, obtaining maximum effectiveness in destroying tumor cells, obtaining minimum cellular toxicity on healthy tissues, or even lack of toxicity. This is a very important result for the practical implementation of SPMHT in vitro, in vivo and in future clinical trials.

By extracting the values of the maximum specific loss power P_{sM} and those of the diameters of nanoparticles D_M corresponding to the maximum powers, for each value of the concentration x in the range 0–1 (Table 1) at the frequencies of 100 kHz, 250 kHz and 500 kHz, the values from Tables 3–5 were obtained. Then, representing the powers P_{sM} and the diameters D_M as a function of the concentration x, the curves shown in Figures 4 and 5 were obtained.

From the curves in Figure 4 it is observed that for all the frequencies considered (100, 250 and 300 kHz) the maximum specific loss power P_{sM} in SPMHT decreases rapidly when the concentration of Co^{2+} ions increases in the range x = 0–0.2, and then the power decreases very slowly until x = 0.8. Then, when the concentration increases in the range x = 0.8–1 the power P_{sM} also increases, but slowly. Thus, in the range of values x = 0.2–1 the variation of maximum loss power P_{sM} presents a very wide minimum, having the lowest value at x = 0.8, depending on the value of frequency (inset of Figure 4). When the frequency decreases from 500 kHz to 100 kHz, the shape of the curves is preserved, only the power values decrease with the decrease of alternating magnetic field frequency (Figure 4, Tables 3–5).

Such a variation is also obtained for the diameter D_M (Figure 5) which determines the maximum specific loss power P_{sM}. From the point of view of magnetic hyperthermia both ranges of Co^{2+} ions concentration, both for x = 0–2 and for x = 0.2–1 are of interest and must be taken into account. If in the range x = 0–0.2 it must be borne in mind that the maximum specific loss power P_{sM} decreases rapidly with increasing concentration of Co^{2+} ions, which could sometimes be a disadvantage in terms of power obtained in magnetic hyperthermia (which it will also be reflected on the heating temperature), in the next interval x = 0.2–1 the specific loss power P_{sM} changes only slightly, which would be an advantage in magnetic hyperthermia. Thus, it results that it could be used in obtaining nanoparticles much different concentrations for Co^{2+} ions, in the range 0.2–1 respectively, without the maximum specific loss power to change too much in SPMHT. In addition, this could be another advantage in terms of the size of magnetic nanoparticles, sizes that are much smaller in this range (5.5–7 nm, depending on the frequency) (inset of Figure 5), and which lead to beneficial effect on reduction of cellular toxicity (due to the small size of the nanoparticles). Moreover, the much smaller size of the nanoparticles for the x = 0.2–1 range is also very beneficial in order to obtain intracellular hyperthermia, which is much more efficient in destroying tumor cells. The nanoparticles, being very small, penetrate much more easily into the cell (cytoplasm or even the nucleus) through the cell membrane, and thus destroying the tumor cells by magnetic hyperthermia much more efficiently inside them. At the same time, in this range of concentrations x = 0.2–1 the size of the nanoparticles does not change much (Figure 5), obtaining practically the same effect by magnetic hyperthermia for very different concentrations of Co^{2+} ions.

However, for the concentration range x = 0–0.2 the diameter of the nanoparticles changes a lot; e.g., at 500 kHz the D_M diameter decreases from ~17 nm to ~7 nm when the x concentration increases from 0 to 0.2. This seems to be a disadvantage in terms of the power obtained in magnetic hyperthermia, and finally, the efficient heating and temperature obtained. However, if the power does not fall below a certain value, which is required in magnetic hyperthermia to heat the nanoparticles sufficiently, then the apparent disadvantage can be turned into a great advantage, namely: by changing the concentration of Co^{2+} ions in the range x = 0–0.2 the different diameters (sizes) of nanoparticles can be obtained in a wide range of values (7–17 nm) which will lead to different maximums of specific loss power in a very wide range of values. Thus, the best conditions can be found regarding the nanoparticle sizes, specific loss power, heating temperature, toxicity on healthy cells, etc., for SPMHT application in optimal conditions, by simply changing the concentration of Co^{2+} ions in the field of x = 0–0.2.

Another important aspect that must take into consideration in the implementation of SPMHT is that the values of nanoparticle diameters D_M that give the maximum specific loss power P_{sM} depend on the frequency of alternating magnetic field besides the concentration of Co^{2+} ions, as shown in Figure 6.

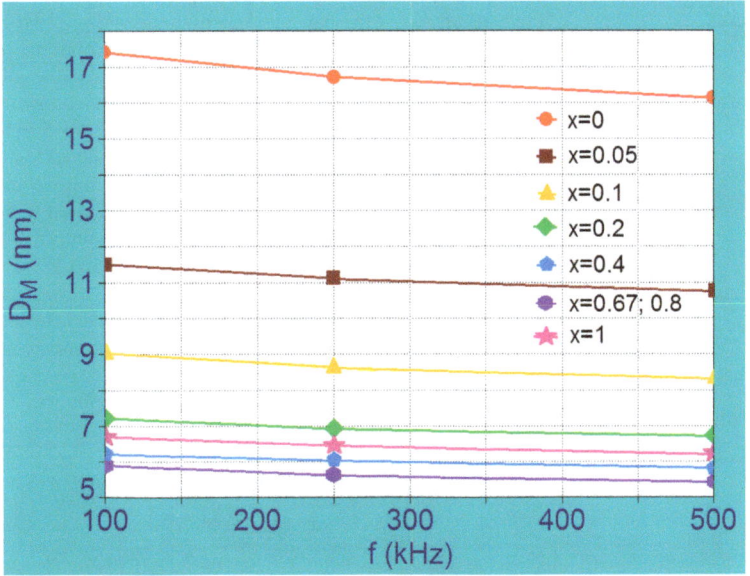

Figure 6. The variation of the nanoparticle diameters corresponding to the maximum specific loss power in the case of $Co_xFe_{3-x}O_4$ ferrimagnetic nanoparticles as a function of frequency for different Co^{2+} ions concentrations in the range x = 0–1.

When the frequency in SPMHT increases from 100 kHz to 500 KHz the diameter of nanoparticles D_M that give the maximum specific loss power (P_{sM}) decreases slightly for each value of the concentration x when it increases from 0 to 1. The decrease in diameter is more pronounced for the concentrations located in the range x = 0–0.2, being the largest at x = 0 where diameter D_M decreases by 1.3 nm (from 17.4 nm to 16.1 nm) (Tables 3 and 5). The D_M values at each concentration must be taken into account for each frequency value used in the SPMHT in order to obtain the maximum loss power and the maximum thermal effect. Otherwise, the diameter being a critical parameter (Figure 3), a value slightly lower or slightly higher than that corresponding to D_M value can greatly reduce the specific loss power, with negative effects on the hyperthermia effect, and consequently on the efficiency of SPMHT in tumor cells destruction.

3.3. Superparamagnetic Hyperthermia Optimization with $Co_xFe_{3-x}O_4$ Ferrite Nanoparticles: The Optimal Conditions Determination for Biologic Limit

Based on our previous results [31,32] we used the range of study for the magnetic field of 10–50 kA/m and the limit frequencies corresponding to these values, which results from the condition [42]:

$$H \times f = 5 \times 10^9 \text{ AHz/m} \tag{11}$$

Using diagrams such as those in Figure 3 for all optimal magnetic fields (H_o) and their corresponding frequencies for the allowable biological limit (f_l), we determined the specific loss power for the allowable biological limit ($P_s)_l$ depending on the concentration of Co^{2+} ions in the considered range (x = 0–1). The diagrams obtained for x = 0; 0.1; 0.8 and 1, and for a field of 30 kA/m, and a limit frequency of 167 kHz, are shown in Figure 7. The maximum values of the specific loss power for the admissible biological limit $(P_{sM})_l$ and those of the nanoparticle diameters (D_{Mo}) that give the maximum loss power $(P_{sM})_l$ under the given conditions were extracted from diagrams like those in Figure 7, for H_o = 10–50 kHz, f_l = 100–500 kHz and x = 0–1. All values obtained for $(P_{sM})_l$ and D_{Mo} are shown in Table 6. The very important result obtained is how the maximum specific loss power $(P_{sM})_l$ depends on the amplitude of the applied magnetic field for the admissible biological limit.

Thus, the variations of power $(P_{sM})_l$ depending on the amplitude of magnetic field for different x concentrations of Co^{2+} ions are shown in Figure 8. The obtained results show a progressive decrease of the power $(P_{sM})_l$ with the increase of the concentration x of the Co^{2+} ions, decrease which is more accentuated for the first part of concentration range x = 0–0.2. Also, for x = 0.67 and x = 0.8 the power values $(P_{sM})_l$ are the lowest for the considered magnetic fields, being approximately the same for the two concentrations (0.67; 0.8) (Table 6), the powers $(P_{sM})_l$ increasing linearly with the magnetic field up to the value of 50 kA/m. Moreover, it is also observed that for the values x = 0.4 and x = 1 the approximately same powers $(P_{sM})_l$ are obtained, but slightly higher than in the previous case.

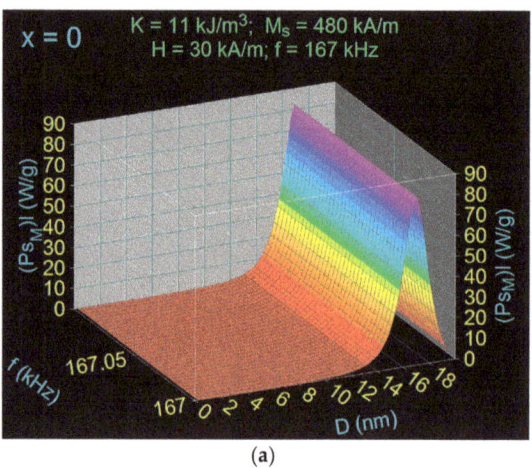

(a)

Figure 7. *Cont.*

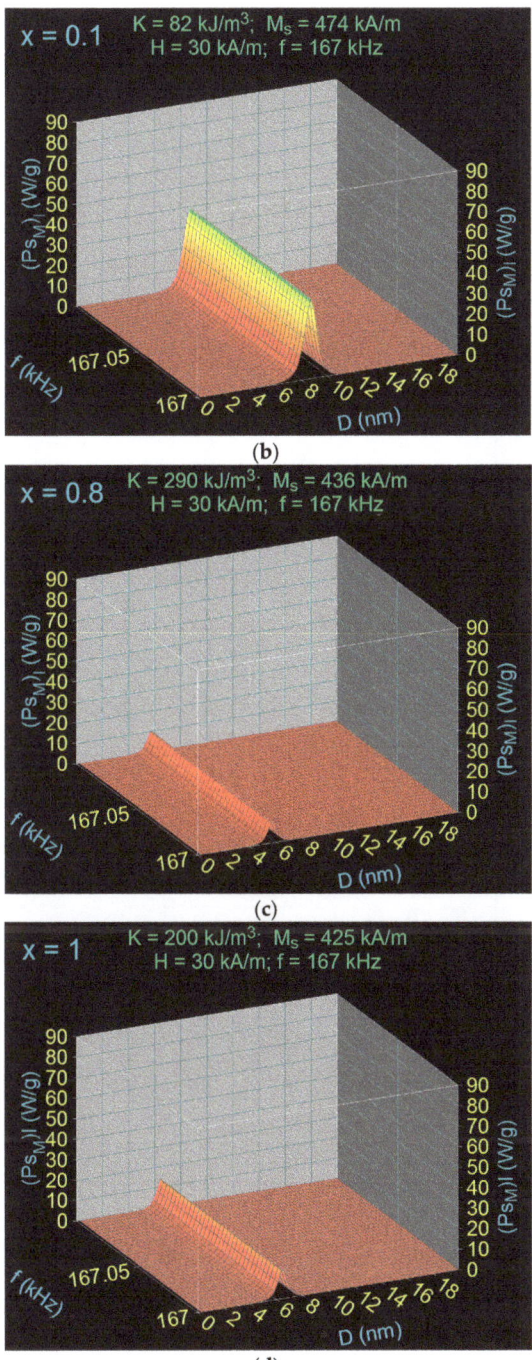

Figure 7. Specific loss power in the case of $Co_xFe_{3-x}O_4$ nanoparticles as a function of diameters for admissible biological limit ($H = 30$ kA/m and $f = 167$ kHz) and different Co^{2+} ions concentration (x): (**a**) 0, (**b**) 0.1, (**c**) 0.8, and (**d**) 1.

Table 6. Maximum specific loss power (P_{sM})$_l$ and corresponding diameter of nanoparticles (D_{Mo}) in the case of Co$_x$Fe$_{3-x}$O$_4$ ferrite nanoparticles for admissible biological limits $H \times f$ and different amplitudes of magnetic field (H_o).

H_o (kA/m)	f_l (kHz)	$H \times f$ AHz/m	x = 0		x = 0.05		x = 0.1		x = 0.2		x = 0.4		x = 0.67		x = 0.8		x = 1	
			(P_{sM})$_l$ (W/g)	D_{Mo} (nm)	(P_{sM})$_l$ (W/g)	D_{Mo} (nm)	(P_{sM})$_l$ (W/g)	D_{Mo} (nm)	(P_{sM})$_l$ (W/g)	D_{Mo} (nm)	(P_{sM})$_l$ (W/g)	D_{Mo} (nm)	(P_{sM})$_l$ (W/g)	D_{Mo} (nm)	(P_{sM})$_l$ (W/g)	D_{Mo} (nm)	(P_{sM})$_l$ (W/g)	D_{Mo} (nm)
10	500	5 × 10^9	62.29	16.1	26.13	10.7	12.47	8.3	6.47	6.7	3.89	5.8	3.06	5.4	2.98	5.4	4.08	6.2
20	250	5 × 10^9	77.60	16.7	48.94	11.1	26.59	8.6	14.23	6.9	8.66	6.0	6.81	5.6	6.63	5.6	9.12	6.4
30	167	5 × 10^9	82.57	17.0	62.52	11.3	39.12	8.7	20.07	7.1	13.75	6.1	10.77	5.7	10.44	5.7	14.41	6.5
40	125	5 × 10^9	84.60	17.2	68.96	11.5	48.92	8.8	29.43	7.2	18.63	6.2	14.82	5.8	14.48	5.8	19.58	6.6
50	100	5 × 10^9	85.94	17.4	74.31	11.5	56.68	8.9	36.59	7.2	23.78	6.2	18.52	5.9	18.42	5.9	24.31	6.7

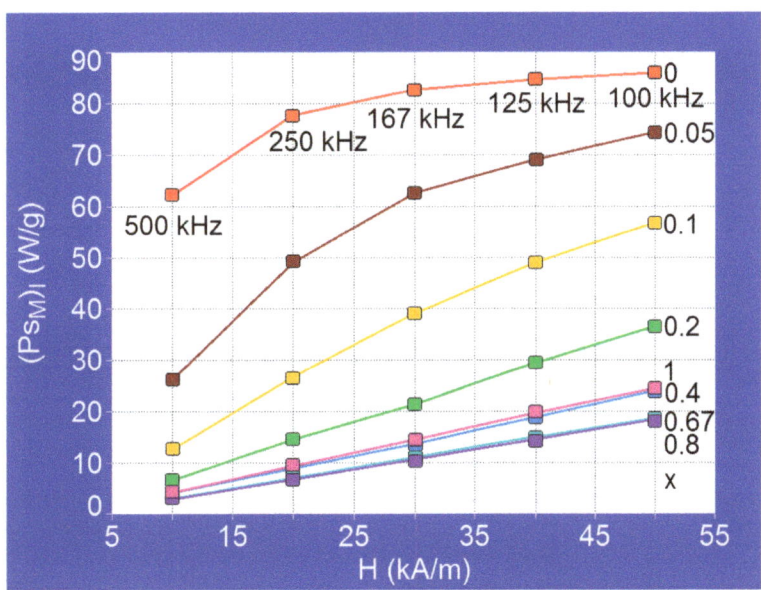

Figure 8. Maximum specific loss power for admissible biological limit $(P_{sM})_l$ in the case of $Co_xFe_{3-x}O_4$ (x = 0–1) nanoparticles as a function of the amplitudes of magnetic field, and for different limit frequencies.

Considering our previous results [32] and considering for the efficient heating of the nanoparticles a value of the power $(P_{sM})_l$ higher of 10–15 W/g, we have established the optimal domains for magnetic field and concentrations which are recommended for the efficient practical implementation of SPMHT in this case. As seen in Figure 8, for x = 0 and magnetic fields greater than 25–30 kA/m the power $(P_{sM})_l$ increases only slightly, reaching a saturation level, so the use of larger magnetic fields is not justified (it does not lead to any significant increase in power). A similar effect is obtained in the case of x = 0.05 for magnetic fields greater than 40 kA/m. For x = 0.1 the power saturation effect occurs at fields greater than 50–60 kA/m. For values of concentration x greater than 0.2 and up to 1 the saturation is obtained at much higher values of the magnetic field, and up to 50 kA/m the variations of the power $(P_{sM})_l$ with concentration x are approximately linear: the power increases proportionally with the concentration of Co^{2+} ions, having low values for these concentrations. However, for concentrations higher than 0.1 we delimited the range for the magnetic field to reasonable values in SPMHT, respectively up to 50 kA/m, because it is practically difficult to obtain large magnetic fields at frequencies of the order of 10^5 Hz, and the magnetization of magnetic nanoparticles still remains in the superparamagnetic range.

In conclusion, taking into account all the above results and observations, in Table 7 we summarize the recommended values for the amplitude and frequency of the magnetic field depending on the concentration of Co^{2+} ions (x) in order to obtain SPMHT in optimal conditions, for maximum efficiency of the method. Thus, as a general observation it can be said that for lower x concentrations (0–0.1) the SPMHT is more suitable to be obtained for higher frequencies and lower magnetic fields, and for x concentrations higher than 0.1 the SPMHT becomes more suitable to be obtained at lower frequencies and higher magnetic fields.

Thus, under these conditions that we found the superparamagnetic hyperthermia with $Co_xFe_{3-x}O_4$ nanoparticles can be applied with maximum efficiency in the destruction of tumor cells. In addition, if necessary in order to further increase the effectiveness of cancer therapy, superparamagnetic hyperthermia can be used in combination with other methods [5,12,16,17,43].

Table 7. Optimum values of the amplitude and frequency of magnetic field for different concentration of Co^{2+} ions.

No.	Observables x	H_o (kA/m)	f_l (kHz)
1	0	10–30	500–167
2	0.05	10–40	500–125
3	0.1	10–50	500–100
4	0.2	20–50	250–100
5	0.4; 1	30–50	167–100
6	0.67; 0.8	40–50	125–100

4. Conclusions

Using $Co_xFe_{3-x}O_4$ nanoparticles in SPMHT, by modifying the concentration x of Co^{2+} ions in the range x = 0–1 an efficient tuning can be obtained in a very wide range of values of observables/parameters of interest in SPMHT: maximum specific loss power (implicitly the heating temperature), the optimal diameter (size) of the nanoparticles corresponding to the maximum of specific loss power, the amplitude and the frequency of magnetic field. Thus, the optimal conditions for the application of SPMHT in the admissible biological limit can be found, depending on the concrete practical situations (tumor therapy in vitro, in vivo or in future clinical trials), to increase its efficiency in destroying tumor cells without affecting healthy tissues. Thus, the results obtained regarding the maximum specific loss power for the allowable biological limit $(P_{sM})_l$, the optimal diameter of the nanoparticles for obtaining the maximum loss power (D_{Mo}), the optimal range for the amplitude of alternating magnetic field (H_o) and the limit frequencies (f_l) (Table 6, Figure 8, Table 7) are effective data/tools for working in the practical implementation of SPMHT in order to obtain an increased efficacy in alternative therapy of tumors with as few toxicity as possible or even without toxicity.

Funding: This work was supported by a grant of the Ministry of Research, Innovation and Digitization, CNCS/CCCDI–UEFISCDI, project number PN-III-P2-2.1-PED-2019-3067, within PNCDI III, and West University of Timisoara from CNFIS-FDI-2020-0253 project.

Institutional Review Board Statement: Not applicable.

Informed Consent Statement: Not applicable.

Data Availability Statement: Not applicable.

Conflicts of Interest: The author declare no conflict of interest.

References

1. Jordan, A.; Scholz, R.; Wust, P.; Schirra, H.; Schiestel, T.; Schmidt, H.; Felix, R.J. Endocytosis of dextran and silan-coated magnetite nanoparticles and the effect of intracellular hyperthermia on human mammary carcinoma cells in vitro. *J. Magn. Magn. Mater.* **1999**, *194*, 185–196. [CrossRef]
2. Ito, A.; Tanaka, K.; Honda, H.; Abe, S.; Yamaguchi, H.; Kobayaschi, T. Complete regression of mouse mammary carcinoma with a size greater than 15 mm by frequent repeated hyperthermia using magnetite nanoparticles. *J. Biosci. Bioeng.* **2003**, *96*, 364–369. [CrossRef]
3. Ito, A.; Shinkai, M.; Honda, H.; Kobayashi, T. Medical application of functionalized magnetic nanoparticles. *J. Biosci. Bioeng.* **2005**, *100*, 1–11. [CrossRef] [PubMed]
4. Hilger, I.; Hergt, R.; Kaiser, W.A. Towards breast cancer treatment by magnetic heating. *J. Magn. Magn. Mater.* **2005**, *293*, 314–319. [CrossRef]
5. Maier-Hauff, K.; Rothe, R.; Scholz, R.; Gneveckow, U.; Wust, P.; Thiesen, B.; Feussner, A.; Deimling, A.; Waldoefner, N.; Felix, R.; et al. Intracranial thermotherapy using magnetic nanoparticles combined with external beam radiotherapy: Results of a feasibility study on patients with glioblastoma multiforme. *J. Neuro-Oncol.* **2007**, *81*, 53–60. [CrossRef] [PubMed]

6. Johannsen, M.; Gneveckow, U.; Thiesen, B.; Taymoorian, K.; Cho, C.H.; Waldofner, N.; Scholz, R.; Jordan, A.; Loening, S.A.; Wust, P. Thermotherapy of prostate cancer using magnetic nanoparticles: Feasibility, imaging, and three-dimensional temperature distribution. *Eur. Urol.* **2007**, *52*, 1653–1662. [CrossRef] [PubMed]
7. Gazeau, F.; Lévy, M.; Wilhelm, C. Optimizing magnetic nanoparticle design for nanothermotherapy. *Nanomedicine* **2008**, *3*, 831–844. [CrossRef] [PubMed]
8. Fortin, J.P.; Gazeau, F.; Wilhelm, C. Intracellular heating of living cells through Néel relaxation of magnetic nanoparticles. *Eur. Biophys. J.* **2008**, *37*, 223–228. [CrossRef]
9. Laurent, S.; Dutz, S.; Hafeli, U.O.; Mahmoudi, M. Magnetic fluid hyperthermia: Focus on superparamagnetic iron oxide nanoparticles. *Adv. Colloid Interface Sci.* **2011**, *166*, 8–23. [CrossRef] [PubMed]
10. Alphandéry, E.; Chebbi, I.; Guyot, F.; Durand-Dubief, M. Use of bacterial magnetosomes in the magnetic hyperthermia treatment of tumours: A review. *Int. J. Hyperth.* **2013**, *29*, 801–809. [CrossRef] [PubMed]
11. Caizer, C. Computational study on superparamagnetic hyperthermia with biocompatible SPIONs to destroy the cancer cells. *J. Phys. Conf. Ser.* **2014**, *521*, 012015. [CrossRef]
12. Di Corato, R.; Béalle, G.; Kolosnjaj-Tabi, J.; Espinosa, A.; Clément, O.; Silva, A.; Ménager, C.; Wilhelm, C. Combining magnetic hyperthermia and photodynamic therapy for tumor ablation with photoresponsive magnetic liposomes. *ACS Nano* **2015**, *9*, 2904–2916. [CrossRef] [PubMed]
13. Wang, F.; Yang, Y.; Ling, Y.; Liu, J.; Cai, X.; Zhou, X.; Tang, X.; Liang, B.; Chen, Y.; Chen, H.; et al. Injectable and thermally contractible hydroxypropyl methyl cellulose/Fe3O4 for magnetic hyperthermia ablation of tumors. *Biomaterials* **2017**, *128*, 84–93. [CrossRef]
14. Caizer, C. Magnetic hyperthermia-using magnetic metal/oxide nanoparticles with potential in cancer therapy. In *Metal Nanoparticles in Pharma*; Rai, M., Shegokar, R., Eds.; Springer: Berlin/Heidelberg, Germany, 2017.
15. Kandasamy, G.; Sudame, A.; Bhati, P.; Chakrabarty, A.; Maity, D. Systematic investigations on heating effects of carboxyl-amine functionalized superparamagnetic iron oxide nanoparticles (SPIONs) based ferrofluids for in vitro cancer hyperthermia therapy. *J. Mol. Liq.* **2018**, *256*, 224–237. [CrossRef]
16. Yan, H.; Shang, W.; Sun, X.; Zhao, L.; Wang, J.; Xiong, Z.; Yuan, J.; Zhang, R.; Huang, Q.; Wang, K.; et al. "All-in-One" Nanoparticles for Trimodality Imaging-Guided Intracellular Photo-magnetic Hyperthermia Therapy under Intravenous Administration. *Adv. Funct. Mater.* **2018**, *28*, 1705710. [CrossRef]
17. Caizer, C. Magnetic/Superparamagnetic hyperthermia as an effective noninvasive alternative method for therapy of malignant tumors. In *Nanotheranostics: Applications and Limitations*; Rai, M., Jamil, B., Eds.; Springer: Berlin/Heidelberg, Germany, 2019; pp. 297–335.
18. Smit, J.; Wijin, H.P.J. *Les Ferites*; Bibliotheque Technique Philips: Paris, France, 1961.
19. Valenzuela, R. *Magnetic Ceramics*; Cambridge University Press: Cambridge, UK, 1994.
20. Rosensweig, R.E. Heating magnetic fluid with alternating magnetic field. *J. Magn. Magn. Mater.* **2002**, *252*, 370–374. [CrossRef]
21. Caizer, C.; Rai, M. Magnetic nanoparticles in alternative tumors therapy: Biocompatibility, toxicity and safety compared with classical methods. In *Magnetic Nanoparticles in Human Health and Medicine: Current Medical Applications and Alternative Therapy of Cancer*; Caizer, C., Rai, M., Eds.; Wiley: Hoboken, NJ, USA, 2021.
22. Hejase, H.; Hayek, S.; Qadri, S.; Haik, Y. MnZnFe nanoparticles for self-controlled magnetic hyperthermia. *J. Magn. Magn. Mater.* **2012**, *324*, 3620–3628. [CrossRef]
23. Caizer, C.; Hadaruga, N.; Hadaruga, D.; Tanasie, G.; Vlazan, P. The Co ferrite nanoparticles/liposomes: Magnetic bionanocomposites for applications in malignant tumors therapy. In Proceedings of the 7th International Conference Inorganic Materials, Biarritz, France, 12–14 September 2010.
24. Kumar, C.S.; Mohammad, F. Magnetic nanomaterials for hyperthermia-based therapy and controlled drug delivery. *Adv. Drug Deliv. Rev.* **2011**, *63*, 789–808. [CrossRef] [PubMed]
25. Pradhan, P.; Giri, J.; Samanta, G.; Sarma, H.D.; Mishra, K.P.; Bellare, J.; Banerjee, R.; Bahadur, D. Comparative evaluation of heating ability and biocompatibility of different ferrite-based magnetic fluids for hyperthermia application. *J. Biomed. Mater. Res. B Appl. Biomater.* **2007**, *81*, 12–22. [CrossRef]
26. Qu, Y.; Li, J.; Ren, J.; Leng, J.; Lin, C.; Shi, D. Enhanced Magnetic Fluid Hyperthermia by Micellar Magnetic Nanoclusters Composed of MnxZn1−xFe2O4 Nanoparticles for Induced Tumor Cell Apoptosis. *ACS Appl. Mater. Interfaces* **2014**, *6*, 16867–16879. [CrossRef]
27. Caizer, C. Magnetic anisotropy of CoxFe3−xO4 nanoparticles for applications in magnetic hyperthermia. In Proceedings of the 19th International Conference on Magnetism (ICM 2012), Busan, Korea, 8–13 July 2012.
28. Saldívar-Ramírez, M.M.G.; Sanchez-Torres, C.G.; Cortés-Hernández, D.A.; Escobedo-Bocardo, J.C.; Almanza-Robles, J.M.; Larson, A.; Reséndiz-Hernández, P.J.; Acuña-Gutiérrez, I.O. Study on the efficiency of nanosized magnetite and mixed ferrites in magnetic hyperthermia. *J. Mater. Sci. Mater. Med.* **2014**, *25*, 2229–2236. [CrossRef]
29. Liu, X.L.; Ng, C.T.; Chandrasekharan, P.; Yang, H.T.; Zhao, L.Y.; Peng, E.; Lv, Y.B.; Xiao, W.; Fang, J.B.; Yi, J.; et al. Synthesis of Ferromagnetic Fe0.6Mn0.4O Nanoflowers as a New Class of Magnetic Theranostic Platform for In Vivo T1-T2Dual-Mode Magnetic Resonance Imaging and Magnetic Hyperthermia Therapy. *Adv. Healthc. Mater.* **2016**, *5*, 2092–2104. [CrossRef] [PubMed]

30. Almaki, J.H.; Nasiri, R.; Idris, A.; Majid, F.A.A.; Salouti, M.; Wong, T.S.; Dabagh, S.; Marvibaigi, M.; Amini, N. Synthesis, characterization and In Vitro evaluation of exquisite targeting SPIONs–PEG–HER in HER2+ human breast cancer cells. *Nanotechnology* **2016**, *27*, 105601. [CrossRef]
31. Caizer, C. Optimization Study on Specific Loss Power in Superparamagnetic Hyperthermia with Magnetite Nanoparticles for High Efficiency in Alternative Cancer Therapy. *Nanomaterials* **2021**, *11*, 40. [CrossRef]
32. Caizer, C. Theoretical Study on Specific Loss Power and Heating Temperature in $CoFe_2O_4$ Nanoparticles as Possible Candidate for Alternative Cancer Therapy by Superparamagnetic Hyperthemia. *Appl. Sci.* **2021**, *11*, 5505. [CrossRef]
33. Caizer, C. Scientific Research Report. *UEFISCDI* **2020**, in press.
34. Néel, L. Théorie du traînage magnétique des ferromagnétiques en grains fins avec application aux terres cuites. *Ann. Geophys.* **1949**, *5*, 99–136.
35. Prasad, N.K.; Rathinasamy, K.; Panda, D.; Bahadur, D. Mechanism of cell death induced by magnetic hyperthermia with nanoparticles of -$MnxFe_2–xO_3$ synthesized by a single step process. *J. Mat. Chem.* **2007**, *17*, 5042–5051. [CrossRef]
36. Pankhurst, Q.A.; Connolly, J.; Jones, S.K.; Dobson, J. Applications of magnetic nanoparticles in biomedicine. *J. Phys. D: Appl. Phys.* **2003**, *36*, R167–R181. [CrossRef]
37. Kneller, E. *Ferromagnetismus*; Springer: Berlin/Heidelberg, Germany, 1962.
38. Shliomis, M. Magnetic fluids. *Sov. Phys. Uspekhi.* **1974**, *17*, 153–169. [CrossRef]
39. Jacobs, I.S.; Bean, C.P. Fine particles, thin films and exchange anisotropy. In *Magnetism*; Rado, G.T., Suhl, H., Eds.; Academic Press: Cambridge, MA, USA, 1963; Volume III, pp. 271–350.
40. Bean, C.P.; Livingston, L.D. Superparamagnetism. *J. Appl. Phys.* **1959**, *30*, S120–S129. [CrossRef]
41. Back, C.H.; Weller, D.; Heidmann, J.; Mauri, D.; Guarisco, D.; Garwin, E.L.; Siegmann, H.C. Magnetization Reversal in Ultrashort Magnetic Field Pulses. *Phys. Rev. Lett.* **1998**, *81*, 3251–3254. [CrossRef]
42. Hergt, R.; Dutz, S. Magnetic particle hyperthermia—Biophysical limitations of a visionary tumour therapy. *J. Magn. Magn. Mater.* **2007**, *311*, 187–192. [CrossRef]
43. Brero, F.; Albino, M.; Antoccia, A.; Arosio, P.; Avolio, M.; Berardinelli, F.; Bettega, D.; Calzolari, P.; Ciocca, M.; Corti, M.; et al. Hadron Therapy, Magnetic Nanoparticles and Hyperthermia: A Promising Combined Tool for Pancreatic Cancer Treatment. *Nanomaterials* **2020**, *10*, 1919. [CrossRef] [PubMed]

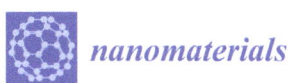

Article

Gold Nanoparticle DNA Damage by Photon Beam in a Magnetic Field: A Monte Carlo Study

Mehwish Jabeen [1] and James C. L. Chow [2,*]

[1] Department of Physics, Ryerson University, Toronto, ON M5B 2K3, Canada; mehwish.jabeen@ryerson.ca
[2] Department of Radiation Oncology, University of Toronto and Radiation Medicine Program, Princess Margaret Cancer Centre, Toronto, ON M5G 1Z5, Canada
* Correspondence: james.chow@rmp.uhn.ca; Tel.: +1-416-946-4501

Abstract: Ever since the emergence of magnetic resonance (MR)-guided radiotherapy, it is important to investigate the impact of the magnetic field on the dose enhancement in deoxyribonucleic acid (DNA), when gold nanoparticles are used as radiosensitizers during radiotherapy. Gold nanoparticle-enhanced radiotherapy is known to enhance the dose deposition in the DNA, resulting in a double-strand break. In this study, the effects of the magnetic field on the dose enhancement factor (DER) for varying gold nanoparticle sizes, photon beam energies and magnetic field strengths and orientations were investigated using Geant4-DNA Monte Carlo simulations. Using a Monte Carlo model including a single gold nanoparticle with a photon beam source and DNA molecule on the left and right, it is demonstrated that as the gold nanoparticle size increased, the DER increased. However, as the photon beam energy decreased, an increase in the DER was detected. When a magnetic field was added to the simulation model, the DER was found to increase by 2.5–5% as different field strengths (0–2 T) and orientations (x-, y- and z-axis) were used for a 100 nm gold nanoparticle using a 50 keV photon beam. The DNA damage reflected by the DER increased slightly with the presence of the magnetic field. However, variations in the magnetic field strength and orientation did not change the DER significantly.

Keywords: gold nanoparticle; nanoparticle-enhanced radiotherapy; MR-guided radiotherapy; DNA damage; Monte Carlo simulation; dose enhancement; magnetic field

1. Introduction

In radiotherapy, the aim is to acquire a conformal dose at the tumor or target as high as possible while, at the same time, sparing the surrounding normal tissues at the minimum dose. One way to achieve this goal is to add a heavy-atom radiosensitizer such as gold nanoparticles to the tumor to increase its compositional atomic number [1–3]. This increase in radiosensitivity is due to a combination of the physical dose enhancement and additional chemical and biological effects associated with the nanoparticle [4]. Gold nanoparticles can be transported to living cells through a liposome-based system. This makes the treatment delivery of gold nanoparticle-enhanced radiotherapy possible [5]. There are two advantages of adding gold nanoparticles to the tumor. First, the increase in the compositional atomic number of the tumor increases the radiation dose absorption through the enhancement of the photoelectric effect. This dose enhancement is particularly significant when photon beam energy in the kilovoltage (kV) range is used, where the photoelectric effect is dominant [6–8]. Moreover, the dose enhancement can increase cancer cell killing. Second, due to the increase in the deviation of beam absorption between the target (with gold nanoparticle addition) and its surrounding tissue (without gold nanoparticle addition), contrast enhancement can be achieved in medical imaging modalities such as computed tomography (CT) using a kV photon beam [9–11]. The increase in target contrast will make it easier for the radiation oncologist to identify the tumor and contour it more accurately in radiation treatment planning. Therefore, gold nanoparticle-enhanced radiotherapy has become popular, resulting in many studies on the basic science and clinical application [12–15]. Many preclinical works have been carried out, and clinical trials are being conducted, building a potential roadmap to clinical implementation [16].

In radiobiology, it is well known that cancer cell killing or control is caused by the energy deposition from the secondary electrons at the deoxyribonucleic acid (DNA). These secondary electrons generated by the ionizing radiation in the tumor medium (water equivalent) would travel to the strands of DNA and damage the molecule, for example, causing a single- and double-strand break [17,18]. The addition of gold nanoparticles to the tumor can enhance the energy deposition because extra secondary electrons are produced by the irradiated nanoparticles. Therefore, more lethal double-strand breaks would be produced in the DNA [19]. Reproduction of the cancer cell is therefore terminated because the DNA has been damaged by the radiation and irradiated gold nanoparticles.

Recently, with advances in magnetic resonance (MR)-guided radiotherapy [20–22], MR images can be acquired during radiation dose delivery. This allows radiation staff to examine the patient's tumor when it is irradiated by photon beams. Moreover, MR imaging can provide an excellent contrast of soft tissue compared to the routine CT imaging. This results in better tumor contouring and targeting [23]. To date, MR-guided radiotherapy has improved soft tissue visualization, management of the intrafraction and interfraction organ motion and online adaptive radiotherapy [24]. However, there is a concern over the dose distribution, affected by the magnetic field from the MR system, in the patient [25]. The absorbed dose contributing to cancer cell killing is determined by the energy deposition in the DNA, due to the secondary electrons generated from the interaction between the radiation beam and tumor medium. Since an electron is a charged particle and its traveling path is affected by the magnetic field, the electron distribution in the tumor can be affected by the presence of a magnetic field, leading to a change in final dose distribution. This may, in turn, affect the treatment outcome of MR-guided gold nanoparticle-enhanced radiotherapy. Although there are macroscopic studies concerning the variation in dose distribution due to the magnetic field in MR-guided radiotherapy [26–28], there is a lack of study on the nanodosimetry regarding the DNA damage, not to say with gold nanoparticle addition.

In this study, we investigated this problem by focusing on the nanodosimetry of a gold nanoparticle and DNA. Using Monte Carlo simulation, we examined the dose enhancement of DNA in the presence of a gold nanoparticle when a magnetic field is or is not added to the beam irradiation. Through determining the dose enhancement factor (DER) at the DNA with different nanoparticle sizes, photon beam energies and magnetic field strengths and orientations, we can find out the relationship between the DNA damage and the presence of the magnetic field when an irradiated gold nanoparticle interacts with a DNA.

2. Materials and Methods

2.1. Monte Carlo Simulation

Monte Carlo simulation was used to investigate the influence of the magnetic field on dose enhancement in the DNA when a gold nanoparticle was irradiated by a photon beam. Monte Carlo simulation is a widely used mathematical method in medical physics to model radiation techniques, assess the dose distribution and analyze radiation effects in a certain environment under different experimental conditions [29,30]. In this study, Geant4 software developed by CREN was used to conduct Monte Carlo simulation [31]. The source code, Geant4-DNA, is an extension of the Geant4 Monte Carlo toolkit used to simulate the irradiation of gold nanoparticles and DNA with a photon beam [32]. The code can construct the environment of a gold nanoparticle near a DNA irradiated by a photon beam at a distance from the nanoparticle in the presence of a magnetic field. Geant4-DNA provides a virtual machine containing CentOS Linux, and the latest version of Geant4 (version 10.7), analysis tools, visualization tools and other utilities were used in the simulation. VMware Workstation 16 player was used for running the virtual machine. This machine consists of a Linux distribution of CentOS 8 64-bit. The virtual machine has pre-installed codes and all the software required to run Geant4. The virtual machine was installed from the CREN website (https://geant4.cenbg.in2p3.fr/ accessed date: 1 January 2021).

The default DNA physics list class, "G4EmDNAPhysics_option2", was implemented in this study, which is recommended for cellular-scale simulations. It includes several physics models that cover physical interactions needed for particle transport in water medium [33]. Different physics models have to be defined in gold nanoparticles for different particles such as photons and electrons. Since the transportation of particles in Geant4-DNA is only valid in water medium, a macroscopic physics list, for example, "G4LivemorePhysics", is defined for physical interactions of photons with gold medium. In this study, the environmental model of the cell was assumed to be water equivalent.

2.2. Simulation Model and Geomtry

A DNA model according to Henthorn et al. [34], alongside a gold nanoparticle, was defined inside a spherical water phantom with a radius of 0.5 µm. The simulation variables were similar to Chun et al. [35]. In this model, the backbones and bases were constructed as tiny spheres with a radius of 0.24 nm and 0.208 nm, respectively. Figure 1 shows the simulation setup for the study. The radiation source was defined as a circular plane source with a radius of twice the radius of the gold nanoparticle. The three photon beam energies considered for this simulation were 50, 100 and 150 keV. The primary photons emitted from the left side of the gold nanoparticle reached the DNA molecule. The most important cause of energy deposition in the DNA is the secondary electrons emitted from the gold nanoparticle. In this study, different nanoparticle diameters (30, 50 and 100 nm) with a nanoparticle-to-DNA distance of 30 nm were used. Photon beam energies of 50, 100 and 150 keV were used with a uniform magnetic field (0, 1 and 2 T) defined along each axis, in order to examine the effect of the magnetic field on the dose enhancement. In Figure 1, three orientations were considered for the magnetic field (B_x, B_y and B_z), separately. Since the primary photons were emitted along the z-axis, the magnetic field orientation parallel to the z-axis was also parallel to the trajectory of the photon, and the magnetic field orientation parallel to the x-axis and y-axis was perpendicular to the trajectory of the photon.

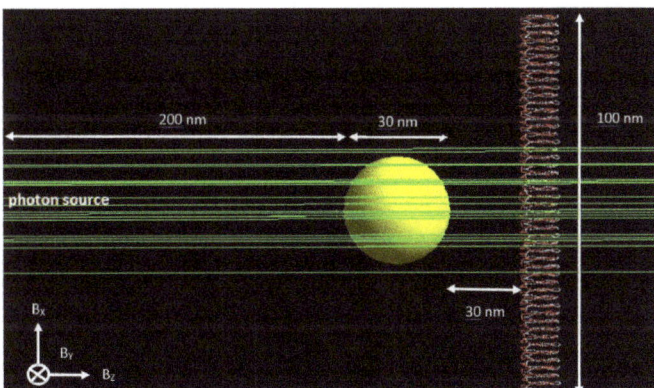

Figure 1. The Monte Carlo model geometry simulated in Geant4-DNA (not to scale). The gold nanoparticle was placed between the photon beam (green) and the DNA molecule. Nanoparticle diameters of 30, 50 and 100 nm were used in the simulation.

Figure 2 shows electron tracks in the simulation model. Energy deposition happened when secondary electrons (yellow dots) were generated along the electron tracks (red). If energy deposition occurred in the DNA (i.e., right-hand side of Figure 2), ionization of the strand of DNA may happen, leading to DNA damage [9,19,36]. The number of histories for the photons interacting with the gold nanoparticle was equal to 300 million in this study, and more photons (~2 billion) were required to achieve a similar uncertainty (2–5% standard deviation) for the simulation model without the gold nanoparticle.

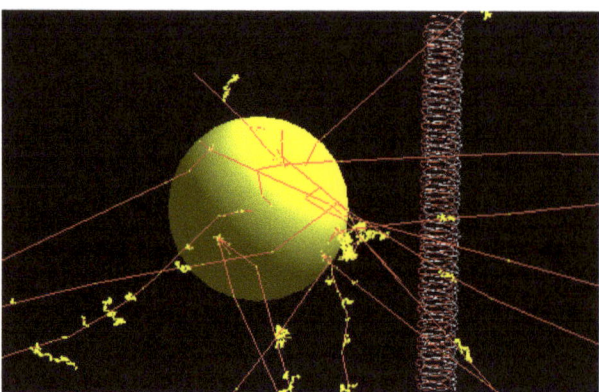

Figure 2. Schematic diagram showing the gold nanoparticle irradiated by the photon beam with electron tracks (red) generated from the nanoparticle. Energy deposition happens when the secondary electrons (yellow dots) are generated along the electron paths. When energy deposition occurs in the DNA, lethal DNA damage such as a double-strand break may be produced, leading to cancer cell killing.

2.3. Dose Enhacnement Ratio

The enhancement of energy deposition in the presence of gold nanoparticles, resulting in DNA damage, can be expressed as the DER [37]:

$$\text{Dose Enhancement Ratio (DER)} = \frac{\text{Dose in the DNA with gold nanoparticle addition}}{\text{Dose in the DNA without gold nanoparticle addition}}$$

When no gold nanoparticle was added to the simulation model, the material of the particle was changed from gold to water. This mimicked the environment of a homogeneous tumor with water equivalent. The DER is therefore equal to one. A DER greater than one shows a dose enhancement due to the gold nanoparticle addition.

3. Results and Discussion

The relationships between the DER and different simulation variables, namely, nanoparticle size and magnetic field strength and orientation for photon beam energies of 50, 100 and 150 keV, are shown in Figure 3a–c, respectively. The gold nanoparticle diameters were equal to 30, 50 and 100 nm, and the magnetic field strengths were equal to 0, 1 and 2 T, with orientations parallel to the x-, y- and z-axis, as shown in Figure 1. The distance between the nanoparticle and DNA was equal to 30 nm.

3.1. Dependence of DER on Nanoparticle Size and Beam Energy

When there was no magnetic field present in the simulation model (i.e., magnetic field strength = 0), the DER was found to increase with the gold nanoparticle size. The rates of increase in the DER were 3.4%, 4.5% and 2.9%/nm for photon beam energies equal to 50, 100 and 150 keV, respectively (Figure 3a–c). The maximum DER was found to be 7.16 for the gold nanoparticle with a diameter equal to 100 nm using the 50 keV photon beam, while the minimum DER was 3.59 for the nanoparticle with a 30 nm diameter using the 150 keV beam. The reason for an increase in the DER with an increase in the nanoparticle size is that the larger particle contains more gold atoms to interact with photons in order to produce secondary electrons, resulting in more energy deposition in the DNA [6]. However, when the nanoparticle size becomes larger, the self-absorption of electrons in the nanoparticle also becomes more significant. This self-absorption effect would decrease the DER when the nanoparticle size increases [38].

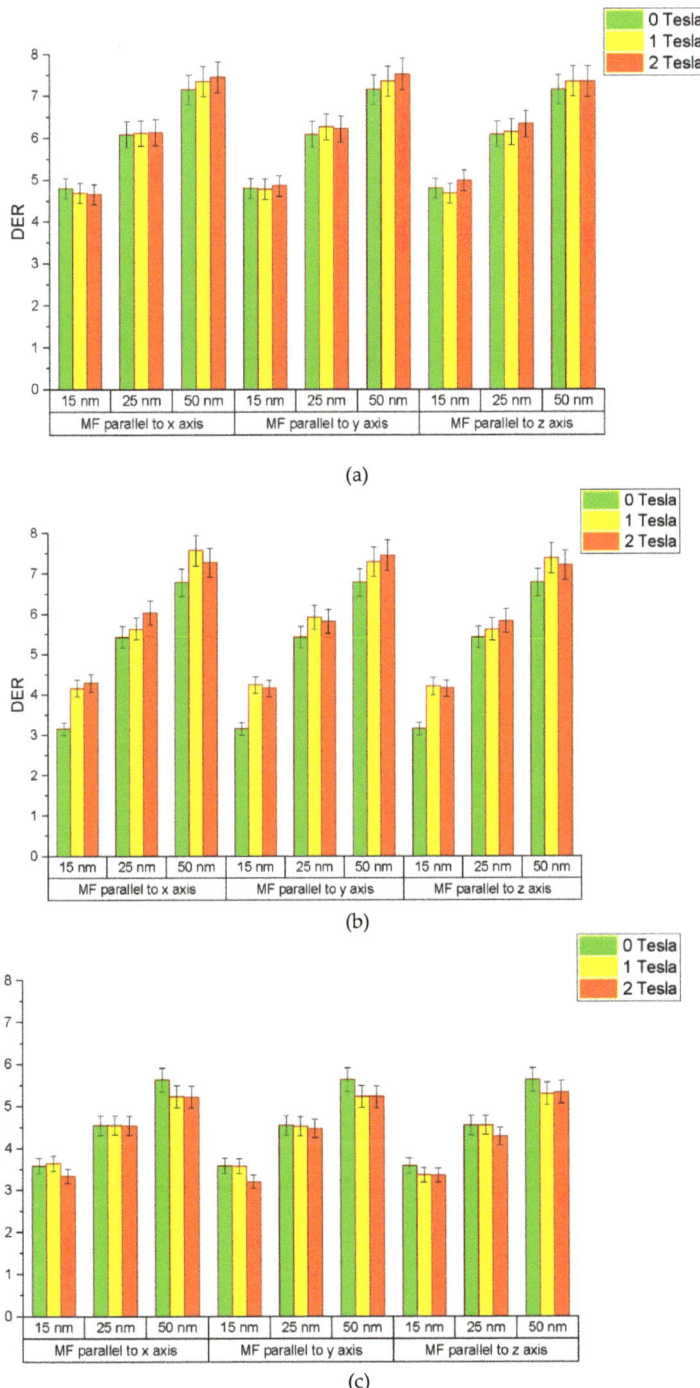

Figure 3. Relationships between the DER and simulation variables of gold nanoparticle size and magnetic field strength and orientation using photon beams with energies equal to (**a**) 50, (**b**) 100 and (**c**) 150 keV.

For the same nanoparticle size with various photon beam energies, it was found that the DER decreased with a beam energy increase. For the nanoparticle with a 50 nm diameter, as shown in Figure 3a–c, the DER was found to decrease from 6.09 to 4.55 when the photon beam energy increased from 50 to 150 keV. This can be explained by the enhancement of the photoelectric effect as the cross-section or attenuation coefficient of the photoelectric interaction decreased with an increase in the photon energy [7–9]. The trends of variation in the DER on the nanoparticle size and photon beam energy agreed with results of our previous work using an older DNA model in the simulation [35].

3.2. Dependence of DER on Magnetic Field Strength and Orientation

For the nanoparticle with a 100 nm diameter using the 50 keV photon beam, as shown in Figure 3a–c, the DER was found to be 7.16, 7.35 and 7.36 when the magnetic field strength was equal to 0, 1 and 2 T along the z-axis. These were increases of about 2.5% and 2.7% in the DER when a magnetic field of 1 and 2 T was added to the simulation model along the z-axis (Figure 1). Similar increases in the DER could be found in the nanoparticles with diameters equal to 30 and 50 nm. It is found that the presence of the magnetic field along the central beam axis would increase the energy deposition in the DNA slightly. However, the increase in the magnetic field strength did not lead to a significant increase in energy deposition in the DNA.

When considering the nanoparticle with a 100 nm diameter using the 50 keV photon beam, with the magnetic field perpendicular to the central beam axis, but parallel to the DNA (i.e., x-axis in Figure 1), the DER was found to be 7.16, 7.36 and 7.46 when the magnetic field strength was equal to 0, 1 and 2 T (Figure 3a–c). These were increases of about 2.7% and 4.0% when a magnetic field of 1 and 2 T was added to the simulation model along the x-axis. Similar increases in the DER were found for nanoparticles of 30 and 50 nm diameter. However, the increase in the DER was in the range of 0.50–1.8%, which was smaller than the nanoparticle with a 100 nm diameter. It is seen that the presence of a magnetic field perpendicular to the central beam axis would increase the energy deposition in the DNA more than along the central beam axis, and the increase was more significant for the larger nanoparticle.

With the same photon beam energy of 50 keV, with the magnetic field along the y-axis (Figure 1), the orientation of the field was perpendicular to the central beam axis and the DNA. This beam and magnetic field geometry was different from placing the magnetic field along the x-axis because the DNA was parallel to the x-axis of the photon beam. For the nanoparticle with a diameter of 100 nm, the DER was found to increase by 2.8% and 4.9% when the magnetic field strength increased by 1 and 2 T, respectively (Figure 3a–c). This increase in energy deposition in the DNA was very similar to the magnetic field orienting in the x-axis. It is seen that the orientation of DNA did not affect its energy deposition significantly regarding the magnetic field orientation.

This work focused on the nanodosimetric change in the DNA interacting with an irradiated gold nanoparticle in the presence of a magnetic field. Based on the results in this study, it is worthwhile to further investigate the dependence of the DER on multiple nanoparticles with different distribution patterns, sizes and shapes. Moreover, macroscopic Monte Carlo simulation [39] can be carried out to investigate the dose enhancement of a tumor in a patient treated with magnetic resonance-guided radiotherapy. This multi-scale study can help us to understand, in detail, the impact of the magnetic field on cancer control from the nanometer to centimeter scales.

4. Conclusions

The DER determined, based on the energy deposition in the DNA, for varying gold nanoparticle diameters (30, 50 and 100 nm), photon beam energies (50, 100 and 150 keV) and magnetic fields (0 T, 1 T and 2 T) in the x, y and z orientations was investigated using Monte Carlo simulation. In general, the DER with no magnetic field present increased as the gold nanoparticle size increased. Moreover, the DER decreased as the photon beam energy increased, since the secondary electrons generated at high energies are less than the electrons generated at lower energies. In the presence of a magnetic field, the DER increased by about 2.5–5% for various field strengths (1 and 2 T) and orientations (x-, y- and z-axis) for the largest nanoparticle (diameter equal to 100 nm) using the lowest photon beam energy (50 keV) in this study. It was found that the increase in the DER was even smaller for smaller gold nanoparticles using a higher photon beam energy.

The results in this work provide important information concerning the variation in energy deposition in DNA when a magnetic field is present in an irradiated gold nanoparticle. Moreover, this single-nanoparticle model can act as a base for the construction of a more complicated multi-nanoparticle model focusing on a more realistic cellular environment for clinical practice.

Author Contributions: Conceptualization, J.C.L.C.; methodology, J.C.L.C.; software, J.C.L.C. and M.J.; validation, J.C.L.C. and M.J.; formal analysis, M.J.; investigation, M.J.; resources, J.C.L.C. and M.J.; data curation, M.J.; writing—original draft preparation, J.C.L.C. and M.J.; writing—review and editing, J.C.L.C.; visualization, J.C.L.C. and M.J.; supervision, J.C.L.C.; project administration, J.C.L.C. All authors have read and agreed to the published version of the manuscript.

Funding: This research received no external funding.

Institutional Review Board Statement: Not applicable.

Informed Consent Statement: Not applicable.

Data Availability Statement: Not applicable.

Acknowledgments: The authors would like to thank Chun He and Kaden Kujanpaa from the University of Toronto, Canada, for their assistance in the Monte Carlo simulation using the Geant4-DNA code.

Conflicts of Interest: The authors declare no conflict of interest.

References

1. Siddique, S.; Chow, J.C.L. Application of nanomaterials in biomedical imaging and cancer therapy. *Nanomaterials.* **2020**, *10*, 1700. [CrossRef]
2. Cui, L.; Her, S.; Borst, G.R.; Bristow, R.G.; Jaffray, D.A.; Allen, C. Radiosensitization by gold nanoparticles: Will they ever make it to the clinic? *Radiother. Oncol.* **2017**, *124*, 344–356. [CrossRef]
3. Chithrani, D.B.; Jelveh, S.; Jalali, F.; Van Prooijen, M.; Allen, C.; Bristow, R.G.; Hill, R.P.; Jaffray, D.A. Gold nanoparticles as radiation sensitizers in cancer therapy. *Radiat. Res.* **2010**, *173*, 719–728. [CrossRef]
4. Her, S.; Jaffray, D.A.; Allen, C. Gold nanoparticles for applications in cancer radiotherapy: Mechanisms and recent advancements. *Adv. Drug Deliv. Rev.* **2017**, *109*, 84–101. [CrossRef]
5. Chithrani, D.B.; Dunne, M.; Stewart, J.; Allen, C.; Jaffray, D.A. Cellular uptake and transport of gold nanoparticles incorporated in a liposomal carrier. *Nanomed. Nanotechnol. Biol. Med.* **2010**, *6*, 161–169. [CrossRef]
6. Chow, J.C.L. Chapter 15 Dose enhancement effect in radiotherapy: Adding gold nanoparticle to tumour in cancer treatment. In *Nanostructures for Cancer Therapy*; Ficai, A., Grumezescu, A.M., Eds.; Elsevier: Amsterdam, The Netherlands, 2017; pp. 383–400.
7. Chow, J.C.L. Chapter 10: Characteristics of secondary electrons from irradiated gold nanoparticle in radiotherapy. In *Handbook of Nanoparticles*; Aliofkhazraei, M., Ed.; Springer International Publishing: Cham, Switzerland, 2015; pp. 1–18.
8. Leung, M.K.K.; Chow, J.C.L.; Chithrani, B.D.; Lee, M.J.; Oms, B.; Jaffray, D.A. Irradiation of gold nanoparticles by x-rays: Monte Carlo simulation of dose enhancements and the spatial properties of the secondary electrons production. *Med. Phys.* **2011**, *38*, 624–631. [CrossRef] [PubMed]
9. Chow, J.C.L. Chapter 2-Photon and electron interactions with gold nanoparticles: A Monte Carlo study on gold nanoparticle-enhanced radiotherapy. In *Nanobiomaterials in Medical Imaging: Applications of Nanobiomaterials*; Grumezescu, A.M., Ed.; Elsevier: Amsterdam, The Netherlands, 2016; Volume 8, pp. 45–70.
10. Mututantri-Bastiyange, D.; Chow, J.C.L. Imaging dose of cone-beam computed tomography in nanoparticle-enhanced image-guided radiotherapy: A Monte Carlo phantom study. *AIMS Bioeng.* **2020**, *7*, 1–11. [CrossRef]
11. Abdulle, A.; Chow, J.C.L. Contrast enhancement for portal imaging in nanoparticle-enhanced radiotherapy: A Monte Carlo phantom evaluation using flattening-filter-free photon beams. *Nanomaterials* **2019**, *9*, 920. [CrossRef] [PubMed]
12. Moore, J.; Chow, J.C.L. Recent progress and applications of gold nanotechnology in medical biophysics using artificial intelligence and mathematical modeling. *Nano EX* **2021**, *2*, 022001. [CrossRef]
13. Siddique, S.; Chow, J.C.L. Gold nanoparticles for drug delivery and cancer therapy. *App Sci.* **2020**, *10*, 3824. [CrossRef]

14. Chow, J.C.L. Synthesis and applications of functionalized nanoparticles in biomedicine and radiotherapy. In *Additive Manufacturing with Functionalized Nanomaterials*; Singh, S., Hussain, C.M., Eds.; Elsevier: Amsterdam, The Netherlands, 2021; pp. 193–214.
15. Chow, J.C.L. Recent progress of gold nanomaterials in cancer therapy. In *Handbook of Nanomaterials and Nanocomposites for Energy and Environmental Applications*; Kharissova, O.V., Torres-Martínez, L.M., Kharisov, B.I., Eds.; Springer Nature: Cham, Switzerland, 2020; pp. 1–30.
16. Ricketts, K.; Ahmad, R.; Beaton, L.; Cousins, B.; Critchley, K.; Davies, M.; Evans, S.; Fenuyi, I.; Gavriilidis, A.; Harmer, Q.J.; et al. Recommendations for clinical translation of nanoparticle-enhanced radiotherapy. *Br. J. Radiol.* **2018**, *91*, 1092. [CrossRef]
17. Ross, G.M. Induction of cell death by radiotherapy. *Endocr. Relat. Cancer* **1999**, *6*, 41–44. [CrossRef] [PubMed]
18. Leenhouts, H.P.; Chadwick, K.H. The crucial role of DNA double-strand breaks in cellular radiobiological effects. In *Advances in Radiation Biology*; Elsevier: Amsterdam, The Netherlands, 1978; Volume 7, pp. 55–101.
19. Chow, J.C.L. Monte Carlo nanodosimetry in gold nanoparticle-enhanced radiotherapy. In *Recent Advancements and Applications in Dosimetry*; Maria, F.C., Ed.; Nova Science Publishers: New York, NY, USA, 2018.
20. Pollard, J.M.; Wen, Z.; Sadagopan, R.; Wang, J.; Ibbott, G.S. The future of image-guided radiotherapy will be MR guided. *Br. J. Radiol.* **2017**, *90*, 1073. [CrossRef]
21. Kurz, C.; Buizza, G.; Landry, G.; Kamp, F.; Rabe, M.; Paganelli, C.; Baroni, G.; Reiner, M.; Keall, P.J.; van den Berg, C.A.; et al. Medical physics challenges in clinical MR-guided radiotherapy. *Radiat. Oncol.* **2020**, *15*, 1–6. [CrossRef]
22. Slotman, B.; Gani, C. Online MR-guided radiotherapy—A new era in radiotherapy. *Clin. Transl. Radiat. Oncol.* **2019**, *18*, 102–103. [CrossRef] [PubMed]
23. Kristensen, B.H.; Laursen, F.J.; Løgager, V.; Geertsen, P.F.; Krarup-Hansen, A. Dosimetric and geometric evaluation of an open low-field magnetic resonance simulator for radiotherapy treatment planning of brain tumours. *Radiother. Oncol.* **2008**, *87*, 100–109. [CrossRef] [PubMed]
24. Corradini, S.; Alongi, F.; Andratschke, N.; Belka, C.; Boldrini, L.; Cellini, F.; Debus, J.; Guckenberger, M.; Hörner-Rieber, J.; Lagerwaard, F.J.; et al. MR-guidance in clinical reality: Current treatment challenges and future perspectives. *Radiat. Oncol.* **2019**, *14*, 1–2. [CrossRef]
25. Raaijmakers, A.J.; Raaymakers, B.W.; Lagendijk, J.J. Magnetic-field-induced dose effects in MR-guided radiotherapy systems: Dependence on the magnetic field strength. *Phys. Med. Biol.* **2008**, *53*, 909. [CrossRef]
26. Xia, W.; Zhang, K.; Li, M.; Tian, Y.; Men, K.; Wang, J.; Yi, J.; Li, Y.; Dai, J. Impact of magnetic field on dose distribution in MR-guided radiotherapy of head and neck cancer. *Front. Oncol.* **2020**, *10*, 1739. [CrossRef]
27. Mohajer, J.K.; Nisbet, A.; Velliou, E.; Ajaz, M.; Schettino, G. Biological effects of static magnetic field exposure in the context of MR-guided radiotherapy. *Br. J. Radiol.* **2019**, *92*, 1094. [CrossRef]
28. Chen, X.; Prior, P.; Chen, G.P.; Schultz, C.J.; Li, X.A. Dose effects of 1.5 T transverse magnetic field on tissue interfaces in MRI-guided radiotherapy. *Med. Phys.* **2016**, *43*, 4797–4802. [CrossRef] [PubMed]
29. Chow, J.C.L. Recent progress in Monte Carlo simulation on gold nanoparticle radiosensitization. *AIMS Biophys.* **2018**, *5*, 231–244. [CrossRef]
30. Rogers, D.W.O. Fifty years of Monte Carlo simulations for medical physics. *Phys. Med. Biol.* **2006**, *51*, R287. [CrossRef] [PubMed]
31. Agostinelli, S.; Allison, J.; Amako, K.A.; Apostolakis, J.; Araujo, H.; Arce, P.; Asai, M.; Axen, D.; Banerjee, S.; Barrand, G.; et al. GEANT4—A simulation toolkit. *Nucl. Instrum. Methods Phys. Res.* **2003**, *506*, 250–303. [CrossRef]
32. Incerti, S.; Baldacchino, G.; Bernal, M.; Capra, R.; Champion, C.; Francis, Z.; Guèye, P.; Mantero, A.; Mascialino, B.; Moretto, P.; et al. The Geant4-DNA project. *Int. J. Model. Simul. Sci. Comput.* **2010**, *1*, 157–178. [CrossRef]
33. Villagrasa, C.; Francis, Z.; Incerti, S. Physical models implemented in the GEANT4-DNA extension of the GEANT-4 toolkit for calculating initial radiation damage at the molecular level. *Radiat. Prot. Dosim.* **2011**, *143*, 214–218. [CrossRef]
34. Henthorn, N.T.; Warmenhoven, J.W.; Sotiropoulos, M.; Mackay, R.I.; Kirkby, K.J.; Merchant, M.J. Nanodosimetric simulation of direct ion-induced DNA damage using different chromatin geometry models. *Radiat. Res.* **2017**, *188*, 690–703. [CrossRef] [PubMed]
35. Chun, H.; Chow, J.C.L. Gold nanoparticle DNA damage in radiotherapy: A Monte Carlo study. *AIMS Bioeng.* **2016**, *3*, 352–361.
36. Chow, J.C.L. Application of nanoparticle materials in radiation therapy. In *Handbook of Ecomaterials*; Martinez, L.M.T., Kharissova, O.V., Kharisov, B.I., Eds.; Springer Nature: Cham, Switzerland, 2017; pp. 3661–3681.
37. Zheng, X.J.; Chow, J.C.L. Radiation dose enhancement in skin therapy with nanoparticle addition: A Monte Carlo study on kilovoltage photon and megavoltage electron beams. *World J. Radiol.* **2017**, *9*, 63–71. [CrossRef] [PubMed]
38. Chow, J.C.L.; Leung, M.K.K.; Jaffray, D.A. Monte Carlo simulation on gold nanoparticle irradiated by electron beams. *Phys. Med. Biol.* **2012**, *57*, 3323–3331. [CrossRef] [PubMed]
39. Martelli, S.; Chow, J.C.L. Dose enhancement for the flattening-filter-free and flattening-filter photon beams in nanoparticle-enhanced radiotherapy: A Monte Carlo phantom study. *Nanomaterials* **2020**, *10*, 637. [CrossRef] [PubMed]

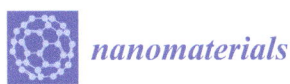

Review

pH-Responsive Nanoparticles for Cancer Immunotherapy: A Brief Review

Yunfeng Yan * and Hangwei Ding

College of Biotechnology and Bioengineering, Zhejiang University of Technology, Hangzhou 310032, China; dhwpao@163.com
* Correspondence: yfyan@zjut.edu.cn

Received: 31 July 2020; Accepted: 15 August 2020; Published: 17 August 2020

Abstract: Immunotherapy has recently become a promising strategy for the treatment of a wide range of cancers. However, the broad implementation of cancer immunotherapy suffers from inadequate efficacy and toxic side effects. Integrating pH-responsive nanoparticles into immunotherapy is a powerful approach to tackle these challenges because they are able to target the tumor tissues and organelles of antigen-presenting cells (APCs) which have a characteristic acidic microenvironment. The spatiotemporal control of immunotherapeutic drugs using pH-responsive nanoparticles endows cancer immunotherapy with enhanced antitumor immunity and reduced off-tumor immunity. In this review, we first discuss the cancer-immunity circle and how nanoparticles can modulate the key steps in this circle. Then, we highlight the recent advances in cancer immunotherapy with pH-responsive nanoparticles and discuss the perspective for this emerging area.

Keywords: nanoparticle; cancer; immunotherapy; pH-responsive; drug delivery

---

1. Introduction

Immunotherapy has revolutionized the cancer treatment by activating the innate and adaptive immune system against tumor cells with immune checkpoint inhibitors (ICIs), agonists, antigens, or engineered T cells. In contrast to the conventional cancer treatment modalities, e.g., chemotherapy, radiotherapy, and surgery, which directly kill cancer cells or resect tumor tissues, immunotherapy aims to restore the antitumor activity of the immune system to attack abnormal cells through natural mechanisms, allowing better potency and fewer off-target effects in the treatment of advanced malignancies [1–4]. Several notable clinical successes in cancer immunotherapy have been made over the past decade, including the FDA approval of the chimeric antigen receptor (CAR) T cell therapy and therapies with monoclonal antibodies (mAbs) targeting cytotoxic T lymphocyte antigen 4 (CTLA4), programmed cell death 1 (PD-1), or its ligand (PD-L1) as the immune checkpoint inhibitors. Due to their contributions in the discovery of cancer therapy through the immune checkpoint blockade, the Nobel Prize in Physiology or Medicine 2018 was awarded to James P. Allison and Tasuku Honjo. Now, there is a large number of active clinical trials worldwide and immunotherapy has become a new pillar of cancer treatment owing to these tremendous achievements [5].

1.1. Modulation of Anticancer Immunity

The generation of endogenous immune response against tumors involves several distinct steps (Figure 1) [1,6,7]. First, tumor-associated antigens (TAAs) are released from cancer cells. The immunogenic signal could be proinflammatory cytokines or factors which are produced in oncogenesis (step 1). Then, TAAs are captured by antigen presenting cells (APCs) (e.g., dendritic cells) and presented on major histocompatibility complex (MHC) class I and class II molecules (step 2). Tumor antigen-loaded dendritic cells migrate to lymph nodes, resulting in the priming and activation of

T cells (step 3). This is a crucial step to generate T cell response against cancer-specific antigens. In the presence of immunogenic stimulators, the antigen presentation elicits effector T cells which are killers to cancer cells. Without such stimulation, dendritic cells will induce T cell deletion and the production of regulatory T cells which relate to the immunosuppression. The activated T cells subsequently leave the lymph node, traffic to tumors through the bloodstream, and infiltrate into tumor parenchyma (steps 4 and 5). Finally, effector T cells recognize cancer cells by the specific binding of T cell receptor (TCR) to the antigen on cancer cell surface (step 6), and kill target cancer cells (step 7). The death of cancer cells further promotes the release of TAAs and elicits the subsequent immune response.

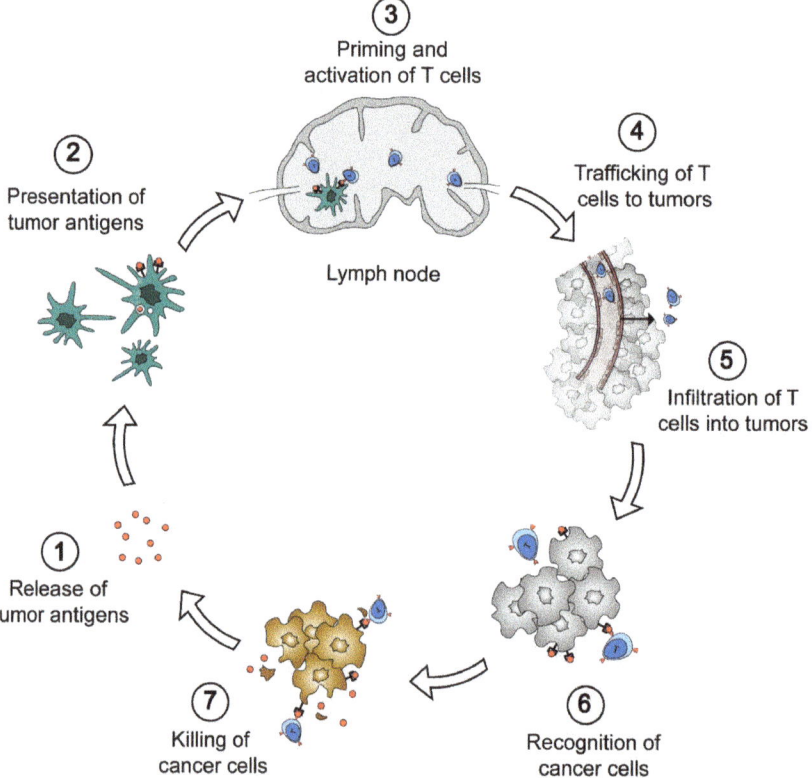

Figure 1. The cancer-immunity cycle. Seven steps are involved in the generation of antitumor immunity, i.e., the release of tumor antigens from cancer cells, the presentation of tumor antigen to antigen-presenting cells (APCs), the priming and activation of T cells in lymph nodes, the trafficking and infiltration of T cells to tumors, the recognition and the killing of cancer cells.

Durable cancer immunotherapy requires the complete cancer-immunity cycle. However, a few factors may waken or suspend the generation and performance of antitumor immunity in cancer patients. The approaches to overcome these obstacles derive the major classes of cancer immunotherapy. The cancer antigens may not be sufficiently released from solid tumors and captured by dendritic cells for the further processing. In this respect, treatments with conventional chemotherapeutics or radiation induce the apoptosis of cancer cells that promotes the release of tumor antigens from dead cells [5]. The immunization could be also initiated with the delivery of exogenous vaccines including conventional protein or peptide antigens, nucleic acids, and dendritic cells. The tumor-associated proteins, peptides, and nucleic acids could be directly administered to cancer patients, then, processed by dendritic cells and cross-presented to T cells in vivo. Alternatively, dendritic cells are engineered with specific antigens ex vivo and injected into patients for personalized immunization [8]. Stimulatory molecules are requisite for dendritic cell maturation, antigen presentation, and T cell activation. For example, agonists of Toll-like receptor (TLR), e.g., cytosine-phosphate-guanine oligonucleotide (CpG-ODN) for TLR9 and Imiquimod for TLR7, and stimulator of interferon genes (STING) are able to promote the maturation of APCs [9,10]. Incubation with interferon-α (IFN-α) and granulocyte-macrophage colony-stimulating factor (GM-CSF) facilitates dendritic cell development and the expression of leukocyte antigen (HLA), B7 co-stimulatory molecules, MHC proteins, and CD40, which benefits the TAAs presentation and immunization [11]. Interleukin-2 (IL-2) is able to stimulate the expanding and activation of T cells in lymph nodes [12]. These cytokines and agonists are legitimately utilized to improve the immune activity of T cells for cancer immunotherapy. To circumvent the elaborate procedures of T cell priming and activation in vivo, T cells are collected from tumors or peripheral blood, selected, genetically engineered, and proliferated in vitro, followed by the reinfusion into the tumor-bearing patient [13]. This strategy of adoptive T cell therapy represents a major advancement of cancer immunotherapy in the past decade. In particular, T cells modified with chimeric antigen receptor (CARs) show exceptional immune activity which have been approved for clinical use to treat B cell acute lymphoblastic leukemia and B cell non-Hodgkin lymphoma [14,15].

Abnormal angiogenesis and proliferation of cancer cells and cancer-associated fibroblasts (CAFs) contribute to the formation of solid tumors with high interstitial fluid pressure (IFP) that hinders the infiltration of all therapeutics into tumor parenchyma from blood vessels [16]. In addition to physical barriers, reduced blood flow and substance exchange further induce the hypoxia and acidity in tumor, resulting in the immunosuppressed tumor microenvironment (TME) that is a major cause of the resistance to the current cancer immunotherapy. The therapeutics for the normalization of TME, e.g., antiangiogenic and CAF-reprogramming agents, have been broadly utilized to improve the tumor perfusion and immunity for cancer immunotherapy [1]. The activity of effector T cells could be suppressed by immunosuppressive macrophages in the TME, including regulatory T cells, M2-like tumor-associated macrophages (TAMs), and myeloid-derived suppressor cells because they are able to secrete a number of immunosuppressive factors (e.g., NO, reactive oxygen species, arginase, iterleukin-10, indoleamine 2,3-dixoygenase, and transforming growth factor-β) and to down-regulate the cytotoxicity of effector T cells [5]. Reprogramming or eliminating immunosuppressive cells has proven to be a complementary approach to augment the antitumor immunity of T cells in solid tumors. Cancer cells usually express immune checkpoint proteins on the surface, leading to the immune resistance when these proteins bind to the specific ligands on T cells. Inhibition of the immune checkpoints with anti-CTLA4, anti-PD-1, or anti-PD-L1 antibodies represents the most notable approach in the current cancer immunotherapy [2]. There are now at least six FDA-approved immune checkpoint inhibitors for the treatment of a wide range of cancers [3].

1.2. Ongoing Challenges in Cancer Immunotherapy

Despite the substantial progress in recent years, the broad implementation of cancer immunotherapy remains challenging. The response rate and magnitude of cancer patients to immunotherapies remains moderate. Only <13% of cancer patients effectively respond to the current immune checkpoint inhibitors because the expression level of checkpoint proteins varies with cancer types and patients [17]. CAR-T cell therapy shows high potency for the treatment of hematologic malignancies. However, its clinical application to solid tumors is still unfulfilled due to the compact and immunosuppressive microenvironment of solid tumors [18]. In addition to the unsatisfactory efficacy, the safety issues further limited the broader clinical use of immunotherapeutics. CAR-T therapy requires successive infusion of CAR-T cells that may cause severe side effects including cytokine-release syndrome (CRS) and CAR-T cell-related encephalopathy syndrome (CRES) [18]. The advance of immune checkpoint inhibitors (ICI) therapy is also associated with some immune-related adverse events (irAEs) including colitis, pneumonitis, hepatitis, myocarditis, and neurotoxic effects [19]. Some immune modulators are toxic and the repeated administration leads to accumulative toxicity for the patients. In addition, the stimulating and activating circulating lymphocytes out of tumors may lead to the attack on normal tissues, causing the off-target side effects [2,19]. The ideal cancer immunotherapy should be capable of precise modulation on the strength and the site of immune response to optimize the clinical outcomes.

2. Cancer Immunotherapy with Nanoparticles

Nanoparticles, particles with a typical size of 1–100 nm in diameter, have been widely utilized in cancer treatments [2,16,20]. Nanoparticle-based delivery offers potent approaches for the spatiotemporal control of immunotherapeutic agents to reduce the adverse effects and maximize the therapeutic index of cancer immunotherapy [1–5]. First, the formulation of immunotherapeutics in nanoparticles can improve the pharmacological properties of drugs, including the solubility and stability. Of particular importance, some biologic drugs, e.g., nucleic acids and antibodies, require protection from degradation and macrophage clearance in blood after systemic administration. Second, nanoparticle platforms enable versatile modification or functionalization to modulate the pharmacokinetic profile of drugs and regulate the interaction between drugs and cells or organs. The level of antibodies or small drugs can be tuned by controlled release to extend the efficacy and avoid the systemic toxicity due to the instantaneous high concentration after systemic administration. In addition, the structure of nanoparticles can be readily designed for the active targeting and the smart response to external stimuli (e.g., light, electronic, and magnetic fields) or the biochemical changes from normal tissues to tumors (e.g., pH, redox potential, and enzymes), resulting in the enhanced tumor accumulation and reduced off-target side effects. For the highly hydrophilic and negatively charged nucleic acid drugs, nanoparticle carriers play significant roles in their cellular uptake, endosomal escape, and release in target cells that are the critical steps for the implementation of nucleic acid-based immunotherapy. Finally, nanoparticle technologies allow feasible combinations of immunotherapy with conventional chemotherapy, radiotherapy, as well as photothermal and photodynamic therapy for the normalization of immunosuppressive TME and improved immunotherapy efficacy.

3. pH-Responsive Nanoparticles for Cancer Immunotherapy

pH-responsive nanoparticles have received intensive attention in cancer immunotherapy because of the distinct acidic features of a tumor microenvironment compared with normal tissues. Deregulated glycolysis in cancer cells results in the high level of lactic acid and consequent acidic pH (6.5–6.9) in tumor tissues [21]. pH-sensitive nanoparticles afford cancer immunotherapy improved pharmacology and enhanced accumulation of immunotherapeutics in tumor tissues. In addition, the intracellular trafficking of drug nanoparticles usually undergoes early endosomes, late endosomes, and fusion with lysosomes with a decreased pH from 6.5 to 4.5 [22,23]. The formulation of biologic drugs with pH-sensitive carriers is able to response to the subtle pH change, facilitating the endosomal escape and avoiding the degradation of nucleic acids or proteins in lysosomes. It is worth noting that pH-responsive nanoparticles have been extensively used in other cancer therapies (e.g., chemotherapy) besides immunotherapy. For these topics, readers may refer to the published reviewer articles [24–26]. This review will focus on the recent advances in cancer immunotherapy using pH-responsive nanoparticles and offer perspectives on this burgeoning field.

Nanoparticles' response to pH change in two typical ways: the protonation/ionization of functional groups and the degradation or the cleavage of acid-labile bonds (Figure 2). pH-dependent protonation/ionization is frequently utilized in the design of pH-triggered delivery systems. In this strategy, various ionizable groups (e.g., amines and carboxyl acids) are incorporated into the delivery carriers, endowing drug-loaded nanoparticles with sensitivity to acid environments. pH variation alters the protonation of amines or the ionization of carboxyl groups that result in the change of the surface charge, the stability, and the interaction with cells or tissues. The pH-dependent protonation of carriers enables the "proton sponge" effect in the intracellular trafficking of nanoparticles which is crucial for the endosomal escape of biological immunotherapeutics (e.g., nucleic acids and proteins) [23].

The protonation of amines increases with the acid degree in endosomes, leading to the extensive influx of water and counterions into the late endosomes, which further results in the rapture of the endosomal membrane and the release of cargoes into the cytoplasm, therefore, avoiding the degradation of the biological drugs in lysosomes. In contrast to the physical changes in pH-responsive protonation/ionization, the increase of acidity may lead to the break of covalent bonds including amide, ester, imine, oxime, acetal, and ketal bonds or the disintegration of inorganic components, altering the physicochemical properties of drug-loaded nanoparticles. For example, acid cleavable PEG segments are incorporated into nanocarriers to shield nanoparticles from protein adsorption and aggregation under physiological conditions. When nanoparticles are circulated to the acidic tumors, the acid-labile linkers break and shielding PEGs are detached from nanoparticles, shifting the surface from a hydrophilic to a hydrophobic one or from a neutral to a positive one that improves the accumulation and retention of nanoparticles in tumor tissues [27,28]. In contrast to changes on the surface, the hydrolysis inside the nanoparticles triggers the degradation and disassembly of nanoparticles under acidic conditions, leading to the rapid release of immune cargoes and facilitating the antigen presentation in the target tissue [29,30]. Several pH-responsive inorganic components have been utilized to construct nanocarriers for cancer immunotherapy because they are highly sensitive to pH change from a physiological to a tumor environment [30,31].

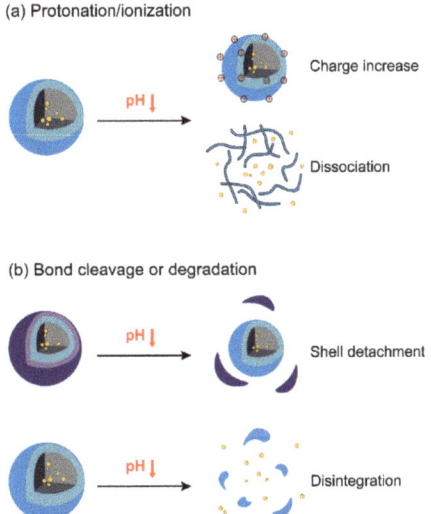

Figure 2. The typical approaches to the pH-response of nanoparticles for cancer immunotherapy. (**a**) Protonation/ionization and (**b**) cleavage of acid-labile shells or degradation of nanoparticles at acid pH enables the significant change of surface properties or the disintegration of nanoparticles.

3.1. Nanoparticles with pH-Responsive Protonation/Ionization for Cancer Immunotherapy

pH-responsive polycations (e.g., poly(2-diethylamino ethyl methacrylate), PDEAEMA) take positive charges upon the protonation of amine groups and enable the proton sponge effect after internalization into cells (Figure 3). Therefore, they could be used to encapsulate negatively charged immunotherapeutic nucleic acids, improve their cellular uptake, and protect intrinsically unstable nucleic acids from degradation in acidic lysosomes in dendritic cells [32]. For example, poly(dimethylaminoethyl methacrylate)-*b*-(dimethylaminoethyl methacrylate-*co*-butyl methacrylate-*co*-propylacrylic acid) (P(DMAEMA)-*b*-(DMAEMA-*co*-BMA-*co*-PAA)) (Figure 3a) was utilized for the delivery of a RNA agonist of the retinoic acid gene (3pRNA) to dendritic cells. The pH-responsive polymer-nucleic acid nanoparticles reduce nuclease degradation and improve cellular uptake and endosomal escape of 3pRNA, enhancing the immunostimulatory activity and the therapeutic efficacy of anti-PD-1 immune checkpoint blockade in a CT26 colon cancer model [33]. Similar pH-responsive polymers, poly(ethylene glycol)-*b*-poly(diisopropanol amino ethyl methacrylate-*co*-hydroxyethyl methacrylate) (PEG-*b*-P(DPA-*co*-HEA)) (Figure 3b) and 1,2-epoxytetradecane alkylated oligoethylenimine (OEI-C14) were utilized to deliver a photosensitizer (PS) and small interfering RNA against PD-L1 (siPD-L1) for combination of photodynamic therapy and RNA interference (RNAi)-based PD-L1 blockade [34]. At physiological pH, the carriers and payloads form stable nanoparticles wherein the fluorescence of photosensitizers is quenched due to the fluorescence resonance energy transfer, implying reduced dark toxicity in the blood circulation upon laser irradiation. After entering the weakly acidic endocytic vesicles in tumor cells (pH 5.0–6.0), the protonation of the tertiary amines of PDPA increases, resulting in the dissociation of nanoparticles and the release of photosensitizers into tumor cells that mediates photodynamic immunotherapy with laser irradiation. Furthermore, the photodynamic treatment induces tumor-specific reactive oxygen species (ROS) and promotes the release of antigens, stimulating the adaptive anti-tumor immunity. The combination of photodynamic immunotherapy and PD-L1 knockdown on the acid-activatable nanoplatform significantly inhibits tumor growth and metastasis in a B16-F10 melanoma xenograft tumor model.

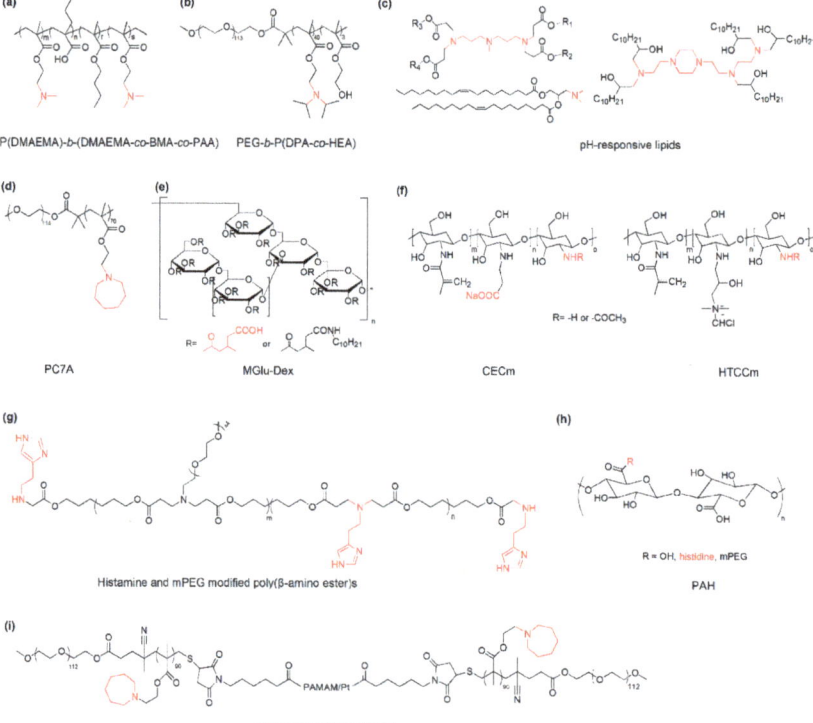

Figure 3. Representative materials with pH-dependent protonation/ionization for cancer immunotherapy. (**a**) P(DMAEMA)-*b*-(DMAEMA-*co*-BMA-*co*-PAA): poly(dimethylaminoethyl methacrylate)-*b*-(dimethylaminoethyl methacrylate-*co*-butyl methacrylate-*co*-propylacrylic acid);

(**b**) PEG-*b*-P(DPA-*co*-HEA): poly(ethylene glycol)-*b*-poly(diisopropanol amino ethyl methacrylate-*co*-hydroxyethyl methacrylate); (**c**) pH-responsive lipids; (**d**) PC7A: poly(ethylene glycol)-*b*-poly(2-(hexamethyleneimino)ethyl methacrylate); (**e**) MGlu-Dex: dextran derivatives having 3-methylglutarylated residues; (**f**) CECm: amphoteric methacrylamide N-carboxyethyl chitosan; HTCCm: methacrylamide N-(2-hydroxy)propyl-3-trmethylammonium chitosan chloride; (**g**) histamine and mPEG modified poly(β-amino ester)s; (**h**) PAH: PEG-histidine modified alginate; and (**i**) PEG-*b*-PAEMA-PAMAM/Pt: platinum (Pt)-prodrug conjugated and poly(ethylene glycol)-*b*-poly(2-azepane ethyl methacrylate)-modified polyamidoamine. The key pH-sensitive groups are indicated in red.

Messenger RNA (mRNA) has great potential in cancer immunotherapy [35]. A successful delivery of TAAs-encoded mRNA into DCs enhances the antigen presentation and the tumor specific immune response. In comparison with a short double-stranded RNA, a single-stranded mRNA is much longer, more flexible, and less stable. Further application of mRNA in cancer immunotherapy requires robust delivery carriers [36]. pH-responsive lipid nanoparticles (Figure 3c) are proven carriers for the cellular uptake and the endosomal escape of mRNA both in vitro and in vivo [17]. There is not a universal carrier for the delivery of any RNAs in different tumor models. In general, a proper content of pH-responsive amines and a delicate balance between hydrophilicity and hydrophobicity is needed to tackle the complicate challenge in RNA delivery. Of particular importance, amines with a pK_a of 6.0–6.5 are crucial for the binding, cellular uptake, and the release of RNAs. A recent research shows that the alteration of the component of lipid nanoparticles changes the global apparent pK_a and the protein corona of nanoparticles that enables the selective delivery of RNAs and proteins to target cells and tissues [37].

Ultra-pH-sensitive nanoparticles consisting of copolymers containing varying tertiary amines have been developed for the delivery of protein antigens to APCs in draining lymph nodes. Due to the robust response to the subtle pH change in organelles, the leading nanoparticle PC7A (Figure 3d) enables excellent cytosolic delivery and efficient surface presentation of tumor antigens, generating a strong cytotoxic T cell response with low systemic cytokine expression [38].

Carboxyl groups have been incorporated into pH-responsive nanoparticles for cancer immunotherapy because their pH-dependent ionization enables the change of hydrophilicity/hydrophobicity of carriers and the modulation of drug release from nanoparticles at varying pHs. For example, dextran was functionalized with carboxyl pendants and C12 alkyl side chains for the fabrication of pH-responsive liposomes for the delivery of a model antigen, ovalbumin (OVA) (Figure 3e). The modified liposomes are stable at neutral pH but destabilized at weakly acidic pH because the solubility of carboxy-bearing dextran decreases with pH, enhancing the release of OVA in the cytosol of dendritic cells. The pH-sensitive OVA-loaded liposomes demonstrate significant suppression of tumors upon subcutaneous injection to E.G7-OVA tumor-bearing mice [39].

In addition to improving the delivery efficacy at a cellular level, pH-responsive nanoparticles benefit cancer immunotherapy by enhancing the accumulation of immunotherapeutic drugs or targeting TAMs in tumor tissues through the charge change in acidic conditions. Paclitaxel (PTX) and interleukin-2 were encapsulated in nanogels composed of hydroxypropyl-β-cyclodextrin acrylate, red blood cell membrane, and two opposite charged chitosan to remodel the immunosuppressive tumor microenvironment (Figure 3f). With the pH decrease in the tumor environment, the ionization of –COOH decreases while the protonation of –NH$_2$ increases, reversing the main driving force in nanogels from electrostatic attraction to repulsion, which further leads to the disintegration of the nanogel and the release of drugs in tumor tissues. The combinational chemotherapy and immunotherapy with the tumor microenvironment responsive nanogel significantly enhance the infiltration of immune effector cells and reduce the immunosuppressive factors in a murine melanoma model [40].

TAM is one of the key targets for the cancer immunotherapy besides tumor cells. Reversing TAMs from a tumor supportive phenotype to a tumoricidal phenotype is an effective way to remodel the immunosuppressive TME and enhance the antitumor immunity of immunotherapy. Histamine and mPEG modified poly(β-amino ester)s (Figure 3g) were prepared for the delivery of IL-12 to re-educate TAMs in TME. The drug-polymer nanoparticles swell under weak acidic conditions (e.g., pH 6.5), resulting in effective accumulation and prolonged release of IL-12 in TME that reverses the tumor-infiltrated macrophage phenotype from M2 to M1. This nanoparticle platform shows great potential in local re-education of TAMs in solid tumors with low systemic side effects in cancer immunotherapy [41]. In another report, pH-sensitive PEG-histidine modified alginate (PAH, $pK_a \sim 6.9$) (Figure 3h) was developed for the delivery of a combination of CpG oligodeoxynucleotide (ODN), anti-IL-10 ODN and anti-IL-10 receptor ODN, to alter the phenotype of TAMs and stimulate their antitumor immunity.

Galactosylated cationic dextran was selected for the fabrication of a ODNs nanocomplex (GDO) for TAM targeting because of high level of galactose-type lectin on TAMs. GDO forms nanoparticles with PAH via electrostatic attraction at physiological pH. After entering the acidic TME, the charge of PAH changes from negative to positive, resulting the detachment of PAH from the GDO complex and the exposure of galactose for TAM targeting. The acidic tumor microenvironment-responsive and TAM-specific approach significantly reduces the systemic side effects of cancer immunotherapy by inhibiting the upregulation of serum proinflammatory cytokines [42].

Cancer therapy can be improved by targeting the delivery of chemotherapeutics and immune modulators to both TAMs and tumor cells. BLZ-945, a small molecule inhibitor of colony stimulating factor 1 receptor (CSF-1R) of TAMs, was encapsulated in ultra-pH-sensitive cluster nanoparticles (SCNs) which was constructed from the self-assembly of platinum (Pt)-prodrug conjugated and poly(ethylene glycol)-*b*-poly(2-azepane ethyl methacrylate)-modified polyamidoamine (PEG-*b*-PAEMA-PAMAM/Pt) (Figure 3i). At neutral pH, PAEMA is hydrophobic and maintains the stable nanoparticles for prolonged blood circulation and reduced systemic toxicity of payloads. PAEMA is rapidly protonated at tumor pH and becomes hydrophilic, leading to instantaneous disintegration of SCNs into small dendrimer nanoparticles (<10 nm) for deep tumor penetration and the release of BLZ-945 for TAM depletion. Comparing with BLZ-945 or Pt-loaded nanoparticles, the spatial targeting nanoparticles demonstrate better tumor growth suppression, metastasis inhibition, and mouse survival in multiple tumor models [43].

Silica nanoparticles with a pH-responsive surface have been used as scaffolds for the controlled release of drugs or enhanced accumulation in tumor tissues [28,31]. Mesoporous silica nanoparticles with pH- and GSH-responsive molecular gates were developed for doxorubicin (DOX) delivery for the treatment of metastatic tumors. The highly integrated nanoplatform demonstrates a robust response to the simultaneously acidic and reductive tumor microenvironment, enabling a precise release of drugs in tumor tissues. The smart nanoparticles not only show good chemotherapy efficacy but also stimulate the maturation of DCs and the release of antitumor cytokines [31]. Hollow silica nanoparticles were coated with PEG and 2-propionic-3-methylmaleic anhydride (CDM)-grafted PEI, enabling prolonged blood circulation and negative-to-positive charge conversion at acidic pH. The catalase and photosensitizer-loaded hybrid nanoparticles show enhanced retention in tumor tissue, leading to greatly relieved tumor hypoxia via decomposition of tumor endogenous H_2O_2 and improving anti-PD-L1 checkpoint blockade therapy [28].

3.2. Nanoparticles with pH-Responsive Bond Cleavage or Degradation for Cancer Immunotherapy

In addition to the physical change induced by protonation/ionization, the break of covalent bonds triggered by pH change can lead to the physicochemical property change on the surface of nanoparticles or the disintegration of the nanoparticle that mediates the targeting or the controlled release of payloads to tumors.

OVA was grafted to alginate (ALG) via pH-sensitive Schiff base bonds and formed nanovaccines with mannose modified ALG by $CaCl_2$ crosslinking (Figure 4a). The nanovaccines are relatively stable at pH 7.4 and release OVA remarkably in the release in the endo/lysosomes (pH 4.5–5.5) due to the detachment of OVA from delivery vehicles after cleavage of a Schiff base linkage at acidic pH. Subcutaneous administration of the nanovaccines enables efficient trafficking of the OVA-bearing nanoparticles from the injection site to the draining lymph nodes, remarkably stimulating the major cytotoxic T lymphocytes (CTL) response and inhibiting E.G7 tumor growth in C57BL/6 mice [44]. Similarly, pH-responsive hydrazone bond has been utilized for the construction of alltrans retinal-loaded nanogels which show long-term stability at physiological pH but dissociate and release antigens in acidic lysosomes in DCs (Figure 4b) [29]. In a recent study, amphiphilic charge-altering releasable transporters (CARTs) (Figure 4c) were developed for mRNA delivery to multiple lymphocytes in which cationic poly(α-amino ester)s bind mRNA at acidic pH but release mRNA after a time-dependent rearrangement of poly(α-amino ester)s to neutral small molecules (diketopiperizine) at pH 7.4, resulting in enhanced lymphocyte transfection in primary T cells and in vivo in mice. In contrast to conventional polycations, CARTs provide a new mechanism for mRNA release and great potential to avoid polycation-associated tolerability issues [45].

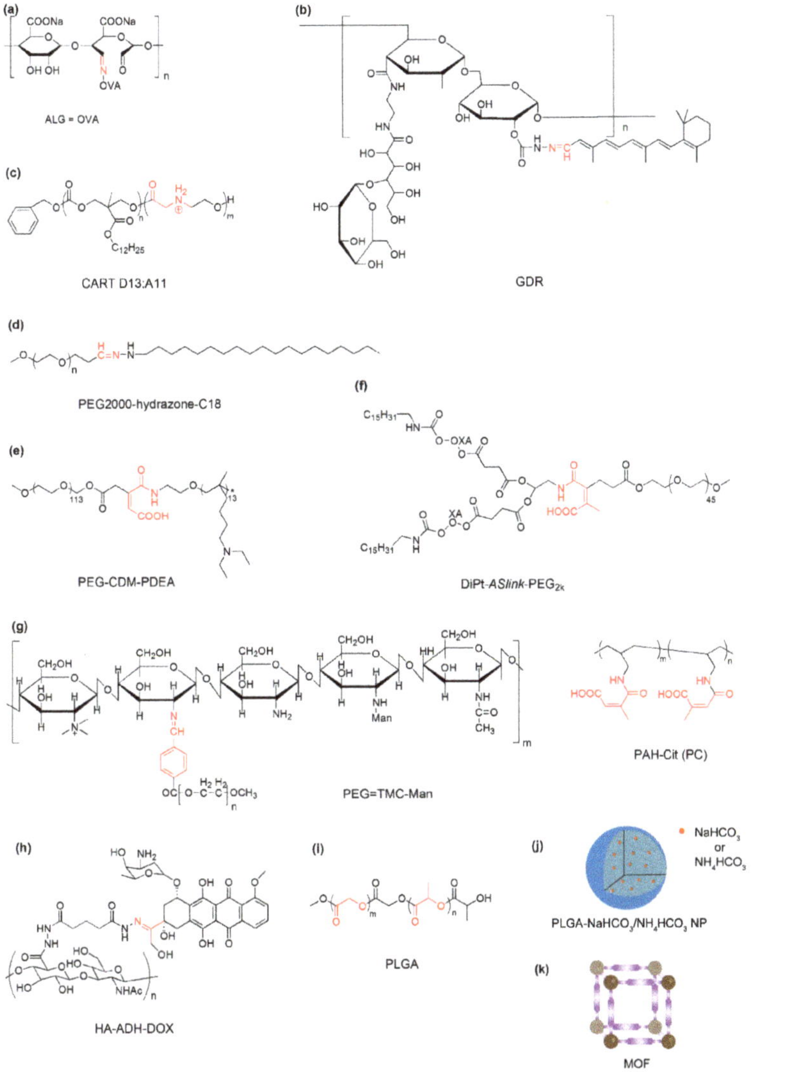

Figure 4. Representative materials with acid-labile bond cleavage or degradation for cancer immunotherapy. (**a**) ALG = OVA: ovalbumin-conjugated alginate; (**b**) GDR: galactosyl dextran-retinal conjugates; (**c**) CART D13:A11: charge-altering releasable transporter with 13 carbonate repeating units and 11 amino ester repeating units; (**d**) PEG2000-hydrazone-C18: conjugates of polyethylene glycol (molecular weight of 2000) and stearic hydrazide; (**e**) PEG-CDM-PDEA: conjugates of PEG and poly(2-(diethylamino) ethyl methacrylate with 2-propionic-3-methylmaleic anhydride linkers; (**f**) DiPt-*ASlink*-PEG$_{2k}$: conjugates of PEG2000 and hexadecyl-oxaliplatin(IV) with 2-propionic-3-methylmaleic anhydride linkers; (**g**) PEG = TMC-Man: PEG and mannose doubly modified trimethyl chitosan; PAH-Cit (PC): citraconic anhydride-grafted poly (allylamine hydrochloride); (**h**) HA-ADH-DOX: conjugates of hyaluronic acid and doxorubicin with hydrazine linkers; (**i**) PLGA: poly(lactic-*co*-glycolic acid); (**j**) PLGA-NaHCO$_3$/NH$_4$HCO$_3$ NP: NaHCO$_3$ or NH$_4$HCO$_3$-encapsulated PLGA nanoparticle; and (**k**) MOF: Metal-organic framework. The acid-labile groups are indicated in red.

Acid liable-PEG has been frequently used in pH-responsive nanoparticles to stabilize nanoparticles in the blood circulation while enhancing the nanoparticle accumulation in acidic tumor tissues. For example, nanoparticles composed of acid liable-PEG-hydrazone-C18 (PHC) (Figure 4d), poly(lactic-*co*-glycolic acid) (PLGA), and *O*-stearoyl mannose (M-C18) enable a decreased accumulation in the mononuclear phagocyte system (MPS) owing to the PEG shielding at normal pH, and thus reduce the off-target immune activation, while they can be effectively accumulated in TAM via mannose-receptor recognition after the hydrolysis of hydrazone bonds and the detachment of PEG in acidic TME [46].

The detachment of the PEG shell also enables the exposure of positively charged groups or negative-to-positive charge conversion on the nanoparticle surface [27,47]. The PEG block was conjugated with poly(2-(diethylamino) ethyl methacrylate) (PDEA) using 2-propionic-3-methylmaleic anhydride (CDM) and formed mix micelles with PEI-PDEA for the delivery of siRNA against PD-L1 and a mitochondrion-targeting photosensitizer (Figure 4e). The detachment of the PEG corona at acidic pH endows nanoparticles with significant size reduction and surface charge increase in TME, facilitating the penetration of nanoparticles to tumors and improving the antitumor immune response in vivo. Using the same pH-sensitive linker, the PEG block was attached to a lipid with two tails (Figure 4f). The nanoparticle is negatively charged at neutral pH due to the partial ionization of carboxyl groups in the side chain. After entering acidic tumor tissue, the acid-labile linker was cleaved, resulting in the detachment of the PEG shell with negative carboxyl groups and the charge conversion from negative to positive. The smart nanoparticle shows enhanced tumor accumulation and deep penetration, consequently enabling efficient delivery of a combination of immunoregulators to suppress tumor growth and metastasis in mice [47].

Moreover, the cleavage of PEG induces simultaneous exposure of targeting ligands and positively charged groups that benefit cancer immunotherapy with enhanced accumulation and specific targeting to M2-TAMs or cancer cells in tumor tissues. For example, nanoparticles composed of PEG and mannose doubly modified trimethyl chitosan and citraconic anhydride-grafted poly (allylamine hydrochloride) (PC) have been developed for the delivery of siRNAs against the vascular endothelial growth factor (VEGF) and placental growth factor (PlGF) to breast cancer cells and M2-TAMs (Figure 4g). The PEG shell is able to mask mannose to reduce the uptake by resident macrophages in the reticuloendothelial system and improve the blood circulation time. When nanoparticles enter acidic tumor tissues, the benzamide bond between PEG and the mannose-modified trimethyl chitosan is cleaved, which results in the detachment of PEG and the exposure of mannose and cationic amines, enabling effective accumulation in tumor tissues and uptake by cancer cells and macrophages. In the more acidic late endosomes or lysosomes (pH 4.5–5.5), the side chains of PC are hydrolyzed, leading to the charge reversal from negative to positive and promoting the endosomal/lysosomal escape of siRNAs. The dual pH-responsive nanoparticle could be a robust platform to reverse TME from pro-oncogenic to anti-tumoral and suppress the tumor growth and metastasis [48].

A combination of an acid-cleavable bond and pH-dependent ionization has been utilized to construct a sequential pH-responsive delivery system for the co-delivery of a TLR7/8 agonist R848 and chemotherapeutic doxorubicin (DOX) (Figure 4h). Hyaluronic acid-DOX (HA-DOX) conjugates were prepared by coupling using acid-cleavable hydrazone bonds. R848 was bound with poly(L-histidine) (PHIS) and the PHIS/R848 nanocomplex were further coated with HA-DOX to form HA-DOX/PHIS/R848 nanoparticles. When pH decreases from neutral to acidic, the mixed nanoparticles undergo two distinguished changes. The ionization of PHIS at pH 6.5 leads to the hydrophobic-to-hydrophilic transition and the release of the encapsulated R848 in TME. The cleavage of the hydrazone bond around pH 5.5 triggers the release of the covalently bound DOX to the cytosol of cancer cells, enabling the synergistic effects of immunotherapy and chemotherapy against breast cancer in 4T1 tumor-bearing mice [49].

In contrast to the cleavage of pH-responsive linkers, the break of acid-liable bonds in the polymer backbone induces the degradation of polymers and the disintegration of nanoparticles that facilitates the release of payloads into an acidic compartment of APCs or tumor tissues. For example, biodegradable PLGA-based nanoparticles have been used for the delivery of protein antigens (Figure 4i) (e.g., gp100, OVA) and JSI-124 (a small molecule inhibitor of activator of transcription-3, STAT3) to protect the immunoregulators and achieve the sustained release of drugs to DCs [50,51]. Biodegradable nanoparticles could be prepared by using acid degradable primary amine monomer and cross-linker in which anti-DEC-205 mABs were encapsulated for cytotoxic T lymphocyte activation [52].

The incorporation of pH-responsive inorganic components into nanoparticles is a robust approach to promote the release of antigens in APCs because they can generate CO_2 and/or NH_3 in acidic conditions which leads to the rupture of antigen-loaded nanoparticles (Figure 4j). In comparison with the degradation of polymers, the disintegration is more readily available for nano-sized inorganic components in mild acidic conditions. For example, ammonium bicarbonate (NH_4HCO_3) was encapsulated in PLGA nanoparticles and could react with hydrogen ions in endosomes and lysosomes that produce NH_3 and CO_2, mediating the dissociation of nanoparticles and the rapid release of encapsulated OVA to cytoplasm [30]. Similarly, PLGA-sodium bicarbonate ($NaHCO_3$) hybrid nanoparticles have been utilized to deliver an agonist 522 to stimulate the maturation of DCs and the secretion of pro-inflammatory cytokines. The incorporation of bicarbonate salts into PLGA nanoparticles enables 33-fold higher loading of the hydrophobic agonist and the rapid rapture of nanoparticles at acidic pH, resulting in an increased expression of co-stimulatory molecules and improved antigen presentation [53].

Metal-organic frameworks (MOFs) have acid-labile metal–ligand bonds and are therefore able to respond to the acidic environment endo/lysosome (Figure 4k). OVA was incorporated into the frameworks during the synthesis of MOF using Eu and guanine monophosphate (GMP). The OVA-loaded MOFs were further coated with CpG as an endosomal-acting oligonucleotide adjuvant. The MOF-based nanocarriers show high loading of antigens. Moreover, the coordination of Eu and GMP is interrupted under pH 5.0 which results in the rapid degradation of MOF and facilitates the endosomal escape and cytosol release of antigens [54].

4. Conclusions and Perspectives

pH-responsive nanoparticles show tremendous potential in cancer immunotherapy because they are capable of targeting the acidic microenvironment of tumor tissues and organelles in cells, therefore, reducing the off-targeting toxic side effects and improving therapeutic efficacy. Current pH-responsive nanoparticles for cancer immunotherapy are constructed via distinct mechanisms involving the protonation/ionization of pH-sensitive groups or the break of acid-labile covalent bonds. The key components of pH-responsive nanoparticles and their delivery payloads as well as the related disease models in this review are summarized in Table 1. The protonation/ionization varies with pH, leading to the change of surface charges or the hydrophilicity/hydrophobicity balance of nanoparticles, consequently promoting the accumulation of nanoparticles and release of payloads in target sides. The acid-cleavable bonds have been incorporated into the backbone of polymers or the linker of PEG and the backbone in pH-responsive nanoparticles. The pH-sensitive linkers are stable at physiological pH, affording nanoparticles' great serum stability upon protection by PEG corona while their cleavage at acidic pH leads to the detachment of the PEG corona and the subsequent exposure of positively charged or targeting groups on nanoparticles, resulting in the enhanced accumulation of nanoparticles in tumors or target cells. The degradation of polymer backbone at acidic pH results in the dissociation of nanoparticles, promoting the release of immunotherapeutic drugs into target sides. Incorporating pH-responsive inorganic components into nanoparticles is a robust approach to the construction of pH-sensitive nanoparticles for cancer immunotherapy because they are able to rapidly respond to the acidic environment and trigger the instant disintegration of nanoparticles at low pH.

Table 1. Selected pH-responsive nanoparticle systems for cancer immunotherapy.

	pH-Responsive Components	Immunotherapeutic Drugs	Disease Models	Refs.
pH-responsive protonation/ionization	Amines	3pRNA	CT26 colon cancer	[33]
		Photosensitizer, siPD-L1	B16-F10 melanoma	[34]
		Luciferase mRNA	C57BL/6 mice	[17]
		OVA	C57BL/6 mice, INF-α/βR$^{-/-}$ mice et al.	[38]
		BLZ-945, Pt-prodrug	B16 melanoma, CT26 colon cancer	[43]
		IL-12	B16-F10 tumor	[41]
		CpG ODN, anti-IL-10 ODN, anti-IL-10 receptor ODN	Hepa 1–6 tumor	[42]
	Carboxyl groups	OVA	E.G7-OVA tumor	[39]
	Amines and Carboxyl groups	PTX and IL-2	Murine melanoma	[40]

Table 1. Cont.

	pH-Responsive Components	Immunotherapeutic Drugs	Disease Models	Refs.
Acid-liable bonds	Schiff base bonds	OVA	E.G7 tumor	[44]
	Hydrazone bonds	OVA	Melanoma	[29]
		TLR7/8 agonist, R848, DOX	4T1 tumor	[49]
		/	C57BL/6 mice	[46]
	Amide bonds	siPD-L1, photosensitizer	B16-F10 tumor	[27]
		Oxaliplatin, NLG919	4T1 tumor	[47]
	Ester bonds	EGFP and luciferase mRNA	Multiple cell lines, BALB/c mice	[45]
		gp100, OVA et al., and JSI-124	B16-F10 tumor	[50], [51]
	Benzamide bonds	siVEGF and siPIGF	4T1, lung metastasis tumor	[48]
	NH_4HCO_3, $NaHCO_3$	OVA, agonist 522	C57BL/6 mice, B16-F10 tumor	[30, 53]
	Metal–ligand bonds	OVA, CpG	B16 melanoma	[54]

The convergence of pH-responsive nanotechnology and immunotherapy provides a promising strategy for improving the unsatisfactory efficacy and reducing the off-target side effects in cancer treatments. Despite the substantial advances in animal models, challenges remain in the clinical translation of cancer immunotherapy with pH-responsive nanoparticles. The therapeutic efficacy should be further evaluated in clinical relevant tumor models. Moreover, clinically translatable materials should be developed for the construction of pH-responsive nanoparticles to meet the strict requirements in clinical use. With the rapid progresses in material chemistry, immunology, and nanotechnology, pH-responsive nanoparticles are expected to exert a significant role in cancer immunotherapy in the near future.

Author Contributions: Y.Y. and H.D. drafted and edited the manuscript. All authors have read and agreed to the published version of the manuscript.

Funding: We gratefully acknowledge the financial support from the National Natural Science Foundation of China (U1932164) and the Zhejiang Provincial Natural Science Foundation (LY19B040004).

Conflicts of Interest: The authors declare that they have no conflict of interest.

References

1. Martin, J.D.; Cabral, H.; Stylianopoulos, T.; Jain, R.K. Improving cancer immunotherapy using nanomedicines: Progress, opportunities and challenges. *Nat. Rev. Clin. Oncol.* **2020**, *17*, 251–266. [CrossRef] [PubMed]
2. Irvine, D.J.; Dane, E.L. Enhancing cancer immunotherapy with nanomedicine. *Nat. Rev. Immunol.* **2020**, *20*, 321–334. [CrossRef] [PubMed]
3. Riley, R.S.; June, C.H.; Langer, R.; Mitchell, M.J. Delivery technologies for cancer immunotherapy. *Nat. Rev. Drug Discov.* **2019**, *18*, 175–196. [CrossRef] [PubMed]
4. Goldberg, M.S. Improving cancer immunotherapy through nanotechnology. *Nat. Rev. Cancer* **2019**, *19*, 587–602. [CrossRef] [PubMed]
5. Nam, J.; Son, S.; Park, K.S.; Zou, W.; Shea, L.D.; Moon, J.J. Cancer nanomedicine for combination cancer immunotherapy. *Nat. Rev. Mater.* **2019**, *4*, 398–414. [CrossRef]
6. Chen, D.S.; Mellman, I. Oncology meets immunology: The cancer-immunity cycle. *Immunity* **2013**, *39*, 1–10. [CrossRef]
7. Mellman, I.; Coukos, G.; Dranoff, G. Cancer immunotherapy comes of age. *Nature* **2011**, *480*, 480–489. [CrossRef]
8. Palucka, K.; Banchereau, J. Dendritic-cell-based therapeutic cancer vaccines. *Immunity* **2013**, *39*, 38–48. [CrossRef]
9. Chi, H.; Li, C.; Zhao, F.S.; Zhang, L.; Ng, T.B.; Jin, G.; Sha, O. Anti-tumor activity of toll-like receptor 7 agonists. *Front. Pharmacol.* **2017**, *8*, 304. [CrossRef]

10. Ramanjulu, J.M.; Pesiridis, G.S.; Yang, J.; Concha, N.; Singhaus, R.; Zhang, S.Y.; Tran, J.L.; Moore, P.; Lehmann, S.; Eberl, H.C.; et al. Design of amidobenzimidazole sting receptor agonists with systemic activity. *Nature* **2018**, *564*, 439–443. [CrossRef]
11. Paquette, R.L.; Hsu, N.C.; Kiertscher, S.M.; Park, A.N.; Tran, L.; Roth, M.D.; Glaspy, J.A. Interferon-alpha and granulocyte-macrophage colony-stimulating factor differentiate peripheral blood monocytes into potent antigen-presenting cells. *J. Leukoc. Biol.* **1998**, *64*, 358–367. [CrossRef] [PubMed]
12. Rosenberg, S.A. Il-2: The first effective immunotherapy for human cancer. *J. Immunol.* **2014**, *192*, 5451–5458. [CrossRef] [PubMed]
13. Rosenberg, S.A.; Restifo, N.P. Adoptive cell transfer as personalized immunotherapy for human cancer. *Science* **2015**, *348*, 62–68. [CrossRef] [PubMed]
14. Neelapu, S.S.; Locke, F.L.; Bartlett, N.L.; Lekakis, L.J.; Miklos, D.B.; Jacobson, C.A.; Braunschweig, I.; Oluwole, O.O.; Siddiqi, T.; Lin, Y.; et al. Axicabtagene ciloleucel car t-cell therapy in refractory large b-cell lymphoma. *N. Engl. J. Med.* **2017**, *377*, 2531–2544. [CrossRef] [PubMed]
15. Maude, S.L.; Laetsch, T.W.; Buechner, J.; Rives, S.; Boyer, M.; Bittencourt, H.; Bader, P.; Verneris, M.R.; Stefanski, H.E.; Myers, G.D.; et al. Tisagenlecleucel in children and young adults with b-cell lymphoblastic leukemia. *N. Engl. J. Med.* **2018**, *378*, 439–448. [CrossRef]
16. Blanco, E.; Shen, H.; Ferrari, M. Principles of nanoparticle design for overcoming biological barriers to drug delivery. *Nat. Biotechnol.* **2015**, *33*, 941–951. [CrossRef]
17. Hajj, K.A.; Ball, R.L.; Deluty, S.B.; Singh, S.R.; Strelkova, D.; Knapp, C.M.; Whitehead, K.A. Branched-tail lipid nanoparticles potently deliver mrna in vivo due to enhanced ionization at endosomal pH. *Small* **2019**, *15*, 1805097. [CrossRef]
18. Neelapu, S.S.; Tummala, S.; Kebriaei, P.; Wierda, W.; Gutierrez, C.; Locke, F.L.; Komanduri, K.V.; Lin, Y.; Jain, N.; Daver, N.; et al. Chimeric antigen receptor t-cell therapy—Assessment and management of toxicities. *Nat. Rev. Clin. Oncol.* **2018**, *15*, 47–62. [CrossRef]
19. Martins, F.; Sofiya, L.; Sykiotis, G.P.; Lamine, F.; Maillard, M.; Fraga, M.; Shabafrouz, K.; Ribi, C.; Cairoli, A.; Guex-Crosier, Y.; et al. Adverse effects of immune-checkpoint inhibitors: Epidemiology, management and surveillance. *Nat. Rev. Clin. Oncol.* **2019**, *16*, 563–580. [CrossRef]
20. Davis, M.E.; Chen, Z.G.; Shin, D.M. Nanoparticle therapeutics: An emerging treatment modality for cancer. *Nat. Rev. Drug Discov.* **2008**, *7*, 771–782. [CrossRef]
21. Zhao, T.; Huang, G.; Li, Y.; Yang, S.C.; Ramezani, S.; Lin, Z.Q.; Wang, Y.G.; Ma, X.P.; Zeng, Z.Q.; Luo, M.; et al. A transistor-like ph nanoprobe for tumour detection and image-guided surgery. *Nat. Biomed. Eng.* **2017**, *1*, UNSP0006. [CrossRef] [PubMed]
22. Ma, X.P.; Wang, Y.G.; Zhao, T.; Li, Y.; Su, L.C.; Wang, Z.H.; Huang, G.; Sumer, B.D.; Gao, J.M. Ultra-ph-sensitive nanoprobe library with broad ph tunability and fluorescence emissions. *J. Am. Chem. Soc.* **2014**, *136*, 11085–11092. [CrossRef] [PubMed]
23. Varkouhi, A.K.; Scholte, M.; Storm, G.; Haisma, H.J. Endosomal escape pathways for delivery of biologicals. *J. Control. Release* **2011**, *151*, 220–228. [CrossRef] [PubMed]
24. Kanamala, M.; Wilson, W.R.; Yang, M.; Palmer, B.D.; Wu, Z. Mechanisms and biomaterials in ph-responsive tumour targeted drug delivery: A review. *Biomaterials* **2016**, *85*, 152–167. [CrossRef] [PubMed]
25. Du, J.; Lane, L.A.; Nie, S. Stimuli-responsive nanoparticles for targeting the tumor microenvironment. *J. Control. Release* **2015**, *219*, 205–214. [CrossRef]
26. Shen, Y.; Tang, H.; Radosz, M.; Van Kirk, E.; Murdoch, W.I. Ph-responsive nanoparticles for cancer drug delivery. In *Drug Delivery Systems*; Jain, K.K., Ed.; Humana Press: Totowa, NJ, USA, 2008; Volume 437, pp. 183–216.
27. Dai, L.; Li, K.; Li, M.; Zhao, X.; Luo, Z.; Lu, L.; Luo, Y.; Cai, K. Size/charge changeable acidity-responsive micelleplex for photodynamic-improved pd-l1 immunotherapy with enhanced tumor penetration. *Adv. Funct. Mater.* **2018**, *28*, 1707249. [CrossRef]
28. Yang, G.B.; Xu, L.G.; Xu, J.; Zhang, R.; Song, G.S.; Chao, Y.; Feng, L.Z.; Han, F.X.; Dong, Z.L.; Li, B.; et al. Smart nanoreactors for ph-responsive tumor homing, mitochondria-targeting, and enhanced photodynamic-immunotherapy of cancer. *Nano Lett.* **2018**, *18*, 2475–2484. [CrossRef]
29. Wang, C.; Li, P.; Liu, L.; Pan, H.; Li, H.; Cai, L.; Ma, Y. Self-adjuvanted nanovaccine for cancer immunotherapy: Role of lysosomal rupture-induced ros in mhc class i antigen presentation. *Biomaterials* **2016**, *79*, 88–100. [CrossRef]

30. Liu, Q.; Chen, X.M.; Jia, J.L.; Zhang, W.F.; Yang, T.Y.; Wang, L.Y.; Ma, G.H. Ph-responsive poly(d,l-lactic-co-glycolic acid) nanoparticles with rapid antigen release behavior promote immune response. *ACS Nano* **2015**, *9*, 4925–4938. [CrossRef]
31. Zheng, D.-W.; Chen, J.-L.; Zhu, J.-Y.; Rong, L.; Li, B.; Lei, Q.; Fan, J.-X.; Zou, M.-Z.; Li, C.; Cheng, S.-X.; et al. Highly integrated nano-platform for breaking the barrier between chemotherapy and immunotherapy. *Nano Lett.* **2016**, *16*, 4341–4347. [CrossRef]
32. Hu, Y.; Litwin, T.; Nagaraja, A.R.; Kwong, B.; Katz, J.; Watson, N.; Irvine, D.J. Cytosolic delivery of membrane-impermeable molecules in dendritic cells using ph-responsive core-shell nanoparticles. *Nano Lett.* **2007**, *7*, 3056–3064. [CrossRef] [PubMed]
33. Jacobson, M.E.; Wang-Bishop, L.; Becker, K.W.; Wilson, J.T. Delivery of 5′-triphosphate rna with endosomolytic nanoparticles potently activates rig-i to improve cancer immunotherapy. *Biomater. Sci.* **2019**, *7*, 547–559. [CrossRef] [PubMed]
34. Wang, D.; Wang, T.; Liu, J.; Yu, H.; Jiao, S.; Feng, B.; Zhou, F.; Fu, Y.; Yin, Q.; Zhang, P.; et al. Acid-activatable versatile micelleplexes for pd-l1 blockade-enhanced cancer photodynamic immunotherapy. *Nano Lett.* **2016**, *16*, 5503–5513. [CrossRef] [PubMed]
35. Xiong, Q.Q.; Lee, G.Y.; Ding, J.X.; Li, W.L.; Shi, J.J. Biomedical applications of mrna nanomedicine. *Nano Res.* **2018**, *11*, 5281–5309. [CrossRef] [PubMed]
36. Yan, Y.F.; Xiong, H.; Zhang, X.Y.; Cheng, Q.; Siegwart, D.J. Systemic mrna delivery to the lungs by functional polyester-based carriers. *Biomacromolecules* **2017**, *18*, 4307–4315. [CrossRef]
37. Cheng, Q.; Wei, T.; Farbiak, L.; Johnson, L.T.; Dilliard, S.A.; Siegwart, D.J. Selective organ targeting (sort) nanoparticles for tissue-specific mrna delivery and crispr-cas gene editing. *Nat. Nanotechnol.* **2020**, *15*, 313–320.
38. Luo, M.; Wang, H.; Wang, Z.; Cai, H.; Lu, Z.; Li, Y.; Du, M.; Huang, G.; Wang, C.; Chen, X.; et al. A sting-activating nanovaccine for cancer immunotherapy. *Nat. Nanotechnol.* **2017**, *12*, 648–654.
39. Yuba, E.; Tajima, N.; Yoshizaki, Y.; Harada, A.; Hayashi, H.; Kono, K. Dextran derivative-based ph-sensitive liposomes for cancer immunotherapy. *Biomaterials* **2014**, *35*, 3091–3101. [CrossRef]
40. Song, Q.; Yin, Y.; Shang, L.; Wu, T.; Zhang, D.; Kong, M.; Zhao, Y.; He, Y.; Tan, S.; Guo, Y.; et al. Tumor microenvironment responsive nanogel for the combinatorial antitumor effect of chemotherapy and immunotherapy. *Nano Lett.* **2017**, *17*, 6366–6375. [CrossRef]
41. Wang, Y.; Lin, Y.X.; Qiao, S.L.; An, H.W.; Ma, Y.; Qiao, Z.Y.; Rajapaksha, R.P.; Wang, H. Polymeric nanoparticles promote macrophage reversal from m2 to m1 phenotypes in the tumor microenvironment. *Biomaterials* **2017**, *112*, 153–163. [CrossRef]
42. Huang, Z.; Zhang, Z.; Jiang, Y.; Zhang, D.; Chen, J.; Dong, L.; Zhang, J. Targeted delivery of oligonucleotides into tumor-associated macrophages for cancer immunotherapy. *J. Control. Release* **2012**, *158*, 286–292. [CrossRef] [PubMed]
43. Shen, S.; Li, H.J.; Chen, K.G.; Wang, Y.C.; Yang, X.Z.; Lian, Z.X.; Du, J.Z.; Wang, J. Spatial targeting of tumor-associated macrophages and tumor cells with a ph-sensitive cluster nanocarrier for cancer chemoimmunotherapy. *Nano Lett.* **2017**, *17*, 3822–3829. [CrossRef] [PubMed]
44. Zhang, C.; Shi, G.; Zhang, J.; Song, H.; Niu, J.; Shi, S.; Huang, P.; Wang, Y.; Wang, W.; Li, C.; et al. Targeted antigen delivery to dendritic cell via functionalized alginate nanoparticles for cancer immunotherapy. *J. Control. Release* **2017**, *256*, 170–181. [CrossRef] [PubMed]
45. McKinlay, C.J.; Benner, N.L.; Haabeth, O.A.; Waymouth, R.M.; Wender, P.A. Enhanced mrna delivery into lymphocytes enabled by lipid-varied libraries of charge-altering releasable transporters. *Proc. Natl. Acad. Sci. USA* **2018**, *115*, E5859–E5866. [CrossRef] [PubMed]
46. Zhu, S.; Niu, M.; O'Mary, H.; Cui, Z. Targeting of tumor-associated macrophages made possible by peg-sheddable, mannose-modified nanoparticles. *Mol. Pharm.* **2013**, *10*, 3525–3530. [CrossRef]
47. Feng, B.; Zhou, F.; Hou, B.; Wang, D.; Wang, T.; Fu, Y.; Ma, Y.; Yu, H.; Li, Y. Binary cooperative prodrug nanoparticles improve immunotherapy by synergistically modulating immune tumor microenvironment. *Adv. Mater.* **2018**, *30*, e1803001. [CrossRef]
48. Song, Y.; Tang, C.; Yin, C. Combination antitumor immunotherapy with vegf and pigf sirna via systemic delivery of multi-functionalized nanoparticles to tumor-associated macrophages and breast cancer cells. *Biomaterials* **2018**, *185*, 117–132. [CrossRef]

49. Liu, Y.; Qiao, L.; Zhang, S.; Wan, G.; Chen, B.; Zhou, P.; Zhang, N.; Wang, Y. Dual ph-responsive multifunctional nanoparticles for targeted treatment of breast cancer by combining immunotherapy and chemotherapy. *Acta Biomater.* **2018**, *66*, 310–324. [CrossRef]
50. Solbrig, C.M.; Saucier-Sawyer, J.K.; Cody, V.; Saltzman, W.M.; Hanlon, D.J. Polymer nanoparticles for immunotherapy from encapsulated tumor-associated antigens and whole tumor cells. *Mol. Pharmaceut.* **2007**, *4*, 47–57. [CrossRef]
51. Molavi, L.; Mahmud, A.; Hamdy, S.; Hung, R.W.; Lai, R.; Samuel, J.; Lavasanifar, A. Development of a poly(d,l-lactic-co-glycolic acid) nanoparticle formulation of stat3 inhibitor jsi-124: Implication for cancer immunotherapy. *Mol. Pharm.* **2010**, *7*, 364–374. [CrossRef]
52. Kwon, Y.J.; James, E.; Shastri, N.; Frechet, J.M.J. In vivo targeting of dendritic cells for activation of cellular immunity using vaccine carriers based on ph-responsive microparticles. *Proc. Natl. Acad. Sci. USA* **2005**, *102*, 18264–18268. [CrossRef] [PubMed]
53. Kim, H.; Sehgal, D.; Kucaba, T.A.; Ferguson, D.M.; Griffith, T.S.; Panyam, J. Acidic ph-responsive polymer nanoparticles as a tlr7/8 agonist delivery platform for cancer immunotherapy. *Nanoscale* **2018**, *10*, 20851–20862. [CrossRef] [PubMed]
54. Duan, F.; Feng, X.; Yang, X.; Sun, W.; Jin, Y.; Liu, H.; Ge, K.; Li, Z.; Zhang, J. A simple and powerful co-delivery system based on ph-responsive metal-organic frameworks for enhanced cancer immunotherapy. *Biomaterials* **2017**, *122*, 23–33. [CrossRef] [PubMed]

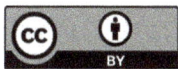

© 2020 by the authors. Licensee MDPI, Basel, Switzerland. This article is an open access article distributed under the terms and conditions of the Creative Commons Attribution (CC BY) license (http://creativecommons.org/licenses/by/4.0/).

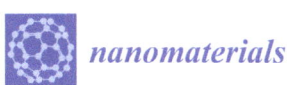

Review

Nanoparticle Systems for Cancer Phototherapy: An Overview

Thais P. Pivetta [1,2,†], **Caroline E. A. Botteon** [3,†], **Paulo A. Ribeiro** [2], **Priscyla D. Marcato** [3] **and Maria Raposo** [2,*]

1. CEFITEC, Department of Physics, NOVA School of Science and Technology, Universidade NOVA de Lisboa, 2829-516 Caparica, Portugal; t.pivetta@campus.fct.unl.pt
2. Laboratory of Instrumentation, Biomedical Engineering and Radiation Physics (LIBPhys-UNL), Department of Physics, NOVA School of Science and Technology, Universidade NOVA de Lisboa, 2829-516 Caparica, Portugal; pfr@fct.unl.pt
3. GNanoBio, School of Pharmaceutical Sciences of Ribeirão Preto, University of São Paulo, Ribeirão Preto 14040-900, Brazil; caroline.botteon@usp.br (C.E.A.B.); pmarcato@fcfrp.usp.br (P.D.M.)
* Correspondence: mfr@fct.unl.pt; Fax: +351-21-294-85-49
† These authors contributed equally to this manuscript.

Abstract: Photodynamic therapy (PDT) and photothermal therapy (PTT) are photo-mediated treatments with different mechanisms of action that can be addressed for cancer treatment. Both phototherapies are highly successful and barely or non-invasive types of treatment that have gained attention in the past few years. The death of cancer cells because of the application of these therapies is caused by the formation of reactive oxygen species, that leads to oxidative stress for the case of photodynamic therapy and the generation of heat for the case of photothermal therapies. The advancement of nanotechnology allowed significant benefit to these therapies using nanoparticles, allowing both tuning of the process and an increase of effectiveness. The encapsulation of drugs, development of the most different organic and inorganic nanoparticles as well as the possibility of surfaces' functionalization are some strategies used to combine phototherapy and nanotechnology, with the aim of an effective treatment with minimal side effects. This article presents an overview on the use of nanostructures in association with phototherapy, in the view of cancer treatment.

Keywords: nanoparticles; phototherapy; cancer; photodynamic therapy; photothermal therapy

1. Introduction

Cancer is a leading cause of death worldwide, with an estimated 19.3 million new cases and nearly 10 million deaths caused by cancer in 2020 [1]. During the 20th century, there was an undeniable technological development aiming to enhance the treatment of cancer, mainly regarding to the discovery of chemotherapy. Nowadays, chemotherapy is one of the pillars for cancer treatment, along with surgery and radiotherapy [2,3]. However, it is known that chemotherapy and radiotherapy have severe side effects to the patient, mainly due to the non-specificity of the treatment [4]. Within this context, phototherapy has gained attention as an alternative treatment with reduced side effects [4].

Photodynamic therapy (PDT) and photothermal therapy (PTT) are photo-mediated therapies with different damage mechanisms that consist in the generation of reactive oxygen species (ROS) and heat, respectively [4,5]. These effects result in the cells' death, thereby, with a potential application for treatment of several types of cancer [6]. PDT requires the application of photosensitizer drugs (PS) that will be triggered by radiation.

These drugs generally present poor solubility in physiological conditions, which can impair therapy's success [7]. For this purpose, it is necessary to find appropriate nanoparticulate systems that can deliver these drugs to the cancer cells. Currently, there is not a unique definition that is accepted internationally, however nanomaterials are often described in the scale of 1–1000 nm [8]. Nanotechnology emerged in order to enhance problems related to drugs' solubility and provide a targeted treatment, enabling to reduce drugs' dosage and

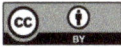

also minimize several side effects in patients [9]. Additionally, through nanotechnology research, there are several types of nanoparticles, particularly metallic nanoparticles such as gold nanoparticles, that can generate heat upon exposition to light, which can be useful for PTT [10] as it induces hyperthermia in the tumor environment, consequently leading to cancer cells' death [11]. PTT is a non-invasive and selective technique which can potentially suppress many kinds of tumors [12]. Cancer treatment with the PTT approach offers many advantages, such as sensitization of hypoxic regions, reinforcement of the immune system, releasing of thermo-sensitive substances and increasing susceptibility of cancer cells to chemotherapeutic agents [13]. The combination of PDT and PTT is also possible through the use of a sensitizing agent able to produce ROS and hyperthermia [5].

NPs for phototherapy have been extensively investigated and reported in the literature [14,15], and in this work, new issues concerning NP systems' design, in view of cancer treatment under photodynamic and photothermal therapies, will be addressed. The referred new issues are intended to exemplify recent approaches related to nanoparticle conditions, such as the targeting of drugs in the tumor site and problems and/or new achievements related to the phototherapy. The overall situation and trend of research in both therapies using nanoparticles is clearly demonstrated in Figure 1, which shows, in the last ten years, both number of publications and number of citations listed in the Web of Science platform using "Photodynamic Therapy AND Nanoparticles" and "Photothermal Therapy AND Nanoparticles" as search topics, where both number of publications and of citations are increasing strongly in recent years.

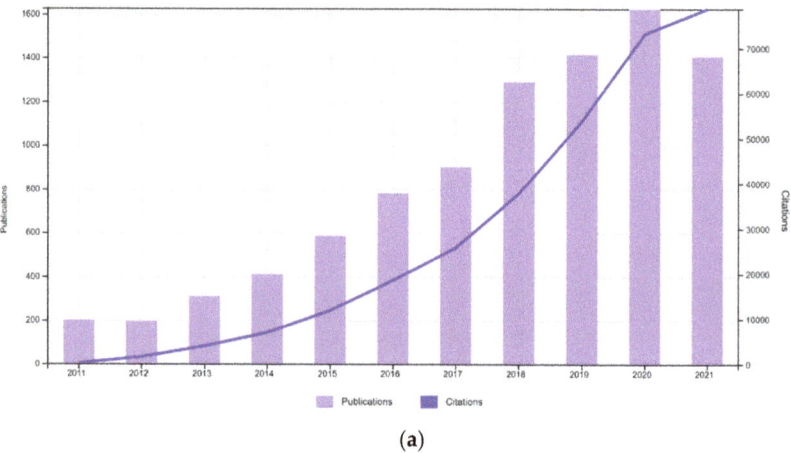

Figure 1. *Cont.*

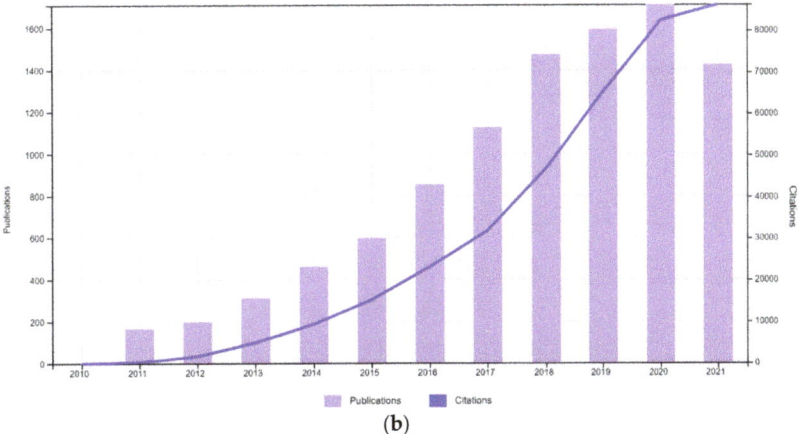

(b)

Figure 1. Updated number of publications and number of citations in the last ten years listed in the Web of Science platform using as search topics: (**a**) "Photodynamic Therapy AND Nanoparticles" and (**b**) "Photothermal Therapy AND Nanoparticles" (November 2021).

2. Photodynamic Therapy

2.1. A Brief Introduction

PDT has been used for centuries, mainly to treat skin disorders, with most treatments involving the intake of extracts of some types of plants followed by exposition to the sun [16]. The main discovery took place in Germany in 1900, where Oscar Raab and Hermann von Tappeiner were investigating the behavior of protozoan *Paramecium* spp. in the presence of the dye acridine orange. They verified that the protozoan died after the exposure to the sunlight coming from an adjacent window. This discovery was important later for the successful achievements on the human skin carcinoma treatment, and by 1904, it was found that the presence of oxygen was important for the treatment, originating the name photodynamic [17]. Currently, PDT is a highly successful and barely or non-invasive type of treatment for several skin disorders, such as psoriasis and cancers [18]. There are three important elements to perform PDT, which are a photosensitizer drug, the light source, and the presence of oxygen. The interaction of these elements results in reactive oxygen species (ROS), which play a key role in the treatment [19]. Upon a specific light wavelength, the photosensitizers (PS) can absorb a photon, which will lead to a conversion from the single basic state to the single excited state, as shown in Figure 2. From there, it can make an intersystem, crossing to a metastable triplet state, which in turn can take two possible paths known as PDT type I or type II. In type I, the activated photosensitizer can trigger a series of reactions with biomolecules generating radicals that interact with oxygen molecules, creating ROS. On the other hand, in PDT type II, the PS by itself can transfer energy directly to oxygen, resulting in ROS molecules [20,21]. Due to their high oxidizing power, ROS molecules have cytotoxic effects, however, due to the short lifetime, the effect of ROS on cell damage will occur around the created species [22].

However, PDT has a limited application that can depend on several factors to achieve a successful treatment. A special mention should be given to the light source. This is an important variable to take into consideration because different light wavelengths have different penetration depths in tissues. For example, ultraviolet (UV) light is known to cause several damages in biomolecules, such as the DNA presents low penetration compared to longer light wavelengths [23–27]. Near-infrared (NIR) light, on the other hand, is capable of higher penetration depths, with the capability of generation of local heat even with low energy input. NIR is also safer than UV, which can cause sunburns, inflammation, and even skin cancer [23,28].

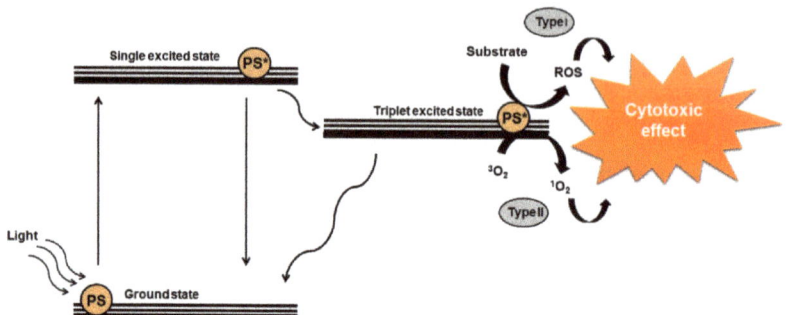

Figure 2. Jablonski diagram representation and the photodynamic therapy mechanism of action.

Another factor that can impair the efficacy of PDT is the hypoxic tumor microenvironment. To overcome this challenge, some strategies involved the elaboration of nanoparticles with molecules such as catalase, that can react and generate oxygen, or hemoglobin and perfluorocarbon, that serve as an oxygen carrier. Therefore, the inclusion of these molecules in nanoparticles is able to improve the PDT efficacy [29].

The photosensitizer drugs themselves are another variable that can interfere with the PDT. For example, some PS can present poor solubility under physiologic conditions and impair the correct distribution of the drug to the target tissue, which of course will interfere with the therapy's success. To circumvent such a drawback, the use of nanoparticulate systems is addressed, enhancing the drug's solubility and the cellular uptake, and consequently the PDT efficacy [7,30]. Many types of nanoparticles for PDT have been attempted for different types of cancers, and some aspects of nanoparticle systems for PDT will be discussed in this section.

2.2. Nanoparticles with Application for PDT

As mentioned before, in phototherapy, the delivery of PS molecules to the target tissue is a relevant issue, as it is in all cases of drug delivery systems. The NP systems to be used should be suitable to release the active components over a defined period of time with control over the nanoparticle size. The raw materials employed, and their biodegradability, is also important to consider for nanoparticles' preparation. The most common NPs used in PDT are not only organic-based but also inorganic, such as silica and magnetic NPs. In the next sections, some of the best achievements with the use of nanocarriers will be presented.

2.2.1. Organic Nanoparticles

Organic nanoparticles are the most used systems to encapsulate molecules which can be used in PDT. There are several categories based on different materials and respective organization. Figure 3 is a representation that summarizes the most common categories of organic nanoparticles, and in Table 1, there is a brief description with examples of nanoparticulate systems that are cited in this review.

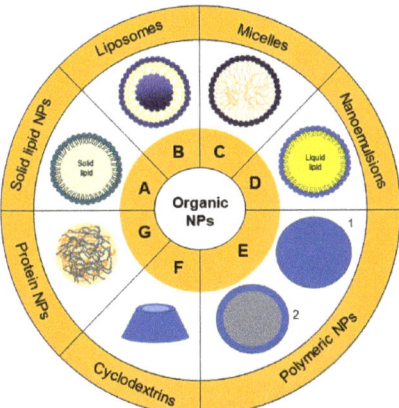

Figure 3. Different organic nanoparticles that can be used for photodynamic therapy: (**A**) solid lipid nanoparticles, (**B**) liposomes, (**C**) micelles, (**D**) nano-emulsions, (**E**) polymeric nanoparticles, (**F**) cyclodextrins and (**G**) protein nanoparticles.

Solid Lipid Nanoparticles

Solid lipid nanoparticles (SLNs) were developed in the 1990s, and ever since, these particles have become the perfect model of safe nanoparticles with an occlusive effect that can also increase the drug permeation in the skin [31]. Generally, these NPs are composed of a surfactant layer, with a lipidic nucleus (Figure 3A, and can be prepared by the Müller and Lucks method based on high-pressure homogenization (1996) or by the microemulsion technique developed by Gasco (1993) [32,33].

Either way, SLNs' production requires lipids that are solid at body temperature, such as some triglycerides or glycerides mixtures. Due to their composition, SLNs are well-tolerated, are biodegradable and can easily be produced on a large scale and at low cost [31,34,35]. However, SLNs present some disadvantages, such as the limited encapsulation efficiency and the possibility of drug release during the storage time. In order to overcome these problems, a second generation of SLNs was developed [34], the so-called nanostructured lipid carriers (NLCs). They consist of SLNs with a less ordered solid matrix based on a mixture of lipids. There are three types of NLCs: imperfect, amorphous and multiple [34]. The imperfect NLCs are composed by a blend of solid lipids with different chain lengths as well as the lipid saturation degree, characteristics that lead to the creation of an imperfect solid matrix. The amorphous type is produced from special solid and liquid lipids, creating a solid particle that does not crystalize. The combination of solid lipids with higher amounts of liquid lipids results in the multiple type, in which there is the creation of oil nano-compartments inside the solid matrix [34,36].

Nanostructured lipid carriers with a photosensitizer precursor (5-aminolevulinic acid) were developed by Qidwai and collaborators [37], aiming for use in basal-cell carcinoma treatment. In their study, the nanoparticles exhibited a sustained release profile, higher retention of the drug in the skin layers and enhanced toxicity. Similarly, solid lipid nanoparticles were used to encapsulate curcumin, a natural product with potential in phototherapy application. Curcumin nanoparticles were revealed to enhance drug uptake into the lung cancerous cells and were able to produce ROS under light exposition, thus presenting potential for phototherapy [38].

Most of the studies employing SLNs and NLCs are intended for skin delivery. For example, Goto et al. [39] developed solid lipid nanoparticles containing aluminum chloride phthalocyanine for melanoma treatment. The developed system showed great stability and the measurements of forced stability indicated that the system would be stable for 12 months. In vitro studies showed no toxicity under dark conditions but, when submitted to a light source, the toxicity was seen dependent on the radiation dose. Almeida et al. [40]

also encapsulated phthalocyanine in lipid nanoparticle formulations and demonstrated an enhancement of the drug penetration in the skin, when compared to the control group. Interestingly, NLC formulation with higher amounts of the liquid lipid oleic acid showed greater retainment (89.5%) in the deeper skin layers when compared to the NLC with less oleic acid and the solid lipid nanoparticle. In vitro studies carried out on melanoma cells revealed that that the free drug did not lead to cell toxicity under light conditions, probably due to poor accumulation in the cells but, on the other hand, drugs encapsulated in NLC showed a significant reduction in cell viability starting from 0.1 µg/mL. Therefore, the composition of solid lipid nanoparticles is a relevant parameter that can directly result in a higher effect in therapeutics.

Liposomes

Liposomes are formed by auto-organization of phospholipids in bilayers that, in an aqueous medium, tend to fold on themselves, creating vesicles (Figure 3B) [41]. Due to the lipid's amphiphilic nature, hydrophilic and hydrophobic drugs can be stored in different compartments of liposomes [42]. These vesicles are usually employed as a model in the study of cell membranes, considering the similarity between them, however, liposomes can also be applied to drug delivery [43,44]. The lipid composition provides great biocompatibility, biodegradability and additionally, does not present toxicity [42,45]. The functionalization of these particles with polyethylene glycol (PEG) can lead to the creation of stealth liposomes, that are able to evade from the immune system and increase their blood circulation [46,47]. Other types of ligands can be used in the functionalization, such as antibodies, which in turn manage a robust targeted drug delivery [48]. Due to the system's versatility, liposomes are great candidates for photodynamic therapy application.

Foscan® is a commercial photosensitizer formulation already approved in Europe for neck and head cancers' application. The active drug of Foscan®, known as temoporfin, also originated Foslip® and Fospeg®, which are liposomes formulations [49]. The temoporfin encapsulation in the lipid carriers presents a similar phototoxicity as Foscan® with significantly lower toxicity. Fospeg®, a derivative from Foslip® and distinguished by a PEGylation, is able to provide enhanced pharmacokinetics with longer circulation in the blood [50,51]. Studies in HeLa spheroids showed that the drug delivery via liposomes is a way to decrease the drug's toxicity in the absence of light, increase the cellular internalization and, consequently, PDT effectiveness [49]. Foslip® and Fospeg® are just examples of formulations developed that are currently approved, however many other liposomal systems containing photosensitizers can be explored targeted to different tumor types.

To overcome issues related with low encapsulation efficiency, drug expulsion and quenching caused by molecules' aggregation, Cai et al. [52] incorporated fluorogens with singular aggregation-induced emission characteristics (AIEgens) in the lipid, creating a conjugate. Liposomes produced from these conjugates (AIEsomes) were able to show a superior ROS production compared to conventional liposomal systems containing photosensitizer molecules. In vitro studies carried out under dark conditions proved that both AIEsomes and conventional liposomes were toxic for a breast cancer cell line, however when irradiated with white light, AIEsomes exhibited more toxicity compared to conventional liposomes. Afterwards, in vivo studies revealed AIEsomes' ability to target and image in the tumor site, factors intrinsically related to their accumulation mainly in tumors. Furthermore, irradiation of animals after injection of AIEsomes was able to suppress tumor growth and induce necrosis in the tissue, which did not happen to other experimental groups, revealing the potential of liposomes prepared with AIEgen-lipid conjugates for targeted PDT.

A similar technique was employed by Kim et al. [53] with liposomes prepared from lipid conjugated with pheophorbide A, which were used as photosensitizers aiming for photo-induced immunotherapy in cholangiocarcinoma. Regardless of whether the technique used to exploit photosensitizer incorporation in liposomes consists in a PS-lipid conjugation or encapsulation, these systems have been studied for PDT in several types of cancer, such as gastric, breast, ovarian, liver, skin and others [45,54–57]. Liposomes' features provide an extensive range of new possibilities to create therapeutic carriers that can improve PDT.

Micelles

Similar to the previous description of liposomes formation, micelles (Figure 3C) are also formed by the self-organization of amphiphilic molecules, and the resultant particle is different from the vesicles because of the different packing parameters [58,59]. The concentration of amphiphilic molecules must reach values above the designated critical micellar concentration (CMC) to form stable micelles, with a confined hydrophobic interior isolated from the aqueous medium. Polymers can also be materials used for micelles' preparation if the polymers present hydrophobic and hydrophilic segments. Therefore, the choice of the amphiphilic molecule that will be used is important due to different CMC values [60].

Aiming at a dual action of chemo- and photo-therapy in melanoma, Zhang et al. [61] investigated the preparation of micelles from block copolymer for the co-delivery of the classical anticancer agents Doxorubicin and pheophorbide A. These compounds were incorporated in the polymer chain, and the prepared micelles were successfully internalized into melanoma cells with ROS formation induced by light observed in vitro and in vivo. Micelles showed high inhibition of tumor growth, almost twice that of micelles without irradiation treatment, and significantly higher than treatment with only Doxorubicin.

To obtain a target system for ovarian cancer and metastatic melanoma cells, Lamch et al. [62] developed micelles with a di-block copolymer mPEG45-PLLA70 conjugated with folic acid for the encapsulation of the photosensitizer zinc (II) phthalocyanine. Wang et al. [63], in turn, used hyaluronic acid functionalization in micelles containing protoporphyrin IX to target cells with overexpression of CD44 receptors. The in vitro application of these micelles in monolayers and spheroids of human lung adenocarcinoma cells suggested that the enhanced cytotoxicity was due to higher internalization, and the effect of the interaction between the ligand hyaluronic acid and the receptor. Therefore, these studies suggest that micelles' functionalization can be an approach to enhance photodynamic therapy using this kind of nanostructure.

Nano-Emulsions

A nano-emulsion is a mixture of oil and surfactant in aqueous phase, which demands energy to form small droplets of 20–200 nm (Figure 3D) [64]. Nano-emulsions can be employed as a strategy to enhance the bioavailability of several lipophilic drugs. For example, studies by Machado et al. [65] on formulations of nano-emulsions containing curcumin, a natural product, as a photosensitizer drug revealed that curcumin-nano-emulsion was highly phototoxic to breast cancer cells and produced high levels of ROS. Mongue-Fuentes et al. [66] also used natural raw materials for the development of nano-emulsions for PDT. In their work, acai oil was used for the nano-emulsion preparation, which, combined with light irradiation, resulted in 85% death of melanoma cells, results which were also confirmed by animal studies in mice, with a decrease of tumor volume.

Polymeric NPs

On the nanotechnology timeline, polymer-based nanoparticles were firstly reported in 1976 [67]. Since then, the great interest in these NPs resulted in the development of several methods to produce polymeric nanoparticles or PNPs (representation of 1-nanospheres and 2-nanocapsules in Figure 3E), such as nanoprecipitation and solvent evaporation. The solvent evaporation method is an example of a two-step procedure where an emulsion is created, homogenized or sonicated, and then an evaporation step is required to remove the organic solvent in which the polymer was dissolved. On the other hand, nanoprecipitation is a one-step procedure where the polymer and drug are dissolved in a solvent miscible in water and dripped in an aqueous solution containing stabilizer. In both methods, organic solvents are employed, and although toxic solvents such as chloroform are no longer used, ether and acetone are currently used for the preparation of nanoparticles. In these cases, evaporation and purification methods are required to remove solvent residues from the dispersion [68–70].

Eltahan and collaborators developed polymeric nanoparticles co-loaded with NVP-BEZ235 and Chlorin-e6 (Ce6), named NVP/Ce6@NPs [71]. Ce6 was the selected photosensitizer and NVP-BEZ235 was used due to its ability to inhibit the PI3K/AKT/mTOR pathway that is related to tumor progression and proliferation and inhibit the repair of DNA damage in tumor cells. This sophisticated system plus irradiation was able to generate ROS by the Singlet Oxygen Sensor Green method, followed by tests in the triple-negative breast cancer cell line, and by flow cytometry, the authors discovered that treatment with NVP/Ce6@NPs and irradiation presented a fluorescence approximately 5 times greater compared to the control and nanoparticles without Ce6. These achievements showed the effect of a biochemical and PDT combination to treat a severe type of cancer.

Polymeric nanoparticles can be used to enhance the solubility of drugs as well as to provide drug's stability and sustained release [72]. PNPs were used to encapsulate the photosensitizer zinc phthalocyanine, and as result, the phototoxicity showed a 500 times increase compared to the free drug in a lung cancer cell line [73]. Polymers' functionalization is another strategy able to achieve multifunctional nanoparticles [74]. The addition of some type of ligand such as an antibody to the nanoparticle surface allows it to bind specifically to sites where there is an overexpression of the receptor (Figure 4). Transferrin receptors, for example, are overexpressed in breast cancer. Regarding this, Jadia and collaborators [75] functionalized polymers with a peptide (hTf) that is able to bind to transferrin receptor and prepared nanoparticles containing the drug benzoporphyrin monoacid. As expected, functionalized nanoparticles exhibited specificity to the cell line in this study and enhanced the phototoxicity compared to non-functionalized nanoparticles. This successful strategy led to the synthesis of polymers containing different ligands, resulting in nanoparticles with different biological activities such as bioimaging and photodynamic therapy [74].

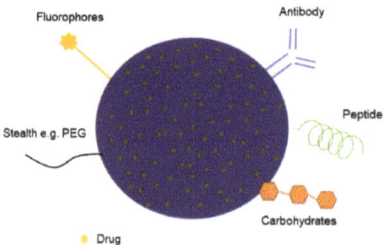

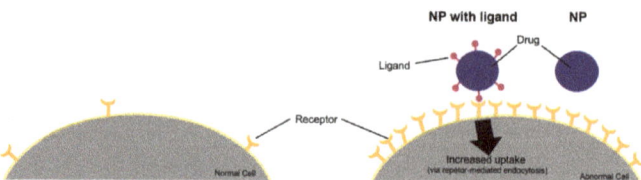

Figure 4. Representation of examples of functionalization to NPs with PEG for stealth NP, with fluorophores for imaging. Functionalization with ligands (e.g., antibody, peptide, carbohydrate and others) can show an advantage in abnormal cells with receptor's overexpression to enhance uptake by the cells mediated by a receptor endocytosis.

Polyethylene glycol (PEG) has gained attention due to its stealth behavior [72]. PEG has shown promising application due to several properties, namely, inertness in biological systems combined with the non-activation of immune components and low adsorption of biomolecules, such as proteins providing a prolonged circulation in the blood [30,76]. The importance of PEG in PDT was investigated by Yang and collaborators [77] using Ce6 as a photosensitizer, a PDT light source based on a 660 nm laser and synthetized polymers with different densities. It was demonstrated that the drug was detected in the circulation for a prolonged time and a higher amount of Ce6 was detected with high-density PEG nanoparticles. On the other hand, the PDT effectiveness was dependent on the cellular internalization, which is maximized when low-density PEG nanoparticles are applied [77]. Therefore, these achievements debate the need of a parameter's balance in the design of the nanoparticles to achieve an effective therapy.

Studies developed by Luo et al. [78] focused on the development of polymeric nanoparticles with co-encapsulation of Doxorubicin and a photosensitizer. To avoid the known toxicity of Doxorubicin, the strategy used was to link DOX to the polymer, a link that can be cleaved by ROS, and thereby the activation of the nanoparticle is ROS-dependent. They encapsulated the catalase enzyme to act on the intracellular H_2O_2 to produce more O_2 and functionalized particles with a peptide IF7 to target the tumor. This versatile and complex system (IF7-ROSPCNP) was shown to be an effective nanoparticle with accurate tumor targeting, that was able to inhibit tumor growth and prolong survival time when submitted to laser irradiation (Figure 5A–D). Mice treated with ROSPCNP and IF7-ROSPCNP, but not irradiated, were also submitted to histopathological studies, which showed that other tissues were no different from the control group, which suggests that the nanoparticles were safe (Figure 5F).

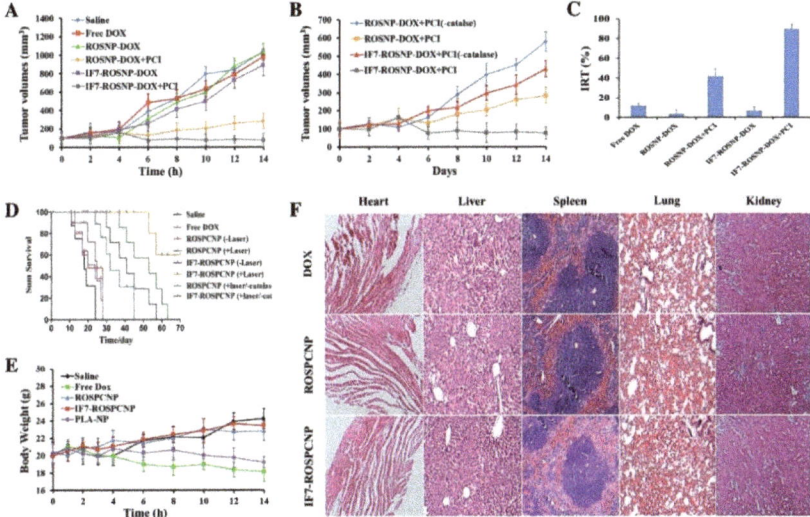

Figure 5. Evaluation of animal studies treated with several samples, such as free DOX, ROSPCNP and IF7-ROSPCNP, in the presence or absence of laser irradiation. (A,B) Evolution of tumor volume, (C) relative inhibition rate of tumor (IRT), (D) survival of the animals along the days of the experiment, (E) evolution of body weight and (F) histopathological analysis of heart, liver, spleen, lung and kidney of animals treated with different approaches (reproduced from Reference [78] with permission from Elsevier. Copyright 2019. Nanomedicine: Nanotechnology, Biology and Medicine).

Deng and collaborators [79] developed systems with tetrakis(4-carboxyphenyl)porphyrin as a photosensitizer, where the drug Doxorubicin was encapsulated forming π-π interactions with PNP to enhance the drug loading. These researchers obtained high drug loading

(17.9%) and encapsulation efficiency (89.3%) associated with π-π interactions, as proven by the fluorescence method. Furthermore, in vivo studies showed that the PNPs developed were able to inhibit the growth of breast tumor in Balb/c mice when exposed to laser irradiation. The studies discussed in this topic were a few examples among many reports of photodynamic therapy exploiting PNPs in several types of cancer, such as in cervical adenocarcinoma, glioblastoma, highly aggressive breast cancer and hepatocellular carcinoma, showing the versatility of combining PNPs and PDT for cancer treatment [72,79–81].

Cyclodextrins

Cyclodextrins (CD) are biodegradable and biocompatible structures composed by oligosaccharides of D(+)-glucose that are able to form nanosized particles by self-organization in aqueous medium [82,83]. As shown in Figure 3F, CD present a conic shape where the hydrophobic cavity provides a way for the solubilization and delivery of hydrophobic drugs [84,85]. The conjugation of the photosensitizer (phthalocyanine) and cyclodextrin was a strategy employed to increase the PS solubility. Assays performed in human bladder cancer cells demonstrated that those conjugates, with higher solubility in water, were more phototoxic to the cells [86]. A similar strategy was adopted by Semeraro and collaborators with a cyclodextrin-chlorophyll α conjugate, with a potential photo-induced toxicity in human colorectal adenocarcinoma cells reiterating the versatility of CD-PS complexation for PDT applications [87].

Protein Nanoparticles

Proteins are polymeric-type macromolecules formed by repeated amino acid monomers. Due to their biodegradability and low toxicity, proteins gained attention as drug delivery systems, as represented in Figure 3G [88,89]. Recently, Ye and Chi [90] published a review about the recent progress in drug and protein encapsulation. This includes a revision on the different encapsulation techniques, namely, emulsion evaporation, self-emulsifying drug delivery system as well as supercritical fluid, and proposed a novel method using foam that can be quite interesting in the encapsulation. Many types of proteins have been explored for the formation of protein-based nanoparticles, such as albumin.

Nanoparticle albumin-bound (NAb™) technology was developed to produce albumin nanoparticles. The success of these NPs has already generated a commercial formulation containing paclitaxel, Abraxane®, which presented advantages mainly with respect to tumor targeting and drugs' toxicity decrease [91,92]. In order to be applied to PDT, the association of protein nanoparticles with photosensitizers such as chlorin e6 was investigated by Phuong and collaborators using NAb™ technology [92]. The treatment with the nanoparticles and submission to 660 nm light radiation resulted in a significantly higher toxicity in breast cancer cells and in vivo tumor suppression of 7 times less than the control group, revealing a promising application of protein nanoparticles in PDT.

Table 1. Brief description of some organic nanostructures cited in this review as well as their materials, methods of preparation and type of cancer used to test the potential photodynamic therapy of the formulation.

Nanostructures	Materials Employed		Drug	Method of Preparation	Investigated for	Ref.
NLC	Lipid Surfactant	Compritol® ATO 888 Oleic acid Tween® 20	5-aminolevulinic acid	Microemulsion technique	Basal-cell carcinoma	[37]
SLN	Lipid Surfactant	Lecithin Stearic acid Myrj52	Curcumin	Emulsification and low-temperature solidification method	Lung cancer	[38]
SLN	Lipid Surfactant	Compritol 888 CG ATO Stearic acid Sorbitan Isostearate Polyoxyethylene-40 hydrogenated	Aluminum chloride Phthalocyanine	Direct emulsification method	Melanoma	[39]
SLN NLC	Lipid Surfactant	Stearic acid Oleic acid Sodium lauryl sulfate	Chloroaluminum Phthalocyanine	Solvent diffusion technique	Lung cancer Melanoma	[40]
Liposome	Lipid	DSPC DSPG TEL	Curcumin	Thin-film hydration and sonication	Ovarian adenocarcinoma	[45]
Liposome	Lipid Modified Lipid	DPPC Cholesterol DOPE DSPE-PEG-Pheophorbide A	Gemcitabine	Thin-film hydration	Biliary tract cancer	[53]
Liposome	Lipid	DMPC DMPG Cholesterol	Photofrin	Thin-film hydration plus sonication and extrusion	Gastric cancer	[54]
Liposome	Lipid Modified lipid	DPPC Cholesterol DSPE-PEG DOTAP (16:0)LysoPC-BPD	Benzoporphyrin derivative	Thin-film hydration with freeze-thaw cycles and extrusion	Breast cancer	[55]
Liposome	Lipid Edge activator	SPC Sodium deoxycholate	Tetra (4-Tiophenyl) sulfonated phthalocyaninatozinc(II)	Thin film hydration and sonication	Liver cancer	[56]

Table 1. Cont.

Nanostructures	Materials Employed		Drug	Method of Preparation	Investigated for	Ref.
Liposome	Lipid Surfactant	DOPC DMPC Tween® 20	Zinc phthalocyanine Ruthenium complex [Ru(NH.NHq)(tpy)NO]3+	Ethanol injection method	Skin melanoma	[57]
Micelle	Modified block copolymer	Pluronic® F127-Pheophorbide A	Doxorubicin Pheophorbide A	Thin-film hydration	Melanoma	[61]
Micelle	Modified block copolymer	FA-PEG-PLLA	Zinc(II) Phthalocyanine	Modified dialysis method	Melanoma Ovarian carcinoma	[62]
Micelle	Modified block copolymer	HA-PLGA	Protoporphyrin IX	Solvent dialysis method	Lung cancer	[63]
Nanoemulsion	Lipid Surfactant	Lipoid S100 Poloxamer 188	Curcumin	Interfacial pre-polymer deposition and spontaneous nano-emulsification	Breast cancer	[65]
PNP	Polymer	PEG-b-PLGA	Synthetized zinc phthalocyanine	-	Lung cancer	[73]
PNP	Polymer	PLGA-PEG PLGA-PEG-methoxy PLGA-PEG-maleimide	Benzoporphyrin monoacid	Nanoprecipitation	Breast cancer	[75]
PNP	Polymer	PLGA PEMA PVA	Curcumin	Nanoprecipitation	Glioblastoma	[80]
PNP	Modified polymer	PEGylated Bodipy	Doxorubicin	-	Breast cancer	[81]

DMPC: 1,2-dimyristoyl-sn-glycero-3-phosphocholine; DMPG: 1,2-dimyristoyl-sn-glycero-3-phospho-(1'-rac-glycerol); DOPC: 1,2-dioleoyl-sn-glycero-3-phosphocholine; DOPE: 1,2-dioleoyl-sn-glycero-3-phosphoethanolamine; DOTAP: 1,2-dioleoyl-1-3-trimethylammonium-propane; DPPC: 1,2-dipalmitoyl-sn-glycero-3-phosphocholine; DSPC: 1,2-distearoyl-sn-glycero-3-phosphocholine; DSPE-PEG(2000): 1,2-distearoyl-sn-glycero-3-phosphoethanolamine-N-[amino(polyethylene glycol)-2000]; DSPG: 1,2-distearoyl-sn-glycero-3-phospho-(1'-rac-glycerol); TEL: tetraether lipids; (16:0)LysoPC: 1-palmitoyl-2-hydroxy-sn-glycero-3-phosphocholine; BDP: Benzoporphyrin derivative; PEG: Poly(ethylene glycol); PLGA: Poly(lactic-co-glycolide); PEG-b-PLGA: poly (ethylene glycol) methyl ether-block-poly (lactide-co-glycolide); PLLA: Poly(L-lactide); FA: Folic acid; HA: Hyaluronic acid; BODIPY: boron dipyrromethene.

2.2.2. Carbon-Based Nanomaterials

Nanotubes, fullerenes and graphenes are among the several carbon-based nanomaterials that became widely explored for medical purposes, mainly due to the π-π interactions in their chemical structure and the ability to produce ROS, as a result of acting as a photosensitizer in PDT [93–95].

The potential of graphitic carbon nitride nanoparticles in PDT using visible light was analyzed by Heo et al. [95] using cervical cancer cells. Their study showed that the PDT allied with nanoparticles selectively killed more cancer cells than the normal cell lines. Other light sources in the NIR region are also found in the literature to carry out PDT with carbon nanoparticles derived from glucose, which resulted in an efficient ROS production [93]. The surface modification technique can also be employed to bind specifically to receptors that are overexpressed in some cancer cells types, as investigated by Xie and collaborators [96]. In their studies, hollow carbon nanospheres with Doxorubicin presented peptide and hyaluronic acid moieties in the surface to enhance the uptake and damage by dual targeting in a lung cancer cell line.

Carbon dots are carbon-based nanomaterials that can be applied for bioimaging, drug delivery and can also be used for PDT [97]. He et al. [98] designed diketopyrrole-based fluorescent carbon dots and the in vitro and in vivo studies showed that they were able to inhibit the tumor growth when irradiated.

2.2.3. Silica Nanoparticles

Silica nanoparticles (SNPs) present several advantages that can be useful for the design of nanoparticles for PDT, such as the easy production, possibility of functionalization and to obtain particles with a controlled size [99]. An efficient anti-tumor effect was achieved by Liu et al. [100] when exploring the complex combination of a photosensitizer (rose Bengal), carbon dots and the drug Doxorubicin in mesoporous silica nanoparticles. In their studies, the developed nanoparticle had high drug loading capacity and the problems related to carbon dots and PS aggregation were prevented. This system was also able to produce a higher amount of singlet oxygen compared to PS rose Bengal, and the combination with Doxorubicin provided a synergy between chemotherapy and phototherapy that resulted in a 90% decrease of cell viability.

The high surface area of silica nanoparticles is another advantage as it allows its modification and functionalization, as demonstrated by the work of Lin and collaborators [101], who developed silica nanoparticles with the PS chlorin e6 encapsulated and a gene plasmid at the surface. Through a photo-induced cleavage of coumarin and detachment of the polycation PDMAEMA, with which the cytocidal gene presented an interaction, the nanoparticles could provide the release of the gene, activation of the PS and therefore a synergistic effect of the gene and phototherapy.

Bretin et al. [102] studied the anticancer potential of the photosensitizer 5-(4-hydroxyphenyl)-10,15,20-triphenylporphyrin (TPPOH) and developed silica nanoparticles coated with the conjugate xylan-TPPOH for photodynamic therapy of cancer. In the xenograft tumor model of colorectal cancer, they studied the biodistribution using Cy5.5-labeled free TPPOH and TPPOH-X SNPs. The fluorescence signal was observed at 24 h post-injection, and as shown in Figure 6A, it was a strong signal for TPPOH-X SNPs, while it showed a minimal accumulation for free TPPOH administration. An ex vivo fluorescence imaging of tumors and organs showed that liver and kidney presented higher intensity compared to the others, but the fluorescence of tumors treated with TPPOH-X SNPs had a superior intensity compared to the other organs when compared to the free TPPOH (Figure 6B). It was also confirmed by a quantitative analysis of fluorescence (Figure 6C).

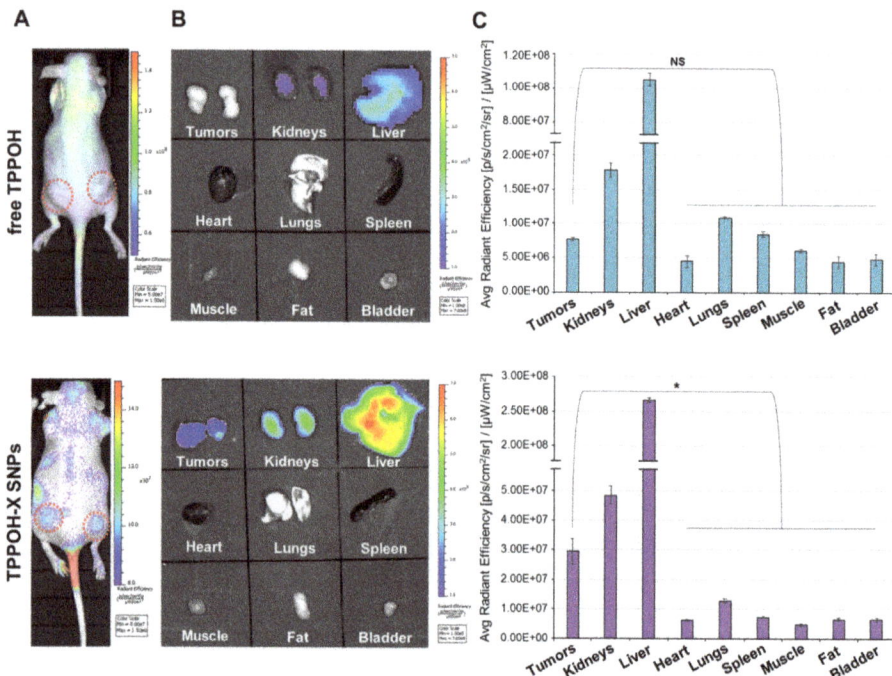

Figure 6. Evaluation of Cy5.5-labeled free TPPOH and TPPOH-X SNPs biodistribution by fluorescence imaging at 24 h post-injection. (**A**) In vivo fluorescence imaging of HT-29 tumor-bearing mice, (**B**) ex vivo fluorescence of tumors and organs, (**C**) fluorescence analysis of tumor and organs. Data are shown as mean ± SEM (n = 3). * $p < 0.05$ and NS: not significant (adapted from Reference [102] with permission from MDPI. Copyright 2019, Cancers).

2.2.4. Magnetic Nanoparticles

Due to their magnetics properties, magnetic nanoparticles can be used in therapy based on the application of an external magnetic field to a targeted tissue. Besides this, it is also possible to attach molecules to it, thus working as a carrier [103].

For example, a delivery system prepared with iron oxide magnetic nanoparticles was employed for the targeted delivery of the anticancer Doxorubicin and PDT therapy using a hematoporphyrin. The synergistic effect of PDT with the anticancer drug was shown to provide an effective inhibition of breast cancer in vivo [104]. Recently, Zhang et al. [105] used nanomotors with iron oxide nanoparticles for the delivery of zinc phthalocyanine, and due to the magnetic properties of the iron nanoparticles, the NPs can be targeted to the desired tumor tissue These nanomotors generate O_2 by catalyzing endogenous H_2O_2 for the creation of O_2 as power to create the nanomotor's displacement. The system allowed an extended distribution of the photosensitizer as well as ROS generation. Additionally, the generation of O_2 also supplied an efficient PDT process.

2.2.5. Hybrid Nanoparticles

The hybrid NPs consist in a combination of two or more types of NPs to achieve a unique multifunctional structure [106]. Hybrid NPs composed by the combination of polymers and lipids is a quite common topic found in the literature over the past few years that can also be applied to PDT, as investigated by Pramual and collaborators [107]. In their study, the polymer-lipid-PEG nanoparticles were used for the encapsulation of a PS molecule that exhibited enhanced ROS production and phototoxicity in thyroid cancer cells.

3. Photothermal Therapy

3.1. A Brief Overview

Photothermal therapy (PTT) is a therapeutic strategy using a near-infrared (NIR) laser/light to heat the tumor region and induce cancer cells' death [108] (Figure 7). Other radiation sources able to generate hyperthermia include visible light, microwaves, radiofrequency and ultrasound waves [109]. PTT has many advantages when compared with conventional therapeutic approaches, including minimal invasiveness and high specificity [110]. In general, PTT approaches explore two mechanisms: The first one involves the exposition of the tumor site to high temperatures (superior to 45 °C) for a few minutes, leading to cellular death by thermal ablation. This approach usually results in stasis in tumor vessels and hemorrhage, which prevent the combination with other treatments. The second one refers to the mild hyperthermia and involves the increasing and setting of temperatures between 42 and 43 °C, prompting cellular damage and enhancing permeability of tumor vessels, which can be used to improve nanoparticles' uptake by tumors [111,112]. Tumor tissues are more hypoxic and acidic than normal tissues [109]. It is believed that these characteristics make them more susceptible to temperature, thus allowing PTT to selectively destroy cancer cells and protect healthy ones around the tumor [113]. Therefore, since the cancer cells are responsive to this temperature range, this procedure allows the union with synergistic therapies.

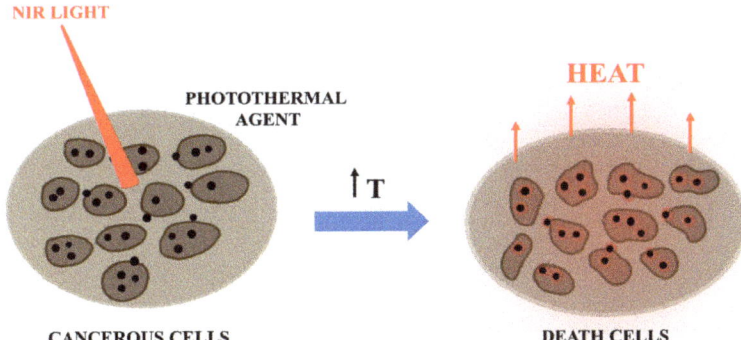

Figure 7. Mechanism of cell death induced by a photothermal agent in the presence of NIR light.

PTT displays promising therapeutic efficacy in the treatment of primary tumors or metastasis, in such a way that it has been studied in animal models with various types of cancer, including bone, lung or lymph metastasis [110]. The photothermal effect can also be enhanced using organic dyes or photothermal nano-agents, including metallic nanoparticles, nanocarbons, metal oxide nanomaterials and organic nanostructures [113,114].

A synergistic way to improve cancer treatment is its combination with current available therapies, such as chemotherapy, immunotherapy and radiotherapy [109]. The combination of hyperthermia therapy and chemotherapy is commonly explored through hydrophobic interactions, in which nanostructures loading antitumor drugs, such as Doxorubicin and paclitaxel, demonstrated anticancer effects. Moreover, imaging-guided PTT is another improvement to minimize adverse effects and to provide better patient outcomes [115,116], making it possible to plan a therapeutic strategy before and during treatment.

In the following sections, attention will be given to the recent developments in nanotechnology for photothermal applications of cancer.

3.2. Nanoparticles with Application in PTT

3.2.1. Metallic Nanoparticles

Gold Nanoparticles

Gold nanoparticles (AuNPs) have attracted great interest as photothermal agents for cancer therapy, as they demonstrate efficient local heating after light irradiation [115]. The photothermal conversion phenomenon in AuNPs is based on the collective oscillations of free electrons at AuNPs surface (Surface Plasmon Resonance, SPR) in the presence of electromagnetic radiation (Figure 8). Due to electron excitation and relaxation, this single physicochemical property supplies high localized heating around AuNPs, resulting in destruction of cancer tissues [113,116].

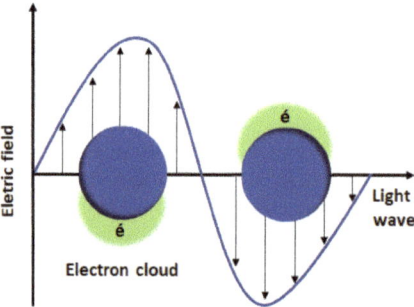

Figure 8. Surface Plasmon Resonance of gold nanoparticles.

It is known that the SPR band of noble metal nanoparticles is much stronger than other metals [117]. Changing AuNPs sizes and shapes, the range of the SPR wavelength of AuNPs is shifted from the visible to the near-infrared (NIR) region, and optical properties can be readily tuned. One of the most interesting parts of the diminished nanoparticles' diameter is due to the fact that decreasing the size (<5 nm) allows them to be excreted by urine, improving their clearance from the body [118].

Moreover, AuNPs size affects the cellular uptake and influences the photothermal conversion efficiency. According to Mie's theory, smaller nanoparticles show superior heat conversion compared to the larger ones. It was reported that 20 nm gold nanospheres exhibited 97–103% of conversion efficiency [119]. Saw et al. [120] studied the use of four sizes of cystine/citric acid-coated confeito-like gold nanoparticles (confeito-AuNPs) (30, 60, 80 and 100 nm) (Figure 9A) in the photothermal treatment of breast cancer cells. The authors observed that the smallest sizes (30 and 60 nm) of confeito-AuNPs showed higher cellular uptake into MDA-MB-231 cells, compared to larger sizes of AuNPs (Figure 9B). This same size range has been reported in the literature [121]. In vitro studies showed that smaller sizes reached the better PTT cytotoxicity activity against cancer cells (Figure 9C). This result is due to the high surface area in relation to the total mass of NPs, which is observed in smaller nanoparticles.

Sun et al. [115] employed gold nanoparticle-coated Pluronic-b-poly(L-lysine) nanoparticles (Pluronic-PLL@AuNPs) for the delivery of paclitaxel (PTX) in PTT of solid tumors. The nanoparticles showed efficient photothermal heating capabilities after exposure to an 808 nm NIR laser irradiation and a synergistic effect of chemo-photothermal treatment. The temperature of the PTX-loaded Pluronic-PLL@Au NP-injected tumors increased to 34 °C, which was adequate to eliminate tumors in vivo.

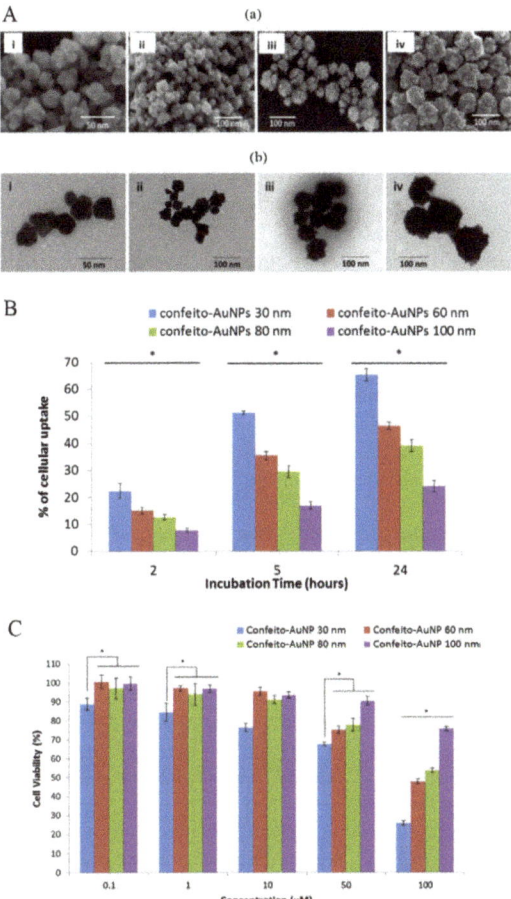

Figure 9. (**A**) Characterization of confeito-AuNPs at (i) 30 nm, (ii) 60 nm, (iii) 80 nm and (iv) 100 nm, by (a) FESEM images and (b) TEM images. (**B**) Evaluation of the cellular uptake of confeito-AuNPs into MDA-MB-231 cells. * $p < 0.05$ (ANOVA). (**C**) In vitro photothermal treatment: MDA-MB-231 cell viability after laser treatment (2 W/cm^2, 1 min of irradiation) with confeito-AuNPs. * $p < 0.05$ (ANOVA) (adapted from Reference [120] with permission from Elsevier. Copyright 2018, Colloids and Surfaces B: Bio-interfaces).

Gold nanoparticles are readily synthesized and allow easy surface modification. Binding a specific ligand on AuNPs surface promotes their targeting to the disease areas and their interactions with cells, such as cancer cells. This procedure increases the effectiveness of the treatment and decreases possible toxic effects in healthy areas of the body [122].

One of the strategies of passive targeting to the tumor site is based on the enhanced permeation and retention mechanism that takes place when gold nanoparticles are intravenously administered. However, the AuNPs presence in the blood can arouse attention of the mononuclear phagocytic system (MPS), leading to the rapid elimination of the nanoparticles from the body [123].

The functionalization with polyethylene glycol (PEG) is one of the most effective strategies to optimize the hydrophilic surface and to improve the blood circulation time of nanoparticles [124]. Wang et al. [125] developed PEGylated hollow gold nanoparticles (mPEG@HGNPs) for combined X-ray radiotherapy and photothermal therapy in cancer cells. The in vitro results using the combination of the 808 nm NIR laser and X-ray radiation demonstrated a synergistic antitumor effect with cell viability decreased to 61% and 65% for HGNPs and mPEG@HGNPs, respectively. The nanoparticle cytotoxicity was decreased after PEGylation, due to less mPEG@HGNPs internalized into the cells. Despite that, the targeting enhanced to the tumor site by the mPEG@HGNPs was confirmed using CT imaging in xenografted breast tumor models, due to the EPR effect.

Cheng et al. [126] reported photolabile AuNPs covalently cross-linkable with a diazirine (DA) terminal group of PEG ligand on the AuNPs surface. The 20.5 nm diazirine-decorated AuNPs (dAuNPs) were obtained after laser excitation at 405 nm. The photothermal therapy in tumor-bearing BALB/c mice was investigated by monitoring the average tumor size in different mice groups. The mice groups that were treated with dAuNPs + λ405 nm and dAuNPs + NIR showed weak tumor inhibition, while the group treated with dAuNPs exhibited a high tumor volume decrease upon 808 nm irradiation (0.75 W cm^{-2}). The tumor region reached 26.7 °C after 10 min of light exposure. The PTT efficacy was further confirmed through tissue analysis, which showed extensive necrosis in dAuNPs + λ405 nm + NIR group.

The extracellular environment of solid tumors has an acidic pH. pH-sensitive AuNPs with potential application in PTT have been reported in the literature [127]. Natural peptides can be used as tumor-targeting agents. Barram et al. [122] used glutathione (GSH), soluble in water, as a coating for AuNPs. GSH is a pH-sensitive polymer, with its isoelectric point (IEP) close to the pH of the cancer cells (~6). Consequently, GSH-AuNPs become responsive to the tumor's acidic environment, improving its targeting to the desired location. In vitro photothermal therapy was applied to rhabdomyosarcoma (RD) cancer cells, using two types of low-power laser (visible green light (532 nm) and infrared light (NIR) (800 nm)). The study observed cell death values of tumor cells for both types of lasers, and these values were proportional to the longer periods of radiation exposure and, even more so, to the highest concentrations of GSH-AuNPs.

From the molecular point of view, several studies on the effect of nanoparticles on DNA molecules and DNA bases have been performed. These studies clearly demonstrate the damage effect of the gold nanoparticles. Recently, Marques et al. [128] analyzed the decomposition of halogenated nucleobases by Surface Plasmon Resonance excitation of gold nanoparticles. In fact, the halogenated uracil derivatives can be of great interest for cancer therapy [129,130] and the authors demonstrated that the presence of irradiated gold nanoparticles decomposes the ring structure of uracil and its halogenated derivatives with similar efficiency. This decomposition is associated with the fragmentation of the pyrimidine ring, for 5-bromouracil, with cleavage of the carbon-halogen bond, whereas for 5-uorouracil, this reaction channel was inhibited. Locally released halogen atoms can react with molecular groups within DNA, and hence this result indicates a specific mechanism by which doping with 5-bromouracil can enhance DNA damage in the proximity of laser-irradiated gold nanoparticles.

Gold Nanorods

Gold nanorods (AuNRs) are one of the many tools employed in cancer photothermal therapy, due to their high capability to transform near-infrared light into heat. The investigation of their aspect ratio allows to adjust a particular SPR band in the NIR [131], consequently reducing damage in normal tissues as these ones have minimal NIR energy absorption. Despite their ability as PTT agents, AuNRs are considered to be toxic to cells, because of the stabilizers, e.g., hexadecyl-trimethylammonium bromide (CTAB), used in their synthesis [132]. Several approaches have been used to minimize the toxicity of AuNRs, such as the binding of polymers to increase their biocompatibility. Kirui et al. [133] improved biocompatibility of AuNRs using poly(acrylic acid) (PAA) for coating of nanoparticles. Liu et al. [134] reduced the toxicity of PEG-AuNRs using multidentate PEG (AuNT-PTP Gm950).

PTT induced by NIR is known to improve chemotherapeutic efficacy by triggering drug release or increasing the cancer cells' sensitivity to chemotherapeutics [135]. Hauck et al. [136] revealed that the heat produced by gold nanorods together with the chemotherapeutic drug cisplatin killed 78% more cancer cells than cisplatin alone. Combination therapy can reduce toxicity associated with chemotherapeutics through reducing the effective drug dosage. Duan et al. [137] developed gold nanorods coated with chitosan (CS) derivatives as a carrier of Doxorubicin (DOX) to combine chemical and photothermal effects. In vitro studies demonstrated that these nanoparticles showed low cytotoxicity and potential against cancer cells. Wang et al. [138] developed gold nanorods coated with polydopamine (PDA) and loaded with thiolated poly(ethylene glycol) tumor-homing peptides (NGR and TAT), as a carrier of Doxorubicin. NGR/TAT-DOX-PDA@GNRs allowed a pH-triggered controlled release of DOX and a synergistic effect with the combination of chemo-photothermal therapy.

Moreover, the efficacy of a targeted synergistic photothermal chemotherapy of breast cancer using gold nanorods (GNRs) functionalized with hyaluronic acid (HA) and folate (FA) to deliver DOX was demonstrated by Xu et al. [139]. The therapeutic system showed a long blood circulation time and high tumor site accumulation. In vitro photothermal chemotherapy was evaluated. Cell viability of MCF-7 cells treated with GNRs-HA-FA-DOX + NIR was reduced to 31%. The authors also investigated the synergistic effect of PTT chemotherapy in vivo and GNRs-HA-FA-DOX exhibited an excellent antitumor effect against MCF-7 breast tumors in nude mice. After 5 min of light exposure, the temperature of MCF-7 breast tumors in nude mice treated with GNRs-HA-FA-DOX reached 67.5 °C (1.5 W/cm^2), leading to irreversible tumor cell death.

In metastasis, cancer cells migrate and invade the surrounding tissues, and therefore collective cell migration is directly related to cancer aggressiveness. This process involves interactions between neighboring cells through the cell junctions and contraction motions of the cytoskeleton filaments [140]. Studying the migration and invasion of cancer cells, Wu et al. [141] developed AuNRs functionalized with PEG and Arg-Gly-Asp (RGD) peptides. These authors found morphological changes of many cytoskeletal and cell junction proteins after PTT treatment, suggesting that interactions between integrin-targeted AuNRs and cells could trigger inhibition of cancer collective migration.

It should also be reported that an effective combined therapy of paclitaxel-loaded gold nanorods against head, neck and lung cancer cells was developed by Ren et al. [142]. Paclitaxel was loaded into a hydrophobic pocket of the polymeric monolayer on the surface of NIR-absorbing AuNRs, which allowed the efficiently direct cellular release of the hydrophobic drug via a cell membrane mimicking two-phase solution. It was demonstrated that the PTT approach with this developed nanocomplex led to total eradication of tumor cells at a dosage of 0.5 nm of nanomaterials with low-intensity (0.55 W/cm^2) NIR light.

Stimuli-responsive materials have attracted attention due to their capability to control the timed release of the entrapped drugs. Near-infrared light (NIR)-responsive polymers have been used for triggered drug delivery in specific tissues [143]. Hribar et al. [144] reported a NIR light-sensitive polymer−nanorod composite for controlled drug release, in the range of body temperature. As the glass transition temperature is near to the physiological temperature, it can be used to control and improve the release of a molecule. The researchers applied this heating system to trigger release of the Doxorubicin from the nano-system. After NIR light exposure, Doxorubicin-encapsulated microspheres were able to decrease 90% of the activity of T6-17 cells.

Gold Hybrid Nanoparticles

Although the research on hybrid nanoparticles to improve the diagnosis and cancer treatment has attracted attention due to its potential use in medicine, its safe application in therapy still remains limited [145,146]. In recent years, it has been reported that the development of iron-gold nanocomplexes are used for the combined PTT with magnetic resonance imaging (MRI). The Au shell composes the light-responsiveness portion, while the iron core can be used to improve the ratio of water molecules' transverse relaxation, leading to strong MRI signals. Additionally, the magnetic center allows the nanocomplex to be directed to the tumor site by means of a magnetic field [147,148].

Dong et al. [149] developed gold-nano-shelled magnetic hybrid nanoparticles functionalized with anti-human epidermal growth factor receptor 2 (Her2) antibodies (Her2-GPH NPs) for multi-modal imaging and cancer treatment. The nanoparticles were produced by loading gold nano-shells with poly (lactic-co-glycolic acid) (PLGA) attached to perfluorooctyl bromide (PFOB) and superparamagnetic iron oxide nanoparticles, and then binding the antibody. Her2-GPH NPs showed high ability as a contrast agent for both ultrasound (US) and magnetic resonance (MR) imaging. The in vitro cytotoxicity studies demonstrated that Her2-GPH NPs specifically promoted Her2-positive human breast cancer SKBR3 cells' death after NIR exposure. Abed et al. [148] directed Iron (III) oxide–gold (Fe_2O_3@Au) core-shell nanoparticles to the tumor site through a magnetic field in Balb/c mice bearing a CT26 colorectal tumor model after intravenous administration of the nanoplatform. The in vivo antitumor studies showed the complete tumor growth eradication after magnetic targeting and subsequent NIR eradication.

The toxicity of Au and magnetic nanocomplexes is still concerning. These nanoparticles can lead, among others, to DNA damage, production of free radicals and modification in cell signaling. Additionally, the toxicity can be caused by nanoparticles' aggregation in biological fluids. Using biocompatible and water-soluble polymers as a coating makes it possible to improve the colloidal stability and decrease nanoparticles' aggregation, thus diminishing the cytotoxicity. Abedin et al. [150] improved the colloidal stability of Au–Fe_3O_4 NPs in aqueous media using poly-l-lysine (PLL) polymer as a surface coating. Additionally, PLL-Au-Fe_3O_4 NPs demonstrated cytocompatibility and NIR light absorption ability.

Mesoporous silica nanoparticles (MSNPs) are highly versatile drug carriers due to their biocompatibility and high surface area, consequences of their well-defined internal mesopore structure, varying from 2 to 10 nm in diameter and with large pore volume. Depending on surface charge and nanoparticle size, the characteristics such as nanoparticle cytotoxicity and cellular uptake can change [151]. Yang et al. [152] designed a system composed of ultra-small gold nanoparticles attached to mesoporous silica nanoparticles (MSN) through Au-S bonds. The in vitro studies showed the fast release of DOX upon NIR light irradiation and synergistic cytotoxic effect against A549 cells.

Gold nanoparticles lose their ability to convert light into heat under repetitive NIR laser irradiation, including gold nanorods that can change their shape and extinction after NIR exposure. Cheng et al. [153] projected gold/mesoporous silica hybrid nanoparticles (GoMe) for lung cancer detection and treatment. This hybrid system has a good photothermal ability and stability, and maintains its capacity of photothermal conversion after repetitive NIR exposures. In addition, ^{64}Cu-labeled GoMe was used to detect lung tumors in vivo through PET imaging, demonstrating to be a potential theranostic system for cancer therapy.

Silver Nanoparticles

Silver nanoparticles (AgNPs) are multifunctional materials which have been used for many applications, such as biosensors, electronic compounds, antimicrobials and medicines [154]. Their general use is due to singular characteristics such as size and shape being controllable, easily modified surface and optical and electrical properties [155]. Additionally, their antibacterial activities are widely known [156].

AgNPs can be produced through various physical and chemical methods [157]. Spherical AgNPs are frequently synthesized using the Turkevich method [158] with citrate as a reducing and stabilizing agent or with $NaBH_4$ as a reducing agent [159]. In recent years, many researchers are using biological methods to produce AgNPs. These techniques utilize plants, fungi, algae and other organic sources to synthesize nanoparticles with great stability [160].

Application of AgNPs in the biomedical field is still limited due to the concern of their intrinsic toxicity. Interactions of AgNPs with the human body are not yet well-understood [161]. Modifying its surface with biodegradable molecules and polymers or incorporating these nanoparticles into hybrid systems are some of the ways that many researchers have found to increase the biocompatibility of AgNPs. Kim and coworkers [162] developed bovine serum albumin (BSA)-coated silver NPs (BSA-silver NPs) by a single-step reduction process.

Similar to gold nanoparticles, SPR of silver nanoparticles can be tuned to the infrared region by altering their size and shape [163]. Boca et al. [164] designed chitosan-coated silver nanotriangles (Chit-AgNTs) for hyperthermia of human non-small lung cancer cells (NCI-H460) using a 800 nm laser. Wu et al. [165] engineered a nanoplatform for fluorescent probe and label-free imaging of cell surface glycans composed of DNA/silver nanoclusters (DNA/AgNCs) via hybridization chain reaction (HCR). The nanoparticles showed a great ability to convert light to heat, reaching 53.6 °C after irradiation with the 808 nm laser at 1 W cm^{-2} for 10 min. The confocal results demonstrated the applicability of the DNA/AgNCs for labeling glycans on the surface of tumor cells. Moreover, in vivo experiments showed that DNA/AgNCs were able to ablate and inhibit tumor growth under the laser exposure.

PEGylated bovine serum albumin (BSA)-coated silver core/shell nanoparticles loaded with ICG ("PEG-BSA-AgNP/ICG") were synthesized by Park et al. [166]. These nanoparticles were tested for anticancer activity in B16F10 cells after light exposure. The cytotoxicity results revealed a cell viability of 6% when temperature reached at 50 °C. PEG-BSA-AgNP/ICG also displayed a long plasma half-life, which led to the higher accumulation in the tumor. At 4 h post-administration of PEG-BSA-AgNP/ICG in a B16F10 nude mice model, the tumor temperature reached 49.6 °C with a laser power of 0.95 W. Furthermore, among the treatment groups, the "PEG-BSA-AgNP/ICG + PTT group" was the only one that exhibited significant inhibition in tumor growth.

3.2.2. Carbon-Based Nanomaterials

Carbon Nanotubes

Carbon nanotubes (CNTs) are cylindrical structures constructed from a sheet of graphene [167]. These NPs are allotropic forms of carbon, with diameter in the nanometric dimension and various millimeters in length [168]. CTNs are classified into two types, according to the number of layers in their structure: single-walled carbon nanotubes (SWCNTs), which consist of a single graphene sheet, and multiwalled carbon nanotubes (MWCNTs), consisting of several sheets forming concentric cylinders [169].

CNTs have a wide range of properties that make them unique nanomaterials, such as excellent electrical, thermal and optical conduction, mechanical strength [170] and high surface areas, which can be easily functionalized [171]. Indeed, CNTs are usually modified with molecules that help to enhance their biocompatibility or enable specific functions [172]. Attachments to PEG is one of the major types of CNTs' functionalization to improve biocompatibility, water solubility and stability [173]. Sobhani et al. [174] successfully attached PEG onto the CNTs's surface.

CNTs have a wide NIR absorption which is dependent on the size and shape of these nanomaterials [175]. Exposing CNTs to NIR light releases vibrational energy in the form of heat, and could be used for cancer cell ablation [176]. The application of CNTs in PTT for the treatment of various kinds of human cancer xenografts in animal models has been investigated in the literature and has been demonstrated to be effective [177].

Li and collaborators [178] designed an interesting system for curcumin (Cur) delivery composed of functionalized single-walled carbon nanotubes by phosphatidylcholine and polyvinylpyrrolidone (SWCNT-Cur). Results of the cellular uptake study showed that SWCNT-Cur effectively improved the delivery of Cur into cells within 4 h. Compared with native Cur, the formulation developed obtained an uptake amount 6-fold higher. Additionally, biodistribution studies demonstrated that SWCNT-Cur could enhance curcumin blood concentration up to 18-fold. Lastly, this system was evaluated for its ability of photothermal ablation in an in vivo model. Among all the groups tested (saline + laser, Cur + laser, SWCNT + laser, SWCNT-Cur + laser), the SWCNT-Cur and laser (808 nm) groups showed the most significant suppression on tumor weight and volume, indicating the synergistic anticancer effect of Cur and PTT.

Waghray et al. [179] synthesized MWCNTs coated with phospholipid-poly(ethylene glycol) and conjugated with an anti-P-glycoprotein (Pgp) antibody, to enhance Pgp-specific cellular uptake. Pgp is an ATP-binding transporter, expressed on tumor cell membranes, and it is related to cancer drug resistance. The phototoxicity of Pab-MWCNTs was investigated in 3T3 and 3T3-MDR1 cells and in a tumor spheroid model (NCI/ADR-RES cells). The nanostructures demonstrated not only Pgp-specific endocytosis by 3T3-MDR1, but they also exhibited dose-dependent phototoxicity only in 3T3-MDR1 cells. Moreover, NCI/ADR-RES spheroids treated with Pab-MWCNTs showed the highest cell death after NIR laser irradiation when compared with control groups.

Zhang and colleagues [180] engineered MWNTs/gemcitabine/lentinan (MWNTs-Ge-Le) to overcome Gemcitabine's clinical application problems related to short plasma half-life and low cellular uptake. It was observed that the MWNTs-Ge-Le conjugated with rhodamine were internalized by MCF-7 cells about 3 h after incubation. Additionally, encouraged by the results in vitro, the authors evaluated the synergistic antitumor effect of MWNTs-Ge-Le on tumor-bearing mice. MWNTs-Ge-Le nanoparticles have reached the tumor site through the EPR effect. After 3 min of NIR irradiation, the temperature of the tumor surface increased to approximately 42.6 °C, while the PBS group only reached about 36.6 °C. Moreover, it was observed that the size of the tumor significantly decreased, confirming the high synergetic effect of chemotherapy and PTT.

Zhao et al. [181] developed SWCNTs and MWCNTs coated with peptide lipid (PL) and sucrose laurate (SL) (denoted as SCNT-PS and MCNT-PS, respectively), which were conjugated with siRNA (anti-survivin siRNA) for synergistic PTT and gene therapy (GT). The engineered CNTs exhibited excellent temperature-sensitivity and biocompatibility. The effective cellular internalization was confirmed after they observed nanoparticles' presence in the cytosol of HeLa cells. The in vitro cytotoxicity after 808 nm laser irradiation was evaluated treating cells with 30 µg/mL of SCNT-PS or MCNT-PS. The results showed that 76.2% ± 4.4% and 75.3% ± 3.5% of the cells were led to death by combined therapy in the SCNT-PS and MCNT-PS, respectively. The PT efficacy of CNTs was also evaluated in vivo. After tumor irradiation (1 W/cm^2 for 5 min), the local temperature reached 42–45 °C. Furthermore, they investigated whether the SCNT-PS/siRNA and MCNT-PS/siRNA complexes could be able to downregulate survivin. The data obtained were promising, indicating that cells that received treatment with SCNT-PS + P + G and MCNT-PS + P + G, followed by PTT, had about a 60% decrease of survivin expression in comparison with GT alone (SCNT-PS + G and MCNT-PS + G).

Besides PTT generating anticancer immune responses, evidence suggests that it could also induce an effect called the abscopal effect [182]. This effect refers to the immune response generated when the primary tumor site is irradiated, which can lead to the regression of metastatic cancer in distant sites that were not irradiated [183]. Nevertheless, some tumors are capable of creating inhibitory binders, which connect to inhibitory co-receptors (immune checkpoints) expressed on tumor immune cells [184]. This activity induces negative regulatory pathways leading to loss of immunological control, allowing tumor growth progression and decreasing immune response to various therapies [185]. New immunotherapeutic approaches are focusing on blocking immune checkpoints in order to recover the suppressed immune response [186]. Among the immune checkpoints, the cytotoxic T-lymphocyte antigen 4 (CTLA-4) is an inhibitory receptor expressed by regulatory and conventional T cells, which suppresses T cell activation via cell intrinsic and extrinsic pathways. Ipilimumab, an antibody against the inhibitory co-receptor CTLA-4, is one of the main targets of immunotherapy [187,188].

CNT-mediated photothermal therapy in combination with checkpoint inhibitors can be used to maximize the abscopal effects of PTT. Li et al. [189] designed SWNT functionalized with glycated chitosan (GC), an immunoadjuvant, for specific treatment of an aggressive 4T1 murine breast cancer model, upon 1064 nm laser irradiation. Putting together

SWNT-GC-laser therapy with anti-CTLA-4, they have achieved synergistic immunomodulatory effects, inducing antitumor immune response and an increase of the survival time of the treated mice group (up to 58 days).

Recently, McKernan and his group [190] presented a delivery nano-system to treat metastatic breast cancer composed of SWCNTs that integrates PT therapy and checkpoint inhibitor immuno-stimulation with anti-CTLA-4. The SWCNTs were functionalized with the protein annexin A5 (ANXA5), which has great affinity to the anionic phospholipid phosphatidylserine expressed on endothelial cells of the tumor vasculature and on tumor cell membranes. The authors noted that PTT with SWCNT-ANXA5 alone was able to destroy primary EMT6 tumors, reaching a temperature of 54 °C at the site, but failed to eliminate the metastasis. On the other hand, the combination of photothermal therapy with SWCNT-ANXA5 and anti-CTLA-4 improved overall survival, leading to 55% of the treated mice surviving at 100 days post-injection. Moreover, in animals who received this combined therapy, increases in the numbers of helper T cells CD4+ and cytotoxic T cells CD8+ were observed, indicating an increase in the immune response.

Hollow Carbon Nanospheres

Hollow carbon nanospheres (HCNs) are mesoporous nanomaterials with high pore volume and surface area [191]. Due the carbon chains, a great amount of a hydrophobic drug can be loaded into their structure, making them a potent drug carrier [192]. Similar to carbon nanotubes, HCNs have a great ability to convert NIR light into heat, which can be used to modulate the drug release at the tumor site [193].

Wang et al. [194] produced biocompatible HCNs for loading and release of paclitaxel (PTX) and PT therapy. The nanoparticles have demonstrated excellent photostability and ability to effectively release the loaded PTX. Additionally, in vitro experiments showed great thermal ablation of HCT116 cells using 50 µg/mL of HCNs and a 3 W/cm^2 laser power density for 180 s.

Xu and his group [195] produced a hollow carbon nanosphere capped with olyethylene glycol-graft-polyethylenimine (HPP) as a photothermal agent. Optical properties were investigated using a 1064 nm laser and power density of 0.6 W/cm^2. After 7 min of laser exposure of the nanoparticle's dispersion, an increased temperature in the range of 17 to 44 °C was observed, indicating an excellent heat conversion efficiency. The photothermal therapeutic effect in vitro (4T1 cells) and in vivo (Balb/c mice inoculated subcutaneously with 4T1 cells) was also evaluated. The percentage of cell death for in vitro experiment varied from 40% up to 95%, using the HPP concentrations of 10, 20, 40, 80 and 160 µg/mL. 4T1 tumor-bearing mice treated with only 40 µg/mL were irradiated. After 14 days, tumors were measured, showing a significant decrease of volume.

3.2.3. Metal Oxide Nanoparticles

Iron Oxide Nanoparticles

Magnetic nanoparticles are mostly formed using magnetite (Fe_3O_4), maghemite (γ-Fe_2O_3) or a combination of both [196]. Due to their intrinsic magnetic properties (superparamagnetism), these nano-systems have emerged as potent contrast agents (CAs) for magnetic resonance imaging (MRI) and biomedical purposes [197].

In the field of cancer therapy, magnetic nanoparticles can be specific delivery drugs by application of alternating magnetic fields to targeting tumor sites and eliminating them using localized moderate heating [198].

Cabana and coworkers [199] compared the application of photothermal (PT) therapy using magnetic multicore nanoflowers versus magnetic hyperthermia (MHT) of magnetic nanospheres. The NPs' performance in MHT and PT was carried out in water and in cancer cells. They found that nanoflowers are heaters that are more effective for both modalities. In the cellular environment, PT showed excellent results at low doses, while MHT was lost for all NPs. Additionally, magnetite nanoflowers demonstrated the highest cellular uptake and the best antitumor activity after the laser exposure (0.3 W/cm^2).

Liu and collaborators [200] synthesized the polyethylene glycol-coated ultrasmall superparamagnetic iron oxide nanoparticle-coupled sialyl Lewis X (USPIO-PEG-sLex) with excellent photothermal conversion properties. The nanoparticles were applied for MRI and PTT in human nasopharyngeal carcinoma (NPC) xenografts on a mouse model. After 808 nm laser exposure, the cytotoxicity results showed a reduction of viability of NPC 5-8F cells at reasonable concentrations of USPIO-PEG-sLex nanoparticles. Moreover, the NPs were able to inhibit xenografts' tumor progression after in vivo post-injection.

Iron oxide NPs exhibit excellent photothermal conversion efficiency, good chemical stability and low toxicity in the biological environment [201]. The in vivo application of iron oxide NPs has been approved by the US Food and Drug Administration (FDA) [202]. However, their use in many clinical approaches is limited due to the low tumor delivery efficiency of the NPs [203].

Aiming to enhance the tumor delivery of iron oxide NPs, Wang and his group [203] developed an Ac-Arg-Val-ArgArg-Cys(StBu)-Lys-CBT probe coupled with monodispersed carboxyl-decorated SPIO NPs to form SPIO@1NPs. When SPIO@1NPs entered tumor cells overexpressing furin, a reaction chain developed, resulting in SPIO NPs' aggregates by cross-linking. The self-aggregation of NPs improved their retention in the tumor site, leading to better T2 imaging results and PTT of cancer cells more effective at low doses.

Surface modification of synthetic nanomaterials with biomimetic cell membranes is a smart strategy to make it harmless and invisible to the immune system [204]. Meng et al. [205] employed vesicles formed from macrophage membranes reconstructed to obtain a biomimetic system for cancer phototherapy. These vesicles coated onto magnetic iron oxide nanoparticles (Fe_3O_4 NPs) resulting in Fe_3O_4@MM NPs exhibited good biocompatibility and light-to-heat conversion efficiency. Cancer targeting of Fe_3O_4@MM NPs was confirmed by cellular uptake in MCF-7 cells. The authors also found that the NPs were able to evade from immune cells, and this activity could be related to the presence of cell membrane components on the nanoparticles' surface. The Fe_3O_4@MM NPs were targeted to the tumor site with application of an external magnetic field, in a breast cancer mouse model. The tumor volume was measured after the laser irradiation, reaching a high tumor regression over time.

Researchers have been employing phytochemical compounds together with magnetic nanoparticles in order to achieve nanomaterials for phototherapy and drug delivery systems [206]. Kharey et al. [207] obtained 15 nm eugenate (4-allyl-2-methoxyphenolate)-capped iron oxide nanoparticles (E-capped IONPs) through green synthesis using a medicinal plant, Pimenta dioica. These NPs showed good biocompatibility in Human cervical cancer (HeLa) and Human embryonic kidney 293 (HEK 293) cell lines, and excellent efficacy of hyperthermia generation upon laser irradiation at NIR wavelength.

A delivery nano-system composed of R837-loaded polyphenols coating ICG-loaded magnetic nanoparticles (MIRDs) was constructed for spatio-temporal PTT/immunotherapy synergism in cancer. This system inhibited tumor growth, metastasis and recurrence, which resulted in potent anticancer therapeutic effects with few side effects [208].

Silica-coated Fe_3O_4 magnetic nanoparticles loaded with curcumin (NC) were synthesized by Ashkbar and colleagues [209] for hyperthermia and singlet oxygen production improvement for in vitro and in vivo experiments. Curcumin (CUR) belongs to the polyphenol class of natural compounds, known for its photosensitizing properties and antitumor activities [210]. The PDT was assessed using diode lasers at 450 nm and PTT was achieved by an 808 nm laser. After injection in a breast tumor mouse model, the results showed that CUR + PDT achieved a tumor volume reduction of about 58%, in comparison with the untreated group, while the NC + PDT + PTT group exhibited more than an 80% reduction compared with other treatment groups. The authors found that the NC + PDT + PTT treatment strategy could interrupt the tumor growth until day ten. This result was related to the synergistic effect achieved by hyperthermia plus ROS generation in the tumor site [209].

Manganese Oxide Nanoparticles

In recent years, manganese oxide nanoparticles (MONs) have emerged as contrast and photothermal agents due to their low toxicity and good T1-weighted contrast signals, constituting a promising alternative to the traditional PTT agents [211].

Xiang and colleagues [212] developed biocompatible and pH-sensitive MnO-loaded carbonaceous nanospheres (MnO@CNSs) for simultaneous PTT and MRI. The mimetic pH-responsive release of Mn^{2+} in the biological environments (pH 7.4, 6.5 and 5.0) was measured. They observed that MnO@CNSs were stable in neutral solution (pH 7.4), while in acidic pH, the nanoparticles quickly released Mn^{2+} ions (pH 6.5 and 5). These data were confirmed in in vivo experiments, which demonstrated that MRT1 signal values were higher in the acid region of the tumors. The MnO@CNSs PTT effect was investigated under irradiation by an 808 nm laser (2 W/cm^2) for 10 min. The results showed an elevated efficiency of the MnO@CNSs for in vivo tumor ablation, making this system a potent nanotheranostic tool.

Molybdenum Oxide Nanoparticles

Molybdenum oxide nanostructures are reported to display good biocompatibility and biodegradability, making them a safe platform for cancer therapy. MoO3 nanoparticles have excellent absorption in the NIR region, and can also generate singlet oxygen under NIR light exposure, which enables their use for both photodynamic and photothermal therapy [213].

Chen et al. [214] synthesized molybdenum oxide (MoOx) nanosheets using the single-pot hydrothermal method and functionalized them with pluronic F127 (MoOX @ F127) to obtain a biocompatible nano-system with pH-dependent degradable properties for chemotherapy and photothermal therapy. It was observed that MoOx @ F127 showed reasonable stability at pH 5.4 and rapid degradation at pH 7.4, indicating that intact nanoparticles could reach the tumor site through the EPR effect. The ability of MoOx @ F127/DOX to kill tumor cells was investigated in MCF-7 cells after 5 min of 808 nm laser irradiation. Cytotoxicity assessment showed that almost 60% of cells died after treatment. Furthermore, in vivo experiments showed that mice injected with MoOx @ F127/DOX had a tumor temperature greater than 50 °C, suggesting high hyperthermic efficiency of the nanoparticles.

Zinc Oxide Nanoparticles

The element zinc has diverse medical applications [215]. Zinc oxide (ZnO) shows high chemical stability, low toxicity, optical, electrical and anticancer properties, becoming a potential alternative for PTT [216]. Production of intracellular reactive oxygen species (ROS) is one of the cytotoxic mechanisms of ZnO NPs [217]. Kim et al. [218] applied hybrid nanoparticles composed of ZnO and berberine (BER) for the chemo-photothermal therapy of lung cancer. The in vitro results revealed an effective antiproliferation activity against A549 (human lung adenocarcinoma) cells without severe toxicity signals observed in rats' blood tests.

Liu et al. [219] designed a core-shell nanoplatform based on a zinc oxide (ZnO) core and a polydopamine (PDA) shell to combine chemotherapy with Doxorubicin (DOX), gene DNAzyme (DZ) and photothermal therapy. The nanoparticles showed good photothermal conversion and stability after application of the 808 nm laser for 500 s. Additionally, confocal microscopy demonstrated that ZnO@PDA-DOX/DZ could be internalized by cells and consequently could deliver DZ to stimulate gene-silencing activity. Moreover, tumor-bearing mice treated with ZnO@PDA-DOX/DZ exhibited an effective NP accumulation in the tumor site. The tumor tissue achieved a temperature of up to 47.3 °C, leading to death of the cancer cells and inhibition of the tumor growth. Lastly, the authors measured the levels of survivin in the tumor tissue by Western blotting. The results found low levels of survivin, suggesting the triggering of DZ for in vivo gene silencing.

3.2.4. Transition Metal Dichalcogenide Nanomaterials

Molybdenum disulfide (MoS_2) nanoparticles display several characteristics that make them excellent photothermal agents for cancer therapy, such as biocompatibility, wide surface plasmon resonance, good light-to-heat conversion efficiency and low cost [220]. In 2014, Liu and collaborators [221] pioneered using PEG-functionalized MoS_2 nanosheets as drug carriers for therapy of cancer. Two-dimensional MoS_2-PEG nanosheets have achieved excellent synergistic anti-tumor effects in in vivo studies, after intravenous administration of MoS_2-PEG/DOX.

Xie and coworkers [222] synthesized egg yolk phospholipid-modified molybdenum disulfide (MoS_2) as a PTT agent and drug delivery system for MCF-7 cells' treatment. The lipid layers on the surface of layered MoS_2 nanosheets were modified to improve the NPs' stability and the accumulation of the nanocarrier in mice tumors. Additionally, Doxorubicin (DOX) was conjugated with MoS_2-lipid nanocomposites for synergistic chemotherapy. Ding et al. [223] produced well-dispersed L-cysteine-modified MoS_2 (MoS_2-Cys) nanospheres measuring 422 nm in size. MoS_2-Cys exhibits biocompatible and good photothermal conversion efficiency (35%) upon 808 nm laser irradiation. The in vitro PTT activity of MoS_2-Cys nanospheres in S180 mouse ascites tumor cells displayed high cytotoxicity, with the IC_{50} value of 2.985 µg/mL. In vivo experiment data demonstrated a remarkable decrease of the tumor volume of the mice treated with MoS_2-Cys nanospheres coupled with NIR irradiation.

Qian et al. [224] developed titanium disulfide (TiS_2) nanosheets functionalized with polyethylene glycol (PEG), obtaining a great PTT agent for in vivo tumor ablation. Balb/c mice bearing 4T1 tumors were treated with TiS_2-PEG, and after 24 h, exposed to an 808 nm laser at 0.8 W cm^{-2} for 5 min. The researchers found that tumors in the mice were completely ablated. Moreover, TiS_2-PEG nanosheets were tested as a contrast agent in photoacoustic imaging. Strong photoacoustic signals were observed around the mice tumor after injection of TiS_2-PEG, indicating the efficient accumulation of these nanoparticles at the targeted site.

Cao et al. [225] produced TiS_2 nanosheets using a human serum albumin (HSA)-assisted exfoliation method, and later, modification with PEGylated folic acid (FA). TiS_2-HSA-FA showed photothermal conversion efficiency of about 58.9% after NIR laser irradiation. In vitro and in vivo experiments demonstrated TiS_2-HSA-FA to have a high biocompatibility and specificity for targeting tumors. In vivo synergistic PTT/radiotherapy (RT) evaluation was assessed in a CT26 tumor xenograft model, under 5 min laser irradiation (808 nm, 0.8 W/cm^2). Researchers found that the highest tumor growth inhibition effect was achieved by TiS_2-HSA-FA + NIR+RT, suggesting the combined therapy effect.

3.2.5. Other Nanoparticles

Over the years, many kinds of inorganic and organic materials have been employed to build an effective PTT system. Graphene quantum dots (GQDs) have excellent photothermal conversion efficiency, incomparable morphology and ease of functionalization [226]. Fang et al. [227] fabricated graphene quantum dots (GQDs) as a pH-sensitive delivery system for chemotherapeutic drugs inside cancer cells. After their cellular uptake, the nanocarriers released Doxorubicin (DOX) upon laser irradiation and upon acidification of the intracellular environment. Studies in vitro and in vivo demonstrated the targeting of HA-functionalized carriers to the CD44 receptor overexpressing human cervical carcinoma HeLa cells and inhibition of tumor growth.

Phase change material (PCM) is a type of storage material that stores and releases energy in the form of heat [228]. An example of this kind of substance, fatty acid, has been studied in the thermal response to release drugs [229]. Yuan and coworkers [230] fabricated CuS-DOX-MBA@PCM nanoparticles by a nanoprecipitation method. The system was composed of copper sulfide (CuS) and DOX, encapsulated with stearic acid and lauric acid. Due to drug release in physiological conditions, this nanocarrier was used as a photothermal and imaging-guided agent. In vivo results exhibited improved inhibition of tumor growth related to the synergistic effect of 808 nm laser irradiation and antitumor therapy with DOX.

The potential anticancer activity of selenium nanoparticles has already been described in the literature [231]. Fang et al. [232] designed a combination of chemo- and PT-therapy based on SeNPs to carry both ICG and Doxorubicin (DOX). Additionally, they conjugated two peptides (RC-12 and PG-6) to SeNPs using chitosan (CS) as the linker. These peptides acted as specific tumor-targeting ligands, which helped to improve the cellular uptake of SeNPs-DOX-ICG-RP. The photothermal effect of NPs was confirmed by the raise of temperature to 78.2 °C after NIR irradiation for 100 s (3 W cm^{-2}). In vitro experiments demonstrated that SeNPs-DOX-ICG-RP generated ROS in HepG2 cells and promoted an efficient anticancer activity. Mohammadi et al. [233] engineered nanostructures of selenium-polyethylene glycol-curcumin (Se-PEG-Cur) for PTT and sonodynamic therapy (SDT). The nanoparticles showed great photothermal conversion efficiency (16.7%) and ability to trigger ROS production in C540 (B16/F10) cancer cells. The percentage of viable cells after irradiation of the 808 nm laser decreased to 33.9%, while ultrasound waves could reduce viability to 22.9%.

4. Final Remarks

This review shows that nanoparticles are being extensively investigated for phototherapies nowadays. Regardless of the type of nanoparticle, there a few characteristics, shown in Figure 10, that can summarize the current state of this technology for medical application. The main advantages include the minimally invasive method of therapy, the minimization of side effects and the possibility to target and enhance accumulation of drugs in the tumor. Therefore, it is possible to achieve a targeted therapy with a reduction of drug dosage and greater drug stability. In conclusion, nanoparticle systems are multifaceted structures that are under extensive investigation to create alternatives for conventional therapies of cancer in combination with phototherapy. There are still parameters such as the hypoxic tumor microenvironment that can be an obstacle for PDT, and for phototherapy in general, the limited penetration depth of the light can hinder the use of these systems in cancer therapy. Finally, scale-up and clinical studies are indeed the main challenges in the next few years, however, the incredible diversity of nanoparticles as well as their multiple qualities allied to phototherapy are a promising combination that can result in a more effective and safer treatment for the patients.

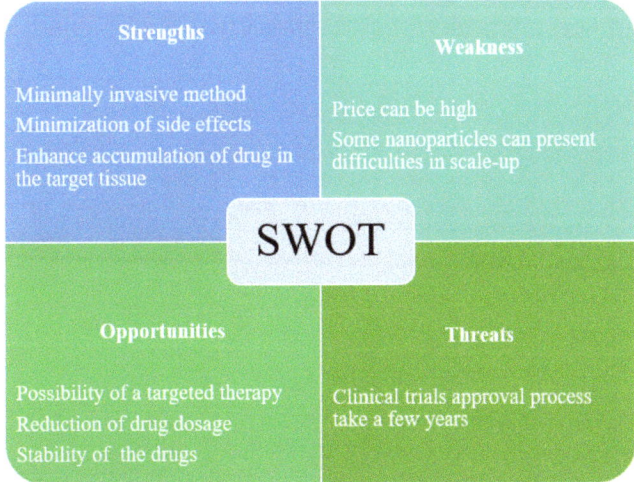

Figure 10. Strengths, weaknesses, opportunities and threats (SWOT) analysis of nanoparticles for Phototherapy.

Author Contributions: Conceptualization, T.P.P., C.E.A.B. and M.R.; methodology, T.P.P., C.E.A.B. and M.R.; investigation, T.P.P., C.E.A.B. and M.R.; writing—original draft preparation, T.P.P., C.E.A.B. and M.R.; writing—review and editing, T.P.P., C.E.A.B., M.R., P.A.R. and P.D.M.; visualization, T.P.P. and C.E.A.B.; supervision, T.P.P., C.E.A.B., M.R., P.A.R. and P.D.M.; project administration, M.R., P.A.R. and P.D.M.; funding acquisition, M.R., P.A.R. and P.D.M. All authors have read and agreed to the published version of the manuscript.

Funding: This research was funded by Fundação para a Ciência e a Tecnologia (FCT-MCTES), Radiation Biology and Biophysics Doctoral Training Programme (RaBBiT, PD/00193/2012), the Applied Molecular Biosciences Unit—UCIBIO (UIDB/04378/2020), the CEFITEC Unit (UIDB/00068/2020), UIDB/04559/2020 (LIBPhys) and UIDP/04559/2020 (LIBPhys) and the scholarship grant number PD/BD/142829/2018, to T.P. Pivetta from the RaBBiT Doctoral Training Programme. C.E.A. Botteon and P.D. Marcato acknowledge the funding from the São Paulo State Research Support Foundation (FAPESP) (grants #2018/13465-5 and #2017/04138-8), the Coordination for the Improvement of Higher Education Personnel (CAPES) and the National Council for Scientific and Technological Development (CNPq, grants #465687/2014-8).

Institutional Review Board Statement: Not applicable.

Informed Consent Statement: Not applicable.

Data Availability Statement: The data presented in this study are available on request from the cited author.

Conflicts of Interest: The authors declare no conflict of interest.

References

1. Sung, H.; Ferlay, J.; Siegel, R.L.; Laversanne, M.; Soerjomataram, I.; Jemal, A.; Bray, F. Global Cancer Statistics 2020: GLOBOCAN Estimates of Incidence and Mortality Worldwide for 36 Cancers in 185 Countries. *CA Cancer J. Clin.* **2021**, *71*, 209–249. [CrossRef]
2. Falzone, L.; Salomone, S.; Libra, M. Evolution of cancer pharmacological treatments at the turn of the third millennium. *Front. Pharmacol.* **2018**, *9*, 1300. [CrossRef]
3. Sivarajakumar, R.; Mallukaraj, D.; Kadavakollu, M.; Neelakandan, N.; Chandran, S.; Bhojaraj, S.; Karri, V.V.S.R. Nanoparticles for the treatment of lung cancers. *J. Young Pharm.* **2018**, *10*, 276–281. [CrossRef]
4. Zhen, X.; Cheng, P.; Pu, K. Recent Advances in Cell Membrane-Camouflaged Nanoparticles for Cancer Phototherapy. *Small* **2019**, *15*, 1804105. [CrossRef] [PubMed]
5. He, Z.; Zhao, L.; Zhang, Q.; Chang, M.; Li, C.; Zhang, H.; Lu, Y.; Chen, Y. An Acceptor–Donor–Acceptor Structured Small Molecule for Effective NIR Triggered Dual Phototherapy of Cancer. *Adv. Funct. Mater.* **2020**, *30*, 1910301. [CrossRef]
6. Liu, P.; Yang, W.; Shi, L.; Zhang, H.; Xu, Y.; Wang, P.; Zhang, G.; Chen, W.R.; Zhang, B.; Wang, X. Concurrent photothermal therapy and photodynamic therapy for cutaneous squamous cell carcinoma by gold nanoclusters under a single NIR laser irradiation. *J. Mater. Chem. B* **2019**, *7*, 6924–6933. [CrossRef] [PubMed]
7. Hong, E.J.; Choi, D.G.; Shim, M.S. Targeted and effective photodynamic therapy for cancer using functionalized nanomaterials. *Acta Pharm. Sin. B* **2016**, *6*, 297–307. [CrossRef] [PubMed]
8. Jeevanandam, J.; Barhoum, A.; Chan, Y.S.; Dufresne, A.; Danquah, M.K. Review on nanoparticles and nanostructured materials: History, sources, toxicity and regulations. *Beilstein J. Nanotechnol.* **2018**, *9*, 1050–1074. [CrossRef]
9. Wolfram, J.; Zhu, M.; Yang, Y.; Shen, J.; Gentile, E.; Paolino, D.; Fresta, M.; Nie, G.; Chen, C.; Shen, H.; et al. Safety of Nanoparticles in Medicine. *Curr. Drug Targets* **2015**, *16*, 1671–1681. [CrossRef] [PubMed]
10. Rodrigues, A.R.O.; Matos, J.O.G.; Nova Dias, A.M.; Almeida, B.G.; Pires, A.; Pereira, A.M.; Araújo, J.P.; Queiroz, M.J.R.P.; Castanheira, E.M.S.; Coutinho, P.J.G. Development of multifunctional liposomes containing magnetic/plasmonic $MnFe_2O_4$/Au core/shell nanoparticles. *Pharmaceutics* **2019**, *11*, 10. [CrossRef]
11. Bunney, P.E.; Zink, A.N.; Holm, A.A.; Billington, C.J.; Kotz, C.M. Orexin activation counteracts decreases in nonexercise activity thermogenesis (NEAT) caused by high-fat diet. *Physiol. Behav.* **2017**, *176*, 139–148. [CrossRef]
12. Nam, J.; Son, S.; Ochyl, L.J.; Kuai, R.; Schwendeman, A.; Moon, J.J. Chemo-photothermal therapy combination elicits anti-tumor immunity against advanced metastatic cancer. *Nat. Commun.* **2018**, *9*, 1074. [CrossRef]
13. Liu, Y.; Crawford, B.M.; Vo-Dinh, T. Gold nanoparticles-mediated photothermal therapy and immunotherapy. *Immunotherapy* **2018**, *10*, 1175–1188. [CrossRef]
14. Hak, A.; Ravasaheb Shinde, V.; Rengan, A.K. A review of advanced nanoformulations in phototherapy for cancer therapeutics. *Photodiagn. Photodyn. Ther.* **2021**, *33*, 102205. [CrossRef]
15. Montaseri, H.; Kruger, C.A.; Abrahamse, H. Review: Organic nanoparticle based active targeting for photodynamic therapy treatment of breast cancer cells. *Oncotarget* **2020**, *11*, 2120–2136. [CrossRef] [PubMed]
16. Hönigsmann, H. History of phototherapy in dermatology. *Photochem. Photobiol. Sci.* **2013**, *12*, 16–21. [CrossRef]

17. Sharma, S.K.; Mroz, P.; Dai, T.; Huang, Y.; St. Denis, T.G.; Hamblin, M.R. Photodynamic Therapy for Cancer and for Infections: What Is the Difference? *Isr. J. Chem.* **2012**, *52*, 691–705. [CrossRef] [PubMed]
18. Agostinis, P.; Berg, K.; Cengel, K.A.; Foster, T.H.; Girotti, A.W.; Gollnick, S.O.; Hahn, S.M.; Hamblin, M.R.; Juzeniene, A.; Kessel, D.; et al. Photodynamic therapy of cancer: An update. *CA Cancer J. Clin.* **2011**, *61*, 250–281. [CrossRef]
19. Oniszczuk, A.; Wojtunik-Kulesza, K.A.; Oniszczuk, T.; Kasprzak, K. The potential of photodynamic therapy (PDT)—Experimental investigations and clinical use. *Biomed. Pharmacother.* **2016**, *83*, 912–929. [CrossRef] [PubMed]
20. Kim, M.; Jung, H.Y.; Park, H.J. Topical PDT in the treatment of benign skin diseases: Principles and new applications. *Int. J. Mol. Sci.* **2015**, *16*, 23259–23278. [CrossRef]
21. Wen, X.; Li, Y.; Hamblin, M.R. Photodynamic therapy in dermatology beyond non-melanoma cancer: An update. *Photodiagn. Photodyn. Ther.* **2017**, *19*, 140–152. [CrossRef] [PubMed]
22. Zhao, B.; He, Y.-Y. Recent advances in the prevention and treatment of skin cancer using photodynamic therapy. *Expert Rev. Anticancer Ther.* **2010**, *10*, 1797–1809. [CrossRef] [PubMed]
23. Costa, D.F.; Mendes, L.P.; Torchilin, V.P. The effect of low-and high-penetration light on localized cancer therapy. *Adv. Drug Deliv. Rev.* **2019**, *138*, 105–116. [CrossRef] [PubMed]
24. Schuch, A.P.; Moreno, N.C.; Schuch, N.J.; Menck, C.F.M.; Garcia, C.C.M. Sunlight damage to cellular DNA: Focus on oxidatively generated lesions. *Free Radic. Biol. Med.* **2017**, *107*, 110–124. [CrossRef]
25. Gomes, P.J.; Ribeiro, P.A.; Shaw, D.; Mason, N.J.; Raposo, M. UV degradation of deoxyribonucleic acid. *Polym. Degrad. Stab.* **2009**, *94*, 2134–2141. [CrossRef]
26. Gomes, P.J.; Coelho, M.; Dionísio, M.; António Ribeiro, P.; Raposo, M. Probing radiation damage by alternated current conductivity as a method to characterize electron hopping conduction in DNA molecules. *Appl. Phys. Lett.* **2012**, *101*, 123702. [CrossRef]
27. Gomes, P.J.; Ferraria, A.M.; Botelho Do Rego, A.M.; Hoffmann, S.V.; Ribeiro, P.A.; Raposo, M. Energy thresholds of DNA damage induced by UV radiation: An XPS study. *J. Phys. Chem. B* **2015**, *119*, 5404–5411. [CrossRef]
28. Vangipuram, R.; Feldman, S.R. Ultraviolet phototherapy for cutaneous diseases: A concise review. *Oral Dis.* **2016**, *22*, 253–259. [CrossRef]
29. Shen, Z.; Ma, Q.; Zhou, X.; Zhang, G.; Hao, G.; Sun, Y.; Cao, J. Strategies to improve photodynamic therapy efficacy by relieving the tumor hypoxia environment. *NPG Asia Mater.* **2021**, *13*, 39. [CrossRef]
30. El Mohtadi, F.; D'Arcy, R.; Yang, X.; Turhan, Z.Y.; Alshamsan, A.; Tirelli, N. Main Chain Polysulfoxides as Active 'Stealth' Polymers with Additional Antioxidant and Anti-Inflammatory Behaviour. *Int. J. Mol. Sci.* **2019**, *20*, 4583. [CrossRef]
31. Müller, R.H.; Radtke, M.; Wissing, S.A. Solid lipid nanoparticles (SLN) and nanostructured lipid carriers (NLC) in cosmetic and dermatological preparations. *Adv. Drug Deliv. Rev.* **2002**, *54*, 131–155. [CrossRef]
32. Müller, R.; Lucks, S. Arzneistoffträger Aus Festen Lipidteilchen, Feste Lipidnanosphären (SLN). European Patent Application No. EP0605497B2, 20 March 1996.
33. Gasco, M.R. Method for Producing Solid Lipid Microspheres Having a Narrow Size Distribution. U.S. Patent Application No. US5250236A, 5 October 1993.
34. Müller, R.H.; Radtke, M.; Wissing, S.A. Nanostructured lipid matrices for improved microencapsulation of drugs. *Int. J. Pharm.* **2002**, *242*, 121–128. [CrossRef]
35. Naseri, N.; Valizadeh, H.; Zakeri-Milani, P. Solid lipid nanoparticles and nanostructured lipid carriers: Structure preparation and application. *Adv. Pharm. Bull.* **2015**, *5*, 305–313. [CrossRef] [PubMed]
36. Üner, M.; Yener, G. Importance of solid lipid nanoparticles (SLN) in various administration routes and future perspective. *Int. J. Nanomed.* **2007**, *2*, 289–300.
37. Qidwai, A.; Khan, S.; Md, S.; Fazil, M.; Baboota, S.; Narang, J.K.; Ali, J. Nanostructured lipid carrier in photodynamic therapy for the treatment of basal-cell carcinoma. *Drug Deliv.* **2016**, *23*, 1476–1485. [CrossRef]
38. Jiang, S.; Zhu, R.; He, X.; Wang, J.; Wang, M.; Qian, Y.; Wang, S. Enhanced photocytotoxicity of curcumin delivered by solid lipid nanoparticles. *Int. J. Nanomed.* **2017**, *12*, 167–178. [CrossRef]
39. Goto, P.L.; Siqueira-Moura, M.P.; Tedesco, A.C. Application of aluminum chloride phthalocyanine-loaded solid lipid nanoparticles for photodynamic inactivation of melanoma cells. *Int. J. Pharm.* **2017**, *518*, 228–241. [CrossRef]
40. Almeida, E.D.P.; Dipieri, L.V.; Rossetti, F.C.; Marchetti, J.M.; Bentley, M.V.L.B.; Nunes, R.D.S.; Sarmento, V.H.V.; Valerio, M.E.G.; Rodrigues Júnior, J.J.; Montalvão, M.M.; et al. Skin permeation, biocompatibility and antitumor effect of chloroaluminum phthalocyanine associated to oleic acid in lipid nanoparticles. *Photodiagn. Photodyn. Ther.* **2018**, *24*, 262–273. [CrossRef]
41. Antonietti, M.; Förster, S. Vesicles and Liposomes: A Self-Assembly Principle Beyond Lipids. *Adv. Mater.* **2003**, *15*, 1323–1333. [CrossRef]
42. Yang, Y.; Yang, X.; Li, H.; Li, C.; Ding, H.; Zhang, M.; Guo, Y.; Sun, M. Near-infrared light triggered liposomes combining photodynamic and chemotherapy for synergistic breast tumor therapy. *Coll. Surf. B Biointerfaces* **2019**, *173*, 564–570. [CrossRef]
43. Matos, C.; Moutinho, C.; Lobão, P. Liposomes as a model for the biological membrane: Studies on Daunorubicin bilayer interaction. *J. Membr. Biol.* **2012**, *245*, 69–75. [CrossRef]
44. Peetla, C.; Stine, A.; Labhasetwar, V. Biophysical Interactions with Model Lipid Membranes: Applications in Drug Discovery and Drug Delivery. *Mol. Pharm.* **2009**, *6*, 1264–1276. [CrossRef]
45. Duse, L.; Pinnapireddy, S.R.; Strehlow, B.; Jedelská, J.; Bakowsky, U. Low level LED photodynamic therapy using curcumin loaded tetraether liposomes. *Eur. J. Pharm. Biopharm.* **2018**, *126*, 233–241. [CrossRef] [PubMed]

46. Immordino, M.L.; Franco, D.; Cattel, L. Stealth liposomes: Review of the basic science, rationale, and clinical applications, existing and potential. *Int. J. Nanomed.* **2006**, *1*, 297–315.
47. Yang, Q.; Jones, S.W.; Parker, C.L.; Zamboni, W.C.; Bear, J.E.; Lai, S.K. Evading immune cell uptake and clearance requires PEG grafting at densities substantially exceeding the minimum for brush conformation. *Mol. Pharm.* **2014**, *11*, 1250–1258. [CrossRef]
48. Ohradanova-Repic, A.; Nogueira, E.; Hartl, I.; Gomes, A.C.; Preto, A.; Steinhuber, E.; Mühlgrabner, V.; Repic, M.; Kuttke, M.; Zwirzitz, A.; et al. Fab antibody fragment-functionalized liposomes for specific targeting of antigen-positive cells. *Nanomed. Nanotechnol. Biol. Med.* **2018**, *14*, 123–130. [CrossRef]
49. Gaio, E.; Scheglmann, D.; Reddi, E.; Moret, F. Uptake and photo-toxicity of Foscan®, Foslip® and Fospeg® in multicellular tumor spheroids. *J. Photochem. Photobiol. B Biol.* **2016**, *161*, 244–252. [CrossRef]
50. Reshetov, V.; Kachatkou, D.; Shmigol, T.; Zorin, V.; D'Hallewin, M.-A.; Guillemin, F.; Bezdetnaya, L. Redistribution of meta-tetra(hydroxyphenyl)chlorin (m-THPC) from conventional and PEGylated liposomes to biological substrates. *Photochem. Photobiol. Sci.* **2011**, *10*, 911–919. [CrossRef] [PubMed]
51. Reshetov, V.; Lassalle, H.-P.; François, A.; Dumas, D.; Hupont, S.; Gräfe, S.; Filipe, V.; Jiskoot, W.; Guillemin, F.; Zorin, V.; et al. Photodynamic therapy with conventional and pegylated liposomal formulations of mTHPC(temoporfin): Comparison of treatment efficacy and distribution characteristics in vivo. *Int. J. Nanomed.* **2013**, *8*, 3817–3831. [CrossRef] [PubMed]
52. Cai, X.; Mao, D.; Wang, C.; Kong, D.; Cheng, X.; Liu, B. Multifunctional Liposome: A Bright AIEgen–Lipid Conjugate with Strong Photosensitization. *Angew. Chem.* **2018**, *57*, 16396–16400. [CrossRef]
53. Kim, D.H.; Im, B.N.; Hwang, H.S.; Na, K. Gemcitabine-loaded DSPE-PEG-PheoA liposome as a photomediated immune modulator for cholangiocarcinoma treatment. *Biomaterials* **2018**, *183*, 139–150. [CrossRef]
54. Igarashi, A.; Konno, H.; Tanaka, T.; Nakamura, S.; Sadzuka, Y.; Hirano, T.; Fujise, Y. Liposomal photofrin enhances therapeutic efficacy of photodynamic therapy against the human gastric cancer. *Toxicol. Lett.* **2003**, *145*, 133–141. [CrossRef]
55. Baglo, Y.; Liang, B.J.; Robey, R.W.; Ambudkar, S.V.; Gottesman, M.M.; Huang, H.-C. Porphyrin-lipid assemblies and nanovesicles overcome ABC transporter-mediated photodynamic therapy resistance in cancer cells. *Cancer Lett.* **2019**, *457*, 110–118. [CrossRef]
56. Abdel Fadeel, D.; Al-Toukhy, G.M.; Elsharif, A.M.; Al-Jameel, S.S.; Mohamed, H.H.; Youssef, T.E. Improved photodynamic efficacy of thiophenyl sulfonated zinc phthalocyanine loaded in lipid nano-carriers for hepatocellular carcinoma cancer cells. *Photodiagn. Photodyn. Ther.* **2018**, *23*, 25–31. [CrossRef] [PubMed]
57. de Lima, R.G.; Tedesco, A.C.; da Silva, R.S.; Lawrence, M.J. Ultradeformable liposome loaded with zinc phthalocyanine and [Ru(NH.NHq)(tpy)NO]$^{3+}$ for photodynamic therapy by topical application. *Photodiagn. Photodyn. Ther.* **2017**, *19*, 184–193. [CrossRef]
58. Salim, M.; Minamikawa, H.; Sugimura, A.; Hashim, R. Amphiphilic designer nano-carriers for controlled release: From drug delivery to diagnostics. *MedChemComm* **2014**, *5*, 1602–1618. [CrossRef]
59. Dutt, S.; Siril, P.F.; Remita, S. Swollen liquid crystals (SLCs): A versatile template for the synthesis of nano structured materials. *RSC Adv.* **2017**, *7*, 5733–5750. [CrossRef]
60. Gaucher, G.; Marchessault, R.H.; Leroux, J.C. Polyester-based micelles and nanoparticles for the parenteral delivery of taxanes. *J. Control. Release* **2010**, *143*, 2–12. [CrossRef]
61. Zhang, C.; Zhang, J.; Qin, Y.; Song, H.; Huang, P.; Wang, W.; Wang, C.; Li, C.; Wang, Y.; Kong, D. Co-delivery of doxorubicin and pheophorbide A by pluronic F127 micelles for chemo-photodynamic combination therapy of melanoma. *J. Mater. Chem. B* **2018**, *6*, 3305–3314. [CrossRef] [PubMed]
62. Lamch, Ł.; Kulbacka, J.; Dubińska-Magiera, M.; Saczko, J.; Wilk, K.A. Folate-directed zinc (II) phthalocyanine loaded polymeric micelles engineered to generate reactive oxygen species for efficacious photodynamic therapy of cancer. *Photodiagn. Photodyn. Ther.* **2019**, *25*, 480–491. [CrossRef]
63. Wang, X.; Wang, J.; Li, J.; Huang, H.; Sun, X.; Lv, Y. Development and evaluation of hyaluronic acid-based polymeric micelles for targeted delivery of photosensitizer for photodynamic therapy in vitro. *J. Drug Deliv. Sci. Technol.* **2018**, *48*, 414–421. [CrossRef]
64. Marzuki, N.H.C.; Wahab, R.A.; Hamid, M.A. An overview of nanoemulsion: Concepts of development and cosmeceutical applications. *Biotechnol. Biotechnol. Equip.* **2019**, *33*, 779–797. [CrossRef]
65. Machado, F.C.; Adum de Matos, R.P.; Primo, F.L.; Tedesco, A.C.; Rahal, P.; Calmon, M.F. Effect of curcumin-nanoemulsion associated with photodynamic therapy in breast adenocarcinoma cell line. *Bioorgan. Med. Chem.* **2019**, *27*, 1882–1890. [CrossRef]
66. Monge-Fuentes, V.; Muehlmann, L.A.; Longo, J.P.F.; Silva, J.R.; Fascineli, M.L.; de Souza, P.; Faria, F.; Degterev, I.A.; Rodriguez, A.; Carneiro, F.P.; et al. Photodynamic therapy mediated by acai oil (*Euterpe oleracea* Martius) in nanoemulsion: A potential treatment for melanoma. *J. Photochem. Photobiol. B Biol.* **2017**, *166*, 301–310. [CrossRef]
67. Langer, R.; Folkman, J. Polymers for the sustained release of proteins and other macromolecules. *Nature* **1976**, *263*, 797–800. [CrossRef] [PubMed]
68. Amoabediny, G.; Haghiralsadat, F.; Naderinezhad, S.; Helder, M.N.; Kharanaghi, E.A.; Arough, J.M.; Zandieh-Doulabi, B. Overview of preparation methods of polymeric and lipid-based (niosome, solid lipid, liposome) nanoparticles: A comprehensive review. *Int. J. Polym. Mater. Polym. Biomater.* **2018**, *67*, 383–400. [CrossRef]
69. Crucho, C.I.C.; Barros, M.T. Polymeric nanoparticles: A study on the preparation variables and characterization methods. *Mater. Sci. Eng. C* **2017**, *80*, 771–784. [CrossRef] [PubMed]
70. Grabnar, P.A.; Kristl, J. The manufacturing techniques of drug-loaded polymeric nanoparticles from preformed polymers. *J. Microencapsul.* **2011**, *28*, 323–335. [CrossRef]

71. Eltahan, A.S.; Liu, L.; Okeke, C.I.; Huang, M.; Han, L.; Chen, J.; Xue, X.; Bottini, M.; Guo, W.; Liang, X.J. NVP-BEZ235/Chlorin-e6 co-loaded nanoparticles ablate breast cancer by biochemical and photodynamic synergistic effects. *Nano Res.* **2018**, *11*, 4846–4858. [CrossRef]
72. Gangopadhyay, M.; Singh, T.; Behara, K.K.; Karwa, S.; Ghosh, S.K.; Singh, N.D.P. Coumarin-containing-star-shaped 4-arm-polyethylene glycol: Targeted fluorescent organic nanoparticles for dual treatment of photodynamic therapy and chemotherapy. *Photochem. Photobiol. Sci.* **2015**, *14*, 1329–1336. [CrossRef]
73. Mehraban, N.; Musich, P.R.; Freeman, H.S. Synthesis and encapsulation of a new zinc phthalocyanine photosensitizer into polymeric nanoparticles to enhance cell uptake and phototoxicity. *Appl. Sci.* **2019**, *9*, 401. [CrossRef]
74. Lin, W.; Zhang, W.; Sun, T.; Liu, S.; Zhu, Y.; Xie, Z. Rational Design of Polymeric Nanoparticles with Tailorable Biomedical Functions for Cancer Therapy. *ACS Appl. Mater. Interfaces* **2017**, *9*, 29612–29622. [CrossRef] [PubMed]
75. Jadia, R.; Kydd, J.; Rai, P. Remotely Phototriggered, Transferrin-Targeted Polymeric Nanoparticles for the Treatment of Breast Cancer. *Photochem. Photobiol.* **2018**, *94*, 765–774. [CrossRef]
76. D'souza, A.A.; Shegokar, R. Polyethylene glycol (PEG): A versatile polymer for pharmaceutical applications. *Expert Opin. Drug Deliv.* **2016**, *13*, 1257–1275. [CrossRef]
77. Yang, X.; Li, J.; Yu, Y.; Wang, J.; Li, D.; Cao, Z.; Yang, X. Engineering of a universal polymeric nanoparticle platform to optimize the PEG density for photodynamic therapy. *Sci. China Chem.* **2019**, *62*, 1379–1386. [CrossRef]
78. Luo, Z.; Li, M.; Zhou, M.; Li, H.; Chen, Y.; Ren, X.; Dai, Y. O_2-evolving and ROS-activable nanoparticles for treatment of multi-drug resistant Cancer by combination of photodynamic therapy and chemotherapy. *Nanomed. Nanotechnol. Biol. Med.* **2019**, *19*, 49–57. [CrossRef]
79. Deng, X.; Liang, Y.; Peng, X.; Su, T.; Luo, S.; Cao, J.; Gu, Z.; He, B. A facile strategy to generate polymeric nanoparticles for synergistic chemo-photodynamic therapy. *Chem. Commun.* **2015**, *51*, 4271–4274. [CrossRef] [PubMed]
80. Jamali, Z.; Khoobi, M.; Hejazi, S.M.; Eivazi, N.; Abdolahpour, S.; Imanparast, F.; Moradi-Sardareh, H.; Paknejad, M. Evaluation of targeted curcumin (CUR) loaded PLGA nanoparticles for in vitro photodynamic therapy on human glioblastoma cell line. *Photodiagn. Photodyn. Ther.* **2018**, *23*, 190–201. [CrossRef]
81. Wang, S.; Li, J.; Ye, Z.; Li, J.; Wang, A.; Hu, J.; Bai, S.; Yin, J. Self-assembly of photosensitive and chemotherapeutic drugs for combined photodynamic-chemo cancer therapy with real-time tracing property. *Coll. Surf. A Physicochem. Eng. Asp.* **2019**, *574*, 44–51. [CrossRef]
82. Datz, S.; Illes, B.; Gößl, D.; Schirnding, C.V.; Engelke, H.; Bein, T. Biocompatible crosslinked β-cyclodextrin nanoparticles as multifunctional carriers for cellular delivery. *Nanoscale* **2018**, *10*, 16284–16292. [CrossRef]
83. Loftsson, T. Self-assembled cyclodextrin nanoparticles and drug delivery. *J. Incl. Phenom. Macrocycl. Chem.* **2014**, *80*, 1–7. [CrossRef]
84. Gidwani, B.; Vyas, A. A Comprehensive Review on Cyclodextrin-Based Carriers for Delivery of Chemotherapeutic Cytotoxic Anticancer Drugs. *BioMed Res. Int.* **2015**, *2015*, 198268. [CrossRef] [PubMed]
85. Lakkakula, J.R.; Krause, R.W.M. A vision for cyclodextrin nanoparticles in drug delivery systems and pharmaceutical applications. *Nanomedicine* **2014**, *9*, 877–894. [CrossRef]
86. Lourenço, L.M.O.; Pereira, P.M.R.; Maciel, E.; Válega, M.; Domingues, F.M.J.; Domingues, M.R.M.; Neves, M.G.P.M.S.; Cavaleiro, J.A.S.; Fernandes, R.; Tomé, J.P.C. Amphiphilic phthalocyanine-cyclodextrin conjugates for cancer photodynamic therapy. *Chem. Commun.* **2014**, *50*, 8363–8366. [CrossRef]
87. Semeraro, P.; Chimienti, G.; Altamura, E.; Fini, P.; Rizzi, V.; Cosma, P. Chlorophyll a in cyclodextrin supramolecular complexes as a natural photosensitizer for photodynamic therapy (PDT) applications. *Mater. Sci. Eng. C* **2018**, *85*, 47–56. [CrossRef]
88. De Frates, K.; Markiewicz, T.; Gallo, P.; Rack, A.; Weyhmiller, A.; Jarmusik, B.; Hu, X. Protein polymer-based nanoparticles: Fabrication and medical applications. *Int. J. Mol. Sci.* **2018**, *19*, 1717. [CrossRef] [PubMed]
89. Lohcharoenkal, W.; Wang, L.; Chen, Y.C.; Rojanasakul, Y. Protein Nanoparticles as Drug Delivery Carriers for Cancer Therapy. *BioMed Res. Int.* **2014**, *2014*, 180549. [CrossRef]
90. Ye, C.; Chi, H. A review of recent progress in drug and protein encapsulation: Approaches, applications and challenges. *Mater. Sci. Eng. C* **2018**, *83*, 233–246. [CrossRef]
91. Lu, C.; Li, X.; Liang, X.; Zhang, X.; Yin, T.; Gou, J.; He, H.; Zhang, Y.; Tang, X. Liver Targeting Albumin-Coated Silybin-Phospholipid Particles Prepared by Nab^{TM} Technology for Improving Treatment Effect of Acute Liver Damage in Intravenous Administration. *AAPS PharmSciTech* **2019**, *20*, 293. [CrossRef]
92. Phuong, P.T.T.; Lee, S.; Lee, C.; Seo, B.; Park, S.; Oh, K.T.; Lee, E.S.; Choi, H.G.; Shin, B.S.; Youn, Y.S. Beta-carotene-bound albumin nanoparticles modified with chlorin e6 for breast tumor ablation based on photodynamic therapy. *Coll. Surf. B Biointerfaces* **2018**, *171*, 123–133. [CrossRef]
93. Kokalari, I.; Gassino, R.; Giovannozzi, A.M.; Croin, L.; Gazzano, E.; Bergamaschi, E.; Rossi, A.M.; Perrone, G.; Riganti, C.; Ponti, J.; et al. Pro-and anti-oxidant properties of near-infrared (NIR) light responsive carbon nanoparticles. *Free Radic. Biol. Med.* **2019**, *134*, 165–176. [CrossRef] [PubMed]
94. Pérez, E.M.; Martín, N. π–π interactions in carbon nanostructures. *Chem. Soc. Rev.* **2015**, *44*, 6425–6433. [CrossRef] [PubMed]
95. Heo, N.S.; Lee, S.U.; Rethinasabapathy, M.; Lee, E.Z.; Cho, H.J.; Oh, S.Y.; Choe, S.R.; Kim, Y.; Hong, W.G.; Krishnan, G.; et al. Visible-light-driven dynamic cancer therapy and imaging using graphitic carbon nitride nanoparticles. *Mater. Sci. Eng. C* **2018**, *90*, 531–538. [CrossRef]

96. Xie, R.; Lian, S.; Peng, H.; Ouyang, C.; Li, S.; Lu, Y.; Cao, X.; Zhang, C.; Xu, J.; Jia, L. Mitochondria and Nuclei Dual-Targeted Hollow Carbon Nanospheres for Cancer Chemophotodynamic Synergistic Therapy. *Mol. Pharm.* **2019**, *16*, 2235–2248. [CrossRef]
97. Nocito, G.; Calabrese, G.; Forte, S.; Petralia, S.; Puglisi, C.; Campolo, M.; Esposito, E.; Conoci, S. Carbon Dots as Promising Tools for Cancer Diagnosis and Therapy. *Cancers* **2021**, *13*, 1991. [CrossRef]
98. He, H.; Zheng, X.; Liu, S.; Zheng, M.; Xie, Z.; Wang, Y.; Yu, M.; Shuai, X. Diketopyrrolopyrrole-based carbon dots for photodynamic therapy. *Nanoscale* **2018**, *10*, 10991–10998. [CrossRef] [PubMed]
99. Jeelani, P.G.; Mulay, P.; Venkat, R.; Ramalingam, C. Multifaceted Application of Silica Nanoparticles. A Review. *Silicon* **2020**, *12*, 1337–1354. [CrossRef]
100. Liu, Y.; Liu, X.; Xiao, Y.; Chen, F.; Xiao, F. A multifunctional nanoplatform based on mesoporous silica nanoparticles for imaging-guided chemo/photodynamic synergetic therapy. *RSC Adv.* **2017**, *7*, 31133–31141. [CrossRef]
101. Lin, X.; Wu, M.; Li, M.; Cai, Z.; Sun, H.; Tan, X.; Li, J.; Zeng, Y.; Liu, X.; Liu, J. Photo-responsive hollow silica nanoparticles for light-triggered genetic and photodynamic synergistic therapy. *Acta Biomater.* **2018**, *76*, 178–192. [CrossRef]
102. Bretin, L.; Pinon, A.; Bouramtane, S.; Ouk, C.; Richard, L.; Perrin, M.; Chaunavel, A.; Carrion, C.; Bregier, F.; Sol, V.; et al. Photodynamic Therapy Activity of New Porphyrin-Xylan-Coated Silica Nanoparticles in Human Colorectal Cancer. *Cancers* **2019**, *11*, 1474. [CrossRef]
103. Matlou, G.G.; Oluwole, D.O.; Prinsloo, E.; Nyokong, T. Photodynamic therapy activity of zinc phthalocyanine linked to folic acid and magnetic nanoparticles. *J. Photochem. Photobiol. B Biol.* **2018**, *186*, 216–224. [CrossRef] [PubMed]
104. Zhang, L.K.; Du, S.; Wang, X.; Jiao, Y.; Yin, L.; Zhang, Y.; Guan, Y.Q. Bacterial cellulose based composites enhanced transdermal drug targeting for breast cancer treatment. *Chem. Eng. J.* **2019**, *370*, 749–759. [CrossRef]
105. Zhang, P.; Wu, G.; Zhao, C.; Zhou, L.; Wang, X.; Wei, S. Magnetic stomatocyte-like nanomotor as photosensitizer carrier for photodynamic therapy based cancer treatment. *Coll. Surf. B Biointerfaces* **2020**, *194*, 111204. [CrossRef] [PubMed]
106. Sailor, M.J.; Park, J.-H. Hybrid Nanoparticles for Detection and Treatment of Cancer. *Adv. Mater.* **2012**, *24*, 3779–3802. [CrossRef]
107. Pramual, S.; Lirdprapamongkol, K.; Svasti, J.; Bergkvist, M.; Jouan-Hureaux, V.; Arnoux, P.; Frochot, C.; Barberi-Heyob, M.; Niamsiri, N. Polymer-lipid-PEG hybrid nanoparticles as photosensitizer carrier for photodynamic therapy. *J. Photochem. Photobiol. B Biol.* **2017**, *173*, 12–22. [CrossRef] [PubMed]
108. Wang, K.; Xiang, Y.; Pan, W.; Wang, H.; Li, N.; Tang, B. Dual-targeted photothermal agents for enhanced cancer therapy. *Chem. Sci.* **2020**, *11*, 8055–8072. [CrossRef] [PubMed]
109. Abadeer, N.S.; Murphy, C.J. Recent Progress in Cancer Thermal Therapy Using Gold Nanoparticles. *J. Phys. Chem. C* **2016**, *120*, 4691–4716. [CrossRef]
110. Zou, L.; Wang, H.; He, B.; Zeng, L.; Tan, T.; Cao, H.; He, X.; Zhang, Z.; Guo, S.; Li, Y. Current approaches of photothermal therapy in treating cancer metastasis with nanotherapeutics. *Theranostics* **2016**, *6*, 762–772. [CrossRef]
111. Wang, J.; Wu, X.; Shen, P.; Wang, J.; Shen, Y.; Shen, Y.; Webster, T.J.; Deng, J. Applications of inorganic nanomaterials in photothermal therapy based on combinational cancer treatment. *Int. J. Nanomed.* **2020**, *15*, 1903–1914. [CrossRef]
112. Fernandes, N.; Rodrigues, C.F.; Moreira, A.F.; Correia, I.J. Overview of the application of inorganic nanomaterials in cancer photothermal therapy. *Biomater. Sci.* **2020**, *8*, 2990–3020. [CrossRef]
113. Mendes, R.; Pedrosa, P.; Lima, J.C.; Fernandes, A.R.; Baptista, P.V. Photothermal enhancement of chemotherapy in breast cancer by visible irradiation of Gold Nanoparticles. *Sci. Rep.* **2017**, *7*, 10872. [CrossRef]
114. Zhao, Y.; He, Z.; Zhang, Q.; Wang, J.; Jia, W.; Jin, L.; Zhao, L.; Lu, Y. 880 nm NIR-Triggered Organic Small Molecular-Based Nanoparticles for Photothermal Therapy of Tumor. *Nanomaterials* **2021**, *11*, 773. [CrossRef] [PubMed]
115. Sun, Y.; Wang, Q.; Chen, J.; Liu, L.; Ding, L.; Shen, M.; Li, J.; Han, B.; Duan, Y. Temperature-sensitive gold nanoparticle-coated Pluronic-PLL nanoparticles for drug delivery and chemo-photothermal therapy. *Theranostics* **2017**, *7*, 4424–4444. [CrossRef] [PubMed]
116. Ferro-Flores, G.; Ocampo-García, B.; Santos-Cuevas, C.; María Ramírez, F.; Azorín-Vega, E.; Meléndez-Alafort, L. Theranostic Radiopharmaceuticals Based on Gold Nanoparticles Labeled with ^{177}Lu and Conjugated to Peptides. *Curr. Radiopharm.* **2015**, *8*, 150–159. [CrossRef]
117. Huang, X.; El-Sayed, M.A. Gold nanoparticles: Optical properties and implementations in cancer diagnosis and photothermal therapy. *J. Adv. Res.* **2010**, *1*, 13–28. [CrossRef]
118. Guo, J.; Rahme, K.; He, Y.; Li, L.L.; Holmes, J.D.; O'Driscoll, C.M. Gold nanoparticles enlighten the future of cancer theranostics. *Int. J. Nanomed.* **2017**, *12*, 6131–6152. [CrossRef]
119. Richardson, H.H.; Carlson, M.T.; Tandler, P.J.; Hernandez, P.; Govorov, A.O. Experimental and theoretical studies of light-to-heat conversion and collective heating effects in metal nanoparticle solutions. *Nano Lett.* **2009**, *9*, 1139–1146. [CrossRef]
120. Saw, W.S.; Ujihara, M.; Chong, W.Y.; Voon, S.H.; Imae, T.; Kiew, L.V.; Lee, H.B.; Sim, K.S.; Chung, L.Y. Size-dependent effect of cystine/citric acid-capped confeito-like gold nanoparticles on cellular uptake and photothermal cancer therapy. *Coll. Surf. B Biointerfaces* **2018**, *161*, 365–374. [CrossRef]
121. Jiang, W.; Kim, B.Y.S.; Rutka, J.T.; Chan, W.C.W. Nanoparticle-mediated cellular response is size-dependent. *Nat. Nanotechnol.* **2008**, *3*, 145–150. [CrossRef]
122. AL-Barram, L.F.A. Laser enhancement of cancer cell destruction by photothermal therapy conjugated glutathione (GSH)-coated small-sized gold nanoparticles. *Lasers Med. Sci.* **2020**, *36*, 325–337. [CrossRef]

123. Kah, J.C.Y.; Wong, K.Y.; Neoh, K.G.; Song, J.H.; Fu, J.W.P.; Mhaisalkar, S.; Olivo, M.; Sheppard, C.J.R. Critical parameters in the pegylation of gold nanoshells for biomedical applications: An in vitro macrophage study. *J. Drug Target.* **2009**, *17*, 181–193. [CrossRef]
124. Santos-Martinez, M.J.; Rahme, K.; Corbalan, J.J.; Faulkner, C.; Holmes, J.D.; Tajber, L.; Medina, C.; Radomski, M.W. Pegylation increases platelet biocompatibility of gold nanoparticles. *J. Biomed. Nanotechnol.* **2014**, *10*, 1004–1015. [CrossRef]
125. Wang, R.; Deng, J.; He, D.; Yang, E.; Yang, W.; Shi, D.; Jiang, Y.; Qiu, Z.; Webster, T.J.; Shen, Y. PEGylated hollow gold nanoparticles for combined X-ray radiation and photothermal therapy in vitro and enhanced CT imaging in vivo. *Nanomed. Nanotechnol. Biol. Med.* **2019**, *16*, 195–205. [CrossRef]
126. Cheng, X.; Sun, R.; Yin, L.; Chai, Z.; Shi, H.; Gao, M. Light-Triggered Assembly of Gold Nanoparticles for Photothermal Therapy and Photoacoustic Imaging of Tumors In Vivo. *Adv. Mater.* **2017**, *29*, 1604894. [CrossRef] [PubMed]
127. Li, Z.; Yu, X.F.; Chu, P.K. Recent advances in cell-mediated nanomaterial delivery systems for photothermal therapy. *J. Mater. Chem. B* **2018**, *6*, 1296–1311. [CrossRef]
128. Marques, T.S.; Śmiałek, M.A.; Schürmann, R.; Bald, I.; Raposo, M.; Eden, S.; Mason, N.J. Decomposition of halogenated nucleobases by surface plasmon resonance excitation of gold nanoparticles. *Eur. Phys. J. D* **2020**, *74*, 222. [CrossRef]
129. Vogel, S.; Ebel, K.; Heck, C.; Schürmann, R.M.; Milosavljević, A.R.; Giuliani, A.; Bald, I. Vacuum-UV induced DNA strand breaks-influence of the radiosensitizers 5-bromouracil and 8-bromoadenine. *Phys. Chem. Chem. Phys.* **2019**, *21*, 1972–1979. [CrossRef] [PubMed]
130. Vodenkova, S.; Buchler, T.; Cervena, K.; Veskrnova, V.; Vodicka, P.; Vymetalkova, V. 5-fluorouracil and other fluoropyrimidines in colorectal cancer: Past, present and future. *Pharmacol. Ther.* **2020**, *206*, 107447. [CrossRef]
131. Knights, O.B.; McLaughlan, J.R. Gold nanorods for light-based lung cancer theranostics. *Int. J. Mol. Sci.* **2018**, *19*, 3318. [CrossRef] [PubMed]
132. Jin, N.; Zhang, Q.; Yang, M.; Yang, M. Detoxification and functionalization of gold nanorods with organic polymers and their applications in cancer photothermal therapy. *Microsc. Res. Tech.* **2019**, *82*, 670–679. [CrossRef]
133. Kirui, D.K.; Krishnan, S.; Strickland, A.D.; Batt, C.A. PAA-Derived Gold Nanorods for Cellular Targeting and Photothermal Therapy. *Macromol. Biosci.* **2011**, *11*, 779–788. [CrossRef]
134. Liu, X.; Huang, N.; Li, H.; Wang, H.; Jin, Q.; Ji, J. Multidentate polyethylene glycol modified gold nanorods for in vivo near-infrared photothermal cancer therapy. *ACS Appl. Mater. Interfaces* **2014**, *6*, 5657–5668. [CrossRef] [PubMed]
135. Liao, J.F.; Li, W.T.; Peng, J.R.; Yang, Q.; Li, H.; Wei, Y.Q.; Zhang, X.N.; Qian, Z.Y. Combined cancer photothermal-chemotherapy based on doxorubicin/gold nanorod-loaded polymersomes. *Theranostics* **2015**, *5*, 345–356. [CrossRef] [PubMed]
136. Hauck, T.S.; Jennings, T.L.; Yatsenko, T.; Kumaradas, J.C.; Chan, W.C.W. Enhancing the toxicity of cancer chemotherapeutics with gold nanorod hyperthermia. *Adv. Mater.* **2008**, *20*, 3832–3838. [CrossRef]
137. Duan, R.; Zhou, Z.; Su, G.; Liu, L.; Guan, M.; Du, B.; Zhang, Q. Chitosan-coated gold nanorods for cancer therapy combining chemical and photothermal effects. *Macromol. Biosci.* **2014**, *14*, 1160–1169. [CrossRef]
138. Wang, J.; Ma, K.; Wang, H.; Hu, Z.; Fu, Y.; Li, F. Peptide Multifunctionalized Gold Nanorods with Dual pH/NIR Responsive Release of Doxorubicin for High-Efficiency Cancer Treatment. *J. Biomed. Nanotechnol.* **2019**, *15*, 2164–2178. [CrossRef]
139. Xu, W.; Qian, J.; Hou, G.; Suo, A.; Wang, Y.; Wang, J.; Sun, T.; Yang, M.; Wan, X.; Yao, Y. Hyaluronic Acid-Functionalized Gold Nanorods with pH/NIR Dual-Responsive Drug Release for Synergetic Targeted Photothermal Chemotherapy of Breast Cancer. *ACS Appl. Mater. Interfaces* **2017**, *9*, 36533–36547. [CrossRef]
140. Chaffer, C.L.; Weinberg, R.A. A perspective on cancer cell metastasis. *Science* **2011**, *331*, 1559–1564. [CrossRef] [PubMed]
141. Wu, Y.; Ali, M.R.K.; Dong, B.; Han, T.; Chen, K.; Chen, J.; Tang, Y.; Fang, N.; Wang, F.; El-Sayed, M.A. Gold Nanorod Photothermal Therapy Alters Cell Junctions and Actin Network in Inhibiting Cancer Cell Collective Migration. *ACS Nano* **2018**, *12*, 9279–9290. [CrossRef]
142. Ren, F.; Bhana, S.; Norman, D.D.; Johnson, J.; Xu, L.; Baker, D.L.; Parrill, A.L.; Huang, X. Gold nanorods carrying paclitaxel for photothermal-chemotherapy of cancer. *Bioconj. Chem.* **2013**, *24*, 376–386. [CrossRef]
143. Timko, B.P.; Dvir, T.; Kohane, D.S. Remotely Triggerable Drug Delivery Systems. *Adv. Mater.* **2010**, *22*, 4925–4943. [CrossRef]
144. Hribar, K.C.; Lee, M.H.; Lee, D.; Burdick, J.A. Enhanced release of small molecules from near-infrared light responsive polymer-nanorod composites. *ACS Nano* **2011**, *5*, 2948–2956. [CrossRef]
145. Liao, J.; Jia, Y.; Chen, L.; Zhou, L.; Li, Q.; Qian, Z.; Niu, D.; Li, Y.; Li, P. Magnetic/Gold Core-Shell Hybrid Particles for Targeting and Imaging-Guided Photothermal Cancer Therapy. *J. Biomed. Nanotechnol.* **2019**, *15*, 2072–2089. [CrossRef] [PubMed]
146. Multari, C.; Miola, M.; Laviano, F.; Gerbaldo, R.; Pezzotti, G.; Debellis, D.; Verné, E. Magnetoplasmonic nanoparticles for photothermal therapy. *Nanotechnology* **2019**, *30*, 255705. [CrossRef]
147. Eyvazzadeh, N.; Shakeri-Zadeh, A.; Fekrazad, R.; Amini, E.; Ghaznavi, H.; Kamran Kamrava, S. Gold-coated magnetic nanoparticle as a nanotheranostic agent for magnetic resonance imaging and photothermal therapy of cancer. *Lasers Med. Sci.* **2017**, *32*, 1469–1477. [CrossRef] [PubMed]
148. Abed, Z.; Beik, J.; Laurent, S.; Eslahi, N.; Khani, T.; Davani, E.S.; Ghaznavi, H.; Shakeri-Zadeh, A. Iron oxide–gold core–shell nano-theranostic for magnetically targeted photothermal therapy under magnetic resonance imaging guidance. *J. Cancer Res. Clin. Oncol.* **2019**, *145*, 1213–1219. [CrossRef]

149. Dong, Q.; Yang, H.; Wan, C.; Zheng, D.; Zhou, Z.; Xie, S.; Xu, L.; Du, J.; Li, F. Her2-Functionalized Gold-Nanoshelled Magnetic Hybrid Nanoparticles: A Theranostic Agent for Dual-Modal Imaging and Photothermal Therapy of Breast Cancer. *Nanoscale Res. Lett.* **2019**, *14*, 235. [CrossRef] [PubMed]
150. Abedin, M.R.; Umapathi, S.; Mahendrakar, H.; Laemthong, T.; Coleman, H.; Muchangi, D.; Santra, S.; Nath, M.; Barua, S. Polymer coated gold-ferric oxide superparamagnetic nanoparticles for theranostic applications. *J. Nanobiotechnol.* **2018**, *16*, 80. [CrossRef] [PubMed]
151. Iturrioz-Rodríguez, N.; Correa-Duarte, M.A.; Fanarraga, M.L. Controlled drug delivery systems for cancer based on mesoporous silica nanoparticles. *Int. J. Nanomed.* **2019**, *14*, 3389–3401. [CrossRef]
152. Yang, Y.; Lin, Y.; Di, D.; Zhang, X.; Wang, D.; Zhao, Q.; Wang, S. Gold nanoparticle-gated mesoporous silica as redox-triggered drug delivery for chemo-photothermal synergistic therapy. *J. Colloid Interface Sci.* **2017**, *508*, 323–331. [CrossRef]
153. Cheng, B.; He, H.; Huang, T.; Berr, S.S.; He, J.; Fan, D.; Zhang, J.; Xu, P. Gold nanosphere gated mesoporous silica nanoparticle responsive to near-infrared light and redox potential as a theranostic platform for cancer therapy. *J. Biomed. Nanotechnol.* **2016**, *12*, 435–449. [CrossRef]
154. Abbasi, E.; Milani, M.; Aval, S.F.; Kouhi, M.; Akbarzadeh, A.; Nasrabadi, H.T.; Nikasa, P.; Joo, S.W.; Hanifehpour, Y.; Nejati-Koshki, K.; et al. Silver nanoparticles: Synthesis methods, bio-applications and properties. *Crit. Rev. Microbiol.* **2016**, *42*, 173–180. [CrossRef] [PubMed]
155. Caro, C.; Castillo, P.M.; Klippstein, R.; Pozo, D.; Zaderenko, A.P. Silver Nanoparticles: Sensing and Imaging Applications. In *Silver Nanoparticles*; IntechOpen: London, UK, 2010. [CrossRef]
156. Yin, I.X.; Zhang, J.; Zhao, I.S.; Mei, M.L.; Li, Q.; Chu, C.H. The antibacterial mechanism of silver nanoparticles and its application in dentistry. *Int. J. Nanomed.* **2020**, *15*, 2555–2562. [CrossRef] [PubMed]
157. Mathur, P.; Jha, S.; Ramteke, S.; Jain, N.K. Pharmaceutical aspects of silver nanoparticles. *Artif. Cells Nanomed. Biotechnol.* **2018**, *46*, 115–126. [CrossRef]
158. Turkevich, J.; Stevenson, P.C.; Hillier, J. A Study of the Nucleation and Growth Processes in the Synthesis of Colloidal Gold. *Discuss. Faraday Soc.* **1951**, *11*, 55–57. [CrossRef]
159. Austin, L.A.; Mackey, M.A.; Dreaden, E.C.; El-Sayed, M.A. The optical, photothermal, and facile surface chemical properties of gold and silver nanoparticles in biodiagnostics, therapy, and drug delivery. *Arch. Toxicol.* **2014**, *88*, 1391–1417. [CrossRef]
160. Mousavi, S.M.; Hashemi, S.A.; Ghasemi, Y.; Atapour, A.; Amani, A.M.; Savar Dashtaki, A.; Babapoor, A.; Arjmand, O. Green synthesis of silver nanoparticles toward bio and medical applications: Review study. *Artif. Cells Nanomed. Biotechnol.* **2018**, *46*, S855–S872. [CrossRef] [PubMed]
161. Dos Santos, C.A.; Seckler, M.M.; Ingle, A.P.; Gupta, I.; Galdiero, S.; Galdiero, M.; Gade, A.; Rai, M. Silver nanoparticles: Therapeutical uses, toxicity, and safety issues. *J. Pharm. Sci.* **2014**, *103*, 1931–1944. [CrossRef]
162. Kim, D.; Amatya, R.; Hwang, S.; Lee, S.; Min, K.A.; Shin, M.C. BSA-silver nanoparticles: A potential multimodal therapeutics for conventional and photothermal treatment of skin cancer. *Pharmaceutics* **2021**, *13*, 575. [CrossRef] [PubMed]
163. Thompson, E.A.; Graham, E.; Macneill, C.M.; Young, M.; Donati, G.; Wailes, E.M.; Jones, B.T.; Levi-Polyachenko, N.H. Differential response of MCF7, MDA-MB-231, and MCF 10A cells to hyperthermia, silver nanoparticles and silver nanoparticle-induced photothermal therapy. *Int. J. Hyperth.* **2014**, *30*, 312–323. [CrossRef]
164. Boca, S.C.; Potara, M.; Gabudean, A.M.; Juhem, A.; Baldeck, P.L.; Astilean, S. Chitosan-coated triangular silver nanoparticles as a novel class of biocompatible, highly effective photothermal transducers for in vitro cancer cell therapy. *Cancer Lett.* **2011**, *311*, 131–140. [CrossRef]
165. Wu, J.; Li, N.; Yao, Y.; Tang, D.; Yang, D.; Ong'Achwa Machuki, J.; Li, J.; Yu, Y.; Gao, F. DNA-Stabilized Silver Nanoclusters for Label-Free Fluorescence Imaging of Cell Surface Glycans and Fluorescence Guided Photothermal Therapy. *Anal. Chem.* **2018**, *90*, 14368–14375. [CrossRef]
166. Park, T.; Lee, S.; Amatya, R.; Cheong, H.; Moon, C.; Kwak, H.D.; Min, K.A.; Shin, M.C. ICG-loaded pegylated BSA-silver nanoparticles for effective photothermal cancer therapy. *Int. J. Nanomed.* **2020**, *15*, 5459–5471. [CrossRef]
167. Negri, V.; Pacheco-Torres, J.; Calle, D.; López-Larrubia, P. Carbon Nanotubes in Biomedicine. *Top. Curr. Chem.* **2020**, *378*, 15. [CrossRef] [PubMed]
168. Sundaram, P.; Abrahamse, H. Phototherapy Combined with Carbon Nanomaterials (1D and 2D) and their Applications in Cancer Therapy. *Materials* **2020**, *13*, 4830. [CrossRef]
169. He, H.; Pham-Huy, L.A.; Dramou, P.; Xiao, D.; Zuo, P.; Pham-Huy, C. Carbon nanotubes: Applications in pharmacy and medicine. *BioMed Res. Int.* **2013**, *2013*, 578290. [CrossRef]
170. Dong, J.; Ma, Q. Integration of inflammation, fibrosis, and cancer induced by carbon nanotubes. *Nanotoxicology* **2019**, *13*, 1244–1274. [CrossRef] [PubMed]
171. Hendler-Neumark, A.; Bisker, G. Fluorescent single-walled carbon nanotubes for protein detection. *Sensors* **2019**, *19*, 5403. [CrossRef] [PubMed]
172. Malarkey, E.B.; Parpura, V. Carbon nanotubes in neuroscience. *Acta Neurochir. Suppl.* **2009**, *106*, 337–341. [CrossRef]
173. Gong, H.; Peng, R.; Liu, Z. Carbon nanotubes for biomedical imaging: The recent advances. *Adv. Drug Deliv. Rev.* **2013**, *65*, 1951–1963. [CrossRef]
174. Sobhani, Z.; Behnam, M.A.; Emami, F.; Dehghanian, A.; Jamhiri, I. Photothermal therapy of melanoma tumor using multiwalled carbon nanotubes. *Int. J. Nanomed.* **2017**, *12*, 4509–4517. [CrossRef] [PubMed]

175. Iancu, C.; Mocan, L. Advances in cancer therapy through the use of carbon nanotube-mediated targeted hyperthermia. *Int. J. Nanomed.* **2011**, *6*, 1675–1684. [CrossRef] [PubMed]
176. Kam, N.W.S.; O'Connell, M.; Wisndon, J.A.; Dai, H. Carbon nanotubes as multifunctional biological transporters and near-infrared agents for selective cancer cell destruction. *Proc. Natl. Acad. Sci. USA* **2005**, *102*, 11600–11605. [CrossRef] [PubMed]
177. Singh, R.; Torti, S.V. Carbon nanotubes in hyperthermia therapy. *Adv. Drug Deliv. Rev.* **2013**, *65*, 2045–2060. [CrossRef]
178. Li, H.; Zhang, N.; Hao, Y.; Wang, Y.; Jia, S.; Zhang, H. Enhancement of curcumin antitumor efficacy and further photothermal ablation of tumor growth by single-walled carbon nanotubes delivery system in vivo. *Drug Deliv.* **2019**, *26*, 1017–1026. [CrossRef] [PubMed]
179. Waghray, D.; Zhang, Q. Inhibit or Evade Multidrug Resistance P-Glycoprotein in Cancer Treatment. *J. Med. Chem.* **2018**, *61*, 5108–5121. [CrossRef]
180. Zhang, P.; Yi, W.; Hou, J.; Yoo, S.; Jin, W.; Yang, Q. A carbon nanotube-gemcitabine-lentinan three-component composite for chemo-photothermal synergistic therapy of cancer. *Int. J. Nanomed.* **2018**, *13*, 3069–3080. [CrossRef]
181. Zhao, Y.; Zhao, T.; Cao, Y.; Sun, J.; Zhou, Q.; Chen, H.; Guo, S.; Wang, Y.; Zhen, Y.; Liang, X.J.; et al. Temperature-Sensitive Lipid-Coated Carbon Nanotubes for Synergistic Photothermal Therapy and Gene Therapy. *ACS Nano* **2021**, *15*, 6517–6529. [CrossRef]
182. Cano-Mejia, J.; Shukla, A.; Ledezma, D.K.; Palmer, E.; Villagra, A.; Fernandes, R. CpG-coated Prussian blue nanoparticles-based photothermal therapy combined with anti-CTLA-4 immune checkpoint blockade triggers a robust abscopal effect against neuroblastoma. *Transl. Oncol.* **2020**, *13*, 100823. [CrossRef]
183. Ngwa, W.; Irabor, O.C.; Schoenfeld, J.D.; Hesser, J.; Demaria, S.; Formenti, S.C. Using immunotherapy to boost the abscopal effect. *Nat. Rev. Cancer* **2018**, *18*, 313–322. [CrossRef]
184. Das, M.; Zhu, C.; Kuchroo, V.K. Tim-3 and its role in regulating anti-tumor immunity HHS Public Access. *Physiol. Behav.* **2016**, *176*, 100–106. [CrossRef]
185. Alsaab, H.O.; Sau, S.; Alzhrani, R.; Tatiparti, K.; Bhise, K.; Kashaw, S.K.; Iyer, A.K. PD-1 and PD-L1 checkpoint signaling inhibition for cancer immunotherapy: Mechanism, combinations, and clinical outcome. *Front. Pharmacol.* **2017**, *8*, 561. [CrossRef]
186. Maruhashi, T.; Sugiura, D.; Okazaki, I.M.; Okazaki, T. LAG-3: From molecular functions to clinical applications. *J. Immunother. Cancer* **2020**, *8*, e001014. [CrossRef] [PubMed]
187. Brunner-Weinzierl, M.C.; Rudd, C.E. CTLA-4 and PD-1 control of T-cell motility and migration: Implications for tumor immunotherapy. *Front. Immunol.* **2018**, *9*, 2737. [CrossRef] [PubMed]
188. Nakamura, Y. Biomarkers for immune checkpoint inhibitor-mediated tumor response and adverse events. *Front. Med.* **2019**, *6*, 119. [CrossRef] [PubMed]
189. Li, Y.; Li, X.; Doughty, A.; West, C.; Wang, L.; Zhou, F.; Nordquist, R.E.; Chen, W.R. Phototherapy using immunologically modified carbon nanotubes to potentiate checkpoint blockade for metastatic breast cancer. *Nanomed. Nanotechnol. Biol. Med.* **2019**, *18*, 44–53. [CrossRef]
190. McKernan, P.; Virani, N.A.; Faria, G.N.F.; Karch, C.G.; Prada Silvy, R.; Resasco, D.E.; Thompson, L.F.; Harrison, R.G. Targeted Single-Walled Carbon Nanotubes for Photothermal Therapy Combined with Immune Checkpoint Inhibition for the Treatment of Metastatic Breast Cancer. *Nanoscale Res. Lett.* **2021**, *16*, 9. [CrossRef]
191. Wang, L.; Sun, Q.; Wang, X.; Wen, T.; Yin, J.J.; Wang, P.; Bai, R.; Zhang, X.Q.; Zhang, L.H.; Lu, A.H.; et al. Using hollow carbon nanospheres as a light-induced free radical generator to overcome chemotherapy resistance. *J. Am. Chem. Soc.* **2015**, *137*, 1947–1955. [CrossRef]
192. Li, X.; Liu, C.; Wang, S.; Jiao, J.; Di, D.; Jiang, T.; Zhao, Q.; Wang, S. Poly(acrylic acid) conjugated hollow mesoporous carbon as a dual-stimuli triggered drug delivery system for chemo-photothermal synergistic therapy. *Mater. Sci. Eng. C* **2017**, *71*, 594–603. [CrossRef]
193. Du, X.; Zhao, C.; Zhou, M.; Ma, T.; Huang, H.; Jaroniec, M.; Zhang, X.; Qiao, S.Z. Hollow Carbon Nanospheres with Tunable Hierarchical Pores for Drug, Gene, and Photothermal Synergistic Treatment. *Small* **2017**, *13*, 1602592. [CrossRef]
194. Wang, X.; Liu, Y.; Liu, Z.; Hu, J.; Guo, H.; Wang, F. Synergistic chemo-photothermal therapy of tumor by hollow carbon nanospheres. *Biochem. Biophys. Res. Commun.* **2018**, *495*, 867–872. [CrossRef]
195. Xu, Z.; Zhang, Y.; Zhou, W.; Wang, L.; Xu, G.; Ma, M.; Liu, F.; Wang, Z.; Wang, Y.; Kong, T.; et al. NIR-II-activated biocompatible hollow nanocarbons for cancer photothermal therapy. *J. Nanobiotechnol.* **2021**, *19*, 137. [CrossRef]
196. Estelrich, J.; Antònia Busquets, M. Iron oxide nanoparticles in photothermal therapy. *Molecules* **2018**, *23*, 1567. [CrossRef]
197. Vangijzegem, T.; Stanicki, D.; Laurent, S. Magnetic iron oxide nanoparticles for drug delivery: Applications and characteristics. *Expert Opin. Drug Deliv.* **2019**, *16*, 69–78. [CrossRef] [PubMed]
198. Alphandéry, E. Bio-synthesized iron oxide nanoparticles for cancer treatment. *Int. J. Pharm.* **2020**, *586*, 119472. [CrossRef]
199. Cabana, S.; Curcio, A.; Michel, A.; Wilhelm, C.; Abou-Hassan, A. Iron oxide mediated photothermal therapy in the second biological window: A comparative study between magnetite/maghemite nanospheres and nanoflowers. *Nanomaterials* **2020**, *10*, 1548. [CrossRef] [PubMed]
200. Liu, Q.; Liu, L.; Mo, C.; Zhou, X.; Chen, D.; He, Y.; He, H.; Kang, W.; Zhao, Y.; Jin, G. Polyethylene glycol-coated ultrasmall superparamagnetic iron oxide nanoparticles-coupled sialyl Lewis X nanotheranostic platform for nasopharyngeal carcinoma imaging and photothermal therapy. *J. Nanobiotechnol.* **2021**, *19*, 171. [CrossRef]

201. Zhu, L.; Zhou, Z.; Mao, H.; Yang, L. Magnetic nanoparticles for precision oncology: Theranostic magnetic iron oxide nanoparticles for image-guided and targeted cancer therapy. *Nanomedicine* **2017**, *12*, 73–87. [CrossRef] [PubMed]
202. Soetaert, F.; Korangath, P.; Serantes, D.; Fiering, S.; Ivkov, R. Cancer therapy with iron oxide nanoparticles: Agents of thermal and immune therapies. *Adv. Drug Deliv. Rev.* **2020**, *163–164*, 65–83. [CrossRef]
203. Wang, Y.; Li, X.; Chen, P.; Dong, Y.; Liang, G.; Yu, Y. Enzyme-instructed self-aggregation of Fe_3O_4 nanoparticles for enhanced MRI T 2 imaging and photothermal therapy of tumors. *Nanoscale* **2020**, *12*, 1886–1893. [CrossRef] [PubMed]
204. Rao, L.; Xu, J.H.; Cai, B.; Liu, H.; Li, M.; Jia, Y.; Xiao, L.; Guo, S.S.; Liu, W.; Zhao, X.Z. Synthetic nanoparticles camouflaged with biomimetic erythrocyte membranes for reduced reticuloendothelial system uptake. *Nanotechnology* **2016**, *27*, 85106. [CrossRef]
205. Meng, Q.F.; Rao, L.; Zan, M.; Chen, M.; Yu, G.T.; Wei, X.; Wu, Z.; Sun, Y.; Guo, S.S.; Zhao, X.Z.; et al. Macrophage membrane-coated iron oxide nanoparticles for enhanced photothermal tumor therapy. *Nanotechnology* **2018**, *29*, 134004. [CrossRef]
206. Bano, S.; Nazir, S.; Nazir, A.; Munir, S.; Mahmood, T.; Afzal, M.; Ansari, F.L.; Mazhar, K. Microwave-assisted green synthesis of superparamagnetic nanoparticles using fruit peel extracts: Surface engineering, T2relaxometry, and photodynamic treatment potential. *Int. J. Nanomed.* **2016**, *11*, 3833–3848. [CrossRef] [PubMed]
207. Kharey, P.; Dutta, S.B.; Manikandan, M.; Palani, I.A.; Majumder, S.K.; Gupta, S. Green synthesis of near-infrared absorbing eugenate capped iron oxide nanoparticles for photothermal application. *Nanotechnology* **2019**, *31*, 095705. [CrossRef] [PubMed]
208. Zhang, F.; Lu, G.; Wen, X.; Li, F.; Ji, X.; Li, Q.; Wu, M.; Cheng, Q.; Yu, Y.; Tang, J.; et al. Magnetic nanoparticles coated with polyphenols for spatio-temporally controlled cancer photothermal/immunotherapy. *J. Control. Release* **2020**, *326*, 131–139. [CrossRef]
209. Ashkbar, A.; Rezaei, F.; Attari, F.; Ashkevarian, S. Treatment of breast cancer in vivo by dual photodynamic and photothermal approaches with the aid of curcumin photosensitizer and magnetic nanoparticles. *Sci. Rep.* **2020**, *10*, 21206. [CrossRef] [PubMed]
210. Ailioaie, L.M.; Litscher, G. Curcumin and photobiomodulation in chronic viral hepatitis and hepatocellular carcinoma. *Int. J. Mol. Sci.* **2020**, *21*, 7150. [CrossRef]
211. Cai, X.; Zhu, Q.; Zeng, Y.; Zeng, Q.; Chen, X.; Zhan, Y. Manganese oxide nanoparticles as mri contrast agents in tumor multimodal imaging and therapy. *Int. J. Nanomed.* **2019**, *14*, 8321–8344. [CrossRef]
212. Xiang, Y.; Li, N.; Guo, L.; Wang, H.; Sun, H.; Li, R.; Ma, L.; Qi, Y.; Zhan, J.; Yu, D. Biocompatible and pH-sensitive MnO-loaded carbonaceous nanospheres (MnO@CNSs): A theranostic agent for magnetic resonance imaging-guided photothermal therapy. *Carbon* **2018**, *136*, 113–124. [CrossRef]
213. Odda, A.H.; Xu, Y.; Lin, J.; Wang, G.; Ullah, N.; Zeb, A.; Liang, K.; Wen, L.P.; Xu, A.W. Plasmonic MoO_3-x nanoparticles incorporated in Prussian blue frameworks exhibit highly efficient dual photothermal/photodynamic therapy. *J. Mater. Chem. B* **2019**, *7*, 2032–2042. [CrossRef]
214. Chen, Y.; Khan, A.R.; Yu, D.; Zhai, Y.; Ji, J.; Shi, Y.; Zhai, G. Pluronic F127-functionalized molybdenum oxide nanosheets with pH-dependent degradability for chemo-photothermal cancer therapy. *J. Colloid Interface Sci.* **2019**, *553*, 567–580. [CrossRef]
215. Zhang, Y.; Nayak, T.R.; Hong, H.; Cai, W. Biomedical applications of zinc oxide nanomaterials. *Curr. Mol. Med.* **2013**, *13*, 1633–1645. [CrossRef]
216. Kolodziejczak-Radzimska, A.; Jesionowski, T. Zinc oxide-from synthesis to application: A review. *Materials* **2014**, *7*, 2833–2881. [CrossRef]
217. Vasuki, K.; Manimekalai, R. NIR light active ternary modified ZnO nanocomposites for combined cancer therapy. *Heliyon* **2019**, *5*, e02729. [CrossRef]
218. Kim, S.; Lee, S.Y.; Cho, H.J. Berberine and zinc oxide-based nanoparticles for the chemo-photothermal therapy of lung adenocarcinoma. *Biochem. Biophys. Res. Commun.* **2018**, *501*, 765–770. [CrossRef] [PubMed]
219. Liu, M.; Peng, Y.; Nie, Y.; Liu, P.; Hu, S.; Ding, J.; Zhou, W. Co-delivery of doxorubicin and DNAzyme using ZnO@polydopamine core-shell nanocomposites for chemo/gene/photothermal therapy. *Acta Biomater.* **2020**, *110*, 242–253. [CrossRef]
220. Li, S.; Tan, L.; Xu, W.; Liu, C.; Wu, Q.; Fu, C.; Meng, X.; Shao, H. Doxorubicin-loaded layered MoS_2 hollow spheres and its photothermo-chemotherapy on hepatocellular carcinoma. *J. Biomed. Nanotechnol.* **2017**, *13*, 1557–1564. [CrossRef] [PubMed]
221. Liu, T.; Wang, C.; Gu, X.; Gong, H.; Cheng, L.; Shi, X.; Feng, L.; Sun, B.; Liu, Z. Drug delivery with PEGylated MoS_2 nano-sheets for combined photothermal and chemotherapy of cancer. *Adv. Mater.* **2014**, *26*, 3433–3440. [CrossRef] [PubMed]
222. Xie, M.; Yang, N.; Cheng, J.; Yang, M.; Deng, T.; Li, Y.; Feng, C. Layered MoS_2 nanosheets modified by biomimetic phospholipids: Enhanced stability and its synergistic treatment of cancer with chemo-photothermal therapy. *Coll. Surf. B Biointerfaces* **2020**, *187*, 110631. [CrossRef]
223. Ding, L.; Chang, Y.; Yang, P.; Gao, W.; Sun, M.; Bie, Y.; Yang, L.; Ma, X.; Guo, Y. Facile synthesis of biocompatible L-cysteine-modified MoS_2 nanospheres with high photothermal conversion efficiency for photothermal therapy of tumor. *Mater. Sci. Eng. C* **2020**, *117*, 111371. [CrossRef]
224. Qian, X.; Shen, S.; Liu, T.; Cheng, L.; Liu, Z. Two-dimensional TiS_2 nanosheets for in vivo photoacoustic imaging and photothermal cancer therapy. *Nanoscale* **2015**, *7*, 6380–6387. [CrossRef]
225. Cao, C.; Zhang, J.; Yang, C.; Xiang, L.; Liu, W. Albumin exfoliated titanium disulfide nanosheet: A multifunctional nanoplatform for synergistic photothermal/radiation colon cancer therapy. *Onco Targets Ther.* **2019**, *12*, 6337–6347. [CrossRef]
226. Xu, Y.; Wang, X.; Zhang, W.L.; Lv, F.; Guo, S. Recent progress in two-dimensional inorganic quantum dots. *Chem. Soc. Rev.* **2018**, *47*, 586–625. [CrossRef] [PubMed]

227. Fang, J.; Liu, Y.; Chen, Y.; Ouyang, D.; Yang, G.; Yu, T. Graphene quantum dots-gated hollow mesoporous carbon nanoplatform for targeting drug delivery and synergistic chemo-photothermal therapy. *Int. J. Nanomed.* **2018**, *13*, 5991–6007. [CrossRef]
228. Šavija, B.; Zhang, H.; Schlangen, E. Influence of microencapsulated phase change material (PCM) addition on (micro) mechanical properties of cement paste. *Materials* **2017**, *10*, 863. [CrossRef] [PubMed]
229. Yuan, Y.; Zhang, N.; Tao, W.; Cao, X.; He, Y. Fatty acids as phase change materials: A review. *Renew. Sustain. Energy Rev.* **2014**, *29*, 482–498. [CrossRef]
230. Yuan, Z.; Qu, S.; He, Y.; Xu, Y.; Liang, L.; Zhou, X.; Gui, L.; Gu, Y.; Chen, H. Thermosensitive drug-loading system based on copper sulfide nanoparticles for combined photothermal therapy and chemotherapy in vivo. *Biomater. Sci.* **2018**, *6*, 3219–3230. [CrossRef] [PubMed]
231. Khurana, A.; Tekula, S.; Saifi, M.A.; Venkatesh, P.; Godugu, C. Therapeutic applications of selenium nanoparticles. *Biomed. Pharmacother.* **2019**, *111*, 802–812. [CrossRef]
232. Fang, X.; Li, C.; Zheng, L.; Yang, F.; Chen, T. Dual-Targeted Selenium Nanoparticles for Synergistic Photothermal Therapy and Chemotherapy of Tumors. *Chem.—Asian J.* **2018**, *13*, 996–1004. [CrossRef]
233. Mohammadi, S.; Soratijahromi, E.; Dehdari, V.R.; Sattarahmady, N. Phototherapy and sonotherapy of melanoma cancer cells using nanoparticles of selenium-polyethylene glycol-curcumin as a dual-mode sensitizer. *J. Biomed. Phys. Eng.* **2020**, *10*, 597–606. [CrossRef]

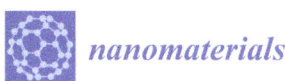

Article

Spiky Gold Nanoparticles for the Photothermal Eradication of Colon Cancer Cells

Paolo Emidio Costantini [1,†], Matteo Di Giosia [2,†], Luca Ulfo [1], Annapaola Petrosino [1], Roberto Saporetti [2], Carmela Fimognari [3], Pier Paolo Pompa [4], Alberto Danielli [1], Eleonora Turrini [3,*], Luca Boselli [4,*] and Matteo Calvaresi [2,*]

[1] Dipartimento di Farmacia e Biotecnologie, Alma Mater Studiorum—Università di Bologna, Via Francesco Selmi 3, 40126 Bologna, Italy; paolo.costantini4@unibo.it (P.E.C.); luca.ulfo2@unibo.it (L.U.); annapaola.petrosino2@unibo.it (A.P.); alberto.danielli@unibo.it (A.D.)
[2] Dipartimento di Chimica "Giacomo Ciamician", Alma Mater Studiorum—Università di Bologna, Via Francesco Selmi 2, 40126 Bologna, Italy; matteo.digiosia2@unibo.it (M.D.G.); roberto.saporetti2@unibo.it (R.S.)
[3] Dipartimento di Scienze per la Qualità della Vita, Alma Mater Studiorum—Università di Bologna, Corso d'Augusto 237, 47921 Rimini, Italy; carmela.fimognari@unibo.it
[4] Nanobiointeractions and Nanodiagnostics, Istituto Italiano di Tecnologia, Via Morego 30, 16163 Genova, Italy; pierpaolo.pompa@iit.it
* Correspondence: eleonora.turrini@unibo.it (E.T.); luca.boselli@iit.it (L.B.); matteo.calvaresi3@unibo.it (M.C.)
† These authors equally contributed to this work.

Abstract: Colorectal cancer (CRC) is a widespread and lethal disease. Relapses of the disease and metastasis are very common in instances of CRC, so adjuvant therapies have a crucial role in its treatment. Systemic toxic effects and the development of resistance during therapy limit the long-term efficacy of existing adjuvant therapeutic approaches. Consequently, the search for alternative strategies is necessary. Photothermal therapy (PTT) represents an innovative treatment for cancer with great potential. Here, we synthesize branched gold nanoparticles (BGNPs) as attractive agents for the photothermal eradication of colon cancer cells. By controlling the NP growth process, large absorption in the first NIR biological window was obtained. The FBS dispersed BGNPs are stable in physiological-like environments and show an extremely efficient light-to-heat conversion capability when irradiated with an 808-nm laser. Sequential cycles of heating and cooling do not affect the BGNP stability. The uptake of BGNPs in colon cancer cells was confirmed using flow cytometry and confocal microscopy, exploiting their intrinsic optical properties. In dark conditions, BGNPs are fully biocompatible and do not compromise cell viability, while an almost complete eradication of colon cancer cells was observed upon incubation with BGNPs and irradiation with an 808-nm laser source. The PTT treatment is characterized by an extremely rapid onset of action that leads to cell membrane rupture by induced hyperthermia, which is the trigger that promotes cancer cell death.

Keywords: photothermal therapy; gold nanoparticles; spiky nanoparticles; phototheranostics; colon cancer cells; NIR triggering

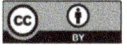

1. Introduction

Colorectal cancer (CRC) is one of the major causes of cancer-related death [1]. Nearly two million new cases and about one million deaths are expected each year worldwide, with an increasing trend in CRC incidence, especially in more economically developed countries [1].

CRC is commonly treated by surgery; however, up to half of patients diagnosed with early-stage CRC experience recurrent disease after a surgical resection and may also develop a metastatic disease. As such, neoadjuvant and adjuvant therapies have a crucial role against CRC [2]. These include chemotherapy, radiotherapy, interventional therapy, and biotherapy [2,3]. Unfortunately, systemic toxic effects, which impair the patient quality of life, and the development of resistance during therapy limit the long-term efficacy of these therapeutic approaches, especially in metastatic cases. A search for alternatives is both timely and necessary in this case.

Thermal ablation and laser-induced thermotherapy are techniques that potentially address these issues [4,5]. These are localized physical treatments that use hyperthermia to damage and kill cancers cells and tumorous tissues and that do not develop resistance in cells [5]. Clinical trials are in progress to evaluate their safety and efficacy and additionally the treatment of metastatic CRC [6].

Similar to the heat-mediated cytotoxicity observed in thermal ablation and in laser-induced thermotherapy, photothermal therapy (PTT) represents an innovative treatment for cancer with great potential [7,8]. The procedure for PTT is based on accumulation of photosensitive molecules/nanoparticles in cancer cells, followed by light irradiation of the target tissue [9]. The irradiation with the appropriate wavelength (usually near-infrared (NIR) light) promotes photosensitizer activation from the ground state to any of their excited states. When they relax back to the ground state via non-radiative de-excitation, the energy dissipation causes a localized release of heat that causes severe damage to nearby cells and tissues [9]. In PTT, the intracellular temperature of cancer cells easily exceeds 50 °C, resulting in rapid cell death [9]. Compared to the traditional treatment methods, PTT has significant advantages including the use of soft and penetrating irradiation sources to activate the photothermal agent (NIR light) and lower collateral damage to healthy tissues because it is possible to focus the irradiation at the desired (localized) site of action.

Gold nanoparticles (GNPs), characterized by a very high light-to-heat conversion efficiency, are among the most important photothermal agents for PTT [9,10] and have shown remarkable results in recent years. Examples include cancer treatments (solid tumor ablation) reaching the clinical trial stage [11], suggesting promise for future applications [12–14]. The unique size and shape-dependent optical properties of GNPs, based on the localized surface plasmon resonance (LSPR) phenomenon, allow for tunable and intense absorption cross-sections and a consequent photothermal conversion ability. According to their size, GNPs present an extinction coefficient up to five order of magnitude larger than other molecular dyes commonly employed in PTT [15–17]. Among other shapes, anisotropic GNPs exist in rod-like, [18,19] prism-like, [19–21] and more recently branched (spiky) nanostructures [22–25], whose geometrical features can be controlled to obtain the LSPR in the near-infrared (NIR) spectrum and appear to be particularly promising due to superior light tissue penetration of NIR light [26].

Branched GNPs (BGNPs) present several advantages. These advantages include the lack of a need to involve highly toxic reagents in the synthesis process (i.e., CTAB, commonly employed for rods), and their complex nanostructure discloses a wider choice of shape-dependent biological and optical properties, which can be carefully tailored by controlling the NPs growth process to obtain the desired average length, width, and tip density, as well as the proper dimension of the central core [27–30]. Changing these parameters not only leads to a spectral shift in the LSPR but also to the modification of their absorption efficiency. While tuning the tip length (and the core-to-tip size ratio) allows modulating the absorption wavelength, the tip density, and the core size mainly impact the LSPR intensity. Here, BGNPs were designed for effective absorbance of NIR light, which is an attractive energy source because human tissues and blood are minimally absorptive in these wavelengths. NIR lasers and fiber optics, which represent minimally invasive and versatile energy delivery systems, are already commercially available, allowing an easy translation to the clinic of NIR based PTT. In the NIR region, two biological windows, i.e., spectral ranges where tissues are partially transparent due to a simultaneous reduction in both absorption and scattering, can be defined. The first biological window (I-BW) extends from 650 nm to 950 nm and corresponds to the spectral range delimited by the absorption of hemoglobin and water. The second biological window (II-BW) extends from 1000 nm to 1350 nm and it is limited by water absorption bands. The I-BW region is characterized by a negligible absorption from tissue and the photothermal agents represent the sole heating sources. In the II-BW window, water absorbs in the whole range, generating background heating upon irradiation, leading to a reduced PPT selectivity and efficiency.

In this work, we design and synthesize highly photostable BGNPs that can be strongly absorbed in the first biological window (I-BW). We develop protocols to ensure the colloidal stability of the BGNPs under physiological conditions and evaluate the BGNP photothermal conversion ability upon irradiation with an 808-nm laser light source. The applicative potential of BGNPs is tested in vitro against a well-established colon cancer cell line, using in vivo-like protein concentration conditions. Hereafter, the biocompatibility, cellular uptake, and ability of the BGNPs to eradicate colon cancer cells following PTT treatment are described.

2. Materials and Methods

2.1. Materials

All chemicals and reagents employed were of the highest technical grade available and stored following the vendor recommendations. Hydrogen tetrachloroaurate(III) hydrate ($\geq$99.9%, Alfa Aesar, Haverhill, MA, USA, 42803), trisodium citrate trihydrate ReagentPlus® ($\geq$99%, SigmaAldrich, St. Louis, MO, USA, 25114), hydroquinone (SigmaAldrich, 605970), and O-(2-carboxyethyl)-O'-(2-mercaptoethyl) heptaethylene glycol (SigmaAldrich, 672688) were used. A PVC calibration standard at 483 nm (PVC000476) was purchased from Analytik Ltd. (Cambridge, UK).

2.2. Synthesis and Characterization of BGNPs

The BGNP colloidal suspension was prepared by slightly modifying previously reported methods [27,31,32]. Briefly, 15-nm gold seeds were first synthesized by adding 4.5 mL of trisodium citrate (34 mM, 0.15 mmol) to 150 mL of $HAuCl_4 \cdot 3H_2O$ (0.038 mmol, 0.25 mM) in a boiling solution. After 30 min, the mixture was let cooled to RT, stirred overnight, and filtered through 0.2-µm syringe filters.

Then, 120 µL of $HAuCl_4 \cdot 3H_2O$ (95 mM), 72 µL of the prepared seeds, 280 µL of trisodium citrate (34 mM), and 280 µL of hydroquinone (140 mM) were subsequently added to 96 mL of ultraclean deionized H_2O under vigorous stirring. After 2 min, 30 µL of O-(2-carboxyethyl)-O'-(2-mercaptoethyl) heptaethylene glycol was added to the colloidal suspension and the mixture was stirred for 6 h. The pegylated BGNPs were finally filtered through 0.4-µm syringe filters and purified from the free ligands by several washing cycles using centrifugal filters.

2.3. UV–Vis–NIR Absorption Spectroscopy

BGNP absorption spectra were examined with a Varian Cary5000 using a 1 cm path length with Hellma quartz cells, measuring in the 400–1200 nm range. Stability tests in serum were performed with a Thermo Fisher NanoDrop® (350–900 nm range) instrument using small-volume PMMA disposable cuvettes (Sarstedt, Nümbrecht, Germany). The samples were diluted prior to analysis to obtain an absorbance of $\leq$1.

2.4. Dynamic Light Scattering (DLS) Analysis

BGNP sample analysis was performed using a Zetasizer Nano Range (Malvern, Worcestershire, UK) instrument and the reported values are an average of three independent measurements (each consisting of an accumulation of 11 runs).

2.5. Differential Centrifugal Sedimentation (DCS) Analysis

The analysis was carried out using the CPS DC24000 UHR ultrahigh resolution particle analyzer (CPS Instrument Inc., Prairieville, LA, USA). DCS measurements were performed using 8–24% sucrose density gradient in ultraclean deionized water (or in PBS when measuring BGNPs stability in FBS) with a disc speed of 18,000 rpm. PVC standard particles (0.483 µm, Analytik Ltd., Jena, Germany) were employed to calibrate the instrument before each sample measurement.

2.6. Transmission Electron Microscopy (TEM) Analysis

The samples were prepared by drop casting 1 µL of a BGNP suspension on a formvar-coated copper grid cleaned with oxygen plasma (200 mesh, Ted Pella, Redding, CA, USA) and were left to dry in air for 2 h. A JEOL JEM 1400 microscope (JEOL, Tokyo, Japan) operating at 120 kV was employed for imaging. The images were analyzed using ImageJ to estimate the mean BGNP diameter (average of the longest tip-to-tip distance).

2.7. Inductively Coupled Plasma (ICP-OES) Elemental Analysis

ICP elemental analysis was performed by inductively coupled plasma optical emission spectroscopy (ICP-OES) using a ThermoScientific (Waltham, MA, USA) iCAP 6300 DUO ICP-OES spectrometer. Chemical analyses by ICP-OES are affected by a systematic error of 5%. Furthermore, 30–50 µL of a BGNP sample was dissolved overnight in 1 mL of aqua regia and then diluted to 10 mL with ultraclean deionized water before analysis.

2.8. BGNPs-Biomolecular Corona Preparation

Next, 50 µL of BGNP stock solution (2.5 mM Au^0) was diluted with 250 µL of fetal bovine serum (FBS) and gently mixed by pipetting. Then, 200 µL of the RPMI cell medium was added to the mixture, obtaining a final concentration of 0.25 mM Au^0 of BGNPs in 50% fetal bovine serum (FBS). Following this, 1% L-glutamine at 200 mM and 1% penicillin/streptomycin solution at 100 U/mL were added for in vitro experiments. The mixture was then incubated at 37 °C under continuous shaking (700 rpm) for 1 h (ThermoMixer HC, S8012-0000; STARLAB, Hamburg, Germany).

2.9. Cell Culture

The authenticated colorectal cancer cells (DLD1) were obtained from LGC Standards (Teddington, Middlesex, United Kingdom), grown in adhesion, and propagated in a RPMI 1640 medium supplemented with 10% heat-inactivated fetal bovine serum (FBS), 1% L-glutamine 200 mM, and 1% penicillin/streptomycin solution 100 U/mL (all purchased by Euroclone, Pero, Italy). Cells were maintained at 37 °C in a humified atmosphere containing 5% CO_2.

2.10. Instrumental Setup for Photothermal Measurements

The photothermal performances of BGNPs were evaluated by measuring the temperature increase during NIR laser irradiation on 96-well plate. A fully automated experimental setup in collaboration with Crisel Instruments (Rome, Italy), integrating a (i) NIR laser source, (ii) XY micropositioning stage, and (iii) thermal camera, was used to perform the treatment.

2.10.1. NIR Laser Source

CW fiber-coupled infrared diode lasers (MDL-F-808; CNI Optoelectronics; Changchun, China) with a nominal power of 2.2 W and emission wavelength of 808 nm were used. A multimode fiber with a core diameter of 400 µm was used to couple the laser with a collimating spherical lens (FOC-01-B, CNI Optoelectronics; Changchun, China), producing a spot size of 6.5 mm at a distance of 10 cm, matching the single well diameter (for 96-well plate). The laser irradiation comes from the top and is perpendicular to the multiwell plate.

2.10.2. XY Micropositioning Stage

The positioning of the plate under the laser spot was performed using the XY micropositioning OptiScan® stage (Prior Scientific, Cambridge, UK), including the XY stage, controller, joystick, and plate holder. The stage was remotely controlled with the Micromanager control software.

2.10.3. Thermal Camera

Real-time temperature changes were recorded by thermal images acquired with an Optris Xi 400 camera (Optris, Berlin, Germany) coupled with a 18° × 14° lens (f = 20 mm) at a framerate of 27 Hz. Data acquisition and analysis were performed with Optrix PIX Connect software.

2.11. Photothermal Treatment in Phantom System

The light to heat conversion performances of the BGNPs were evaluated using the abovementioned integrated setup. Volumes of 200 µL of the different solutions was used to carry out all the PTT measurements. Different concentrations of BGNPs (0.25, 0.1, 0.05, 0.025 mM Au^0) were prepared by diluting the stock solution with milliQ water.

2.12. Cell Treatment

About 15,000 cells were seeded in each well in a 96-well plate. After overnight incubation, cells were treated with FBS-dispersed BGNPs for 24 h. Cells were washed twice with RPMI supplemented with 50% FBS in order to remove free BGNPs, and then were irradiated with an 808 nm NIR laser at 3.3 and 6.6 W cm^{-2} for 1 or 3 min. At the end of irradiation, the medium was removed and cells were incubated for 3, 6, or 24 h according to experimental exigences for the analysis.

2.13. BGNP Uptake by Flow Cytometry

After 24 h of BGNP exposure, cells were trypsinized, centrifuged at 1200 rpm for 5 min, and resuspended with PBS for the uptake analysis via flow cytometry. A side scattering setting associated with a 488-nm excitation laser was used to detect BGNPs uptake [33,34]. The median fold-increase was used to quantify the SSC of BGNP-treated cells compared to not treated cells. All the flow cytometric analyses were performed using an EasyCyte 6-2L (Guava Technologies, Merck, Darmstadt, Germany) instrument. At least 10,000 events were evaluated for each analyzed sample.

2.14. BGNP Uptake by Confocal Microscopy

Following the cell treatment, cells were fixed on 12-mm glass coverslips with 4% paraformaldehyde (PFA) in PBS for 15 min at RT, then washed three times with PBS. The coverslips were mounted with an antifade mounting medium (vectashield H-1000, Vector Laboratories, Burlingame, CA, USA) on a glass microscopy slide. Images were acquired by a confocal microscope (Leica SP8 TCS, Leica Microsystems GmbH, Wetzlar, Germany) with 63× and 100× oil immersion objectives. Z-stacks were acquired by using a 1024 × 1024 scan format and 400 msec speed.

2.15. Cell Viability and Analysis of Cell Death Mechanism

To assess DLD1 viability, a MTT test was performed. Briefly, after cell treatment with BGNPs and 24 h after irradiation, the media were removed from each well and cells were incubated with a 0.5 mg/mL MTT solution for 90 min at 37 °C with 5% CO_2. At the end of the incubation, the MTT solution was removed and formazan salts were dissolved in 100 µL of DMSO. The absorbance was measured at 570 nm using an EnSpire multimode microplate reader (Perkin Elmer, Waltham, MA, USA). To investigate if the recorded cytotoxic effects were triggered by regulated mechanisms, such as the apoptotic cell death, the Guava Nexin Reagent (Merck, Dramstadt, Germany) was used while containing 7-aminoactinomycin (7-AAD) and annexin V-phycoerythrin. Early events in regulated cell death are characterized by the exposure of phosphatidylserine on the cell membrane, whose integrity remains preserved. Exposed phosphatidylserine is detected by the binding protein annexin V. On the contrary, necrotic cells suffer from the loss of membrane integrity, resulting in being permeable to the dye 7-AAD, which is a DNA intercalator. Accordingly, by using the Guava Nexin Reagent it is possible to distinguish three cell populations, i.e., (i) living cells (annexin V −/7-AAD −), (ii) cells undergoing early phases of regulated cell death (annexin

V +/7-AAD −), (iii) and necrotic cells (annexin V +/7-AAD +). Cell viability was analyzed at 3, 6, and 24 h post-irradiation. According to manufacturer instructions, 2×10^4 cells were stained with the reagent for 20 min in the dark at room temperature and analyzed via flow cytometry.

2.16. Statistical Analyses

Results are expressed as the mean ± SEM of at least three independent experiments. The analysis of variance for reported measures and Bonferroni as posttest were used. The statistical software GraphPad InStat 5.0 version (GraphPad Prism, San Diego, CA, USA) was used. In this work, $p < 0.05$ was considered significant.

3. Results and Discussion

3.1. Synthesis and Characterization of BGNPs

A BGNP colloidal suspension was prepared by seed-mediated synthesis [31,32] (see experimental section) to guarantee good shape control [27,30,35,36], despite the irregular (non-geometrical) shape. This aspect is crucial when aiming for a biological application, since different shapes can lead to different biomolecular corona, uptake, biodistribution, and immune response characteristics [27,37–40]. The BGNPs were functionalized with O-(2-carboxyethyl)-O′-(2-mercaptoethyl) heptaethylene glycol (HS-PEG$_7$-COOH) to gain better colloidal stability and strong surface anchoring, which are essential to maintain and stabilize the shape. The short length of the thiol ligand was selected to allow high-density coating, potentially providing better resistance of the nanostructure (and therefore of the optical properties) to thermal annealing and laser irradiation [41]. Furthermore, compared to the bare NPs, the negatively charged PEG ligand coating helps reduce the strength of protein interactions with the surface [42,43], while a positive charge can lead to stronger interactions with proteins [44].

BGNPs were fully characterized (see Figure 1). TEM analysis showed a monodistributed sample with an average size (calculated measuring the particle longest tip-to-tip distance) of 180 ± 10 nm (Figure 1a,b); the nanostructures presented a large core with a multitude of tips, which are the main responsible for the characteristic NIR-LSPR band centered near 800 nm (Figure 1c). The DLS and DCS analyses confirmed the high quality of the prepared BGNPs and the monodisperse size distribution (Figure 1d,e). Only the apparent size of BGNPs could be obtained by DCS in this case, as the technique estimates the diameter considering the object analyzed as a solid sphere of a specific density. The technique is nevertheless suitable to spot the presence of multiple populations or aggregation. In addition, it allows performing direct analysis of the BGNPs in the biological media with no need for purification/isolation steps to remove the excess of proteins. The stability test of the BGNPs in cell culture media showed excellent stability of the sample, with only a slight shift towards smaller sizes due to protein adsorption (biomolecular corona), which leads to a minor total density of the particles (Figure 1e,f) [45]. Further tests in 50% FBS (the in vivo-like conditions employed in our in vitro studies) were performed by absorption spectroscopy, confirming the stability of BGNPs. The slight DCS shift (3 nm) and the absence of a significant shift in the LSPR suggested a limited strength of the NP–proteins interaction, as expected (see Figure 1f). Nevertheless, the observed protein corona formation can actually lead to improved colloidal stability and biocompatibility [46,47] and might still play an essential role in the particle interaction with cells (i.e., specific interactions with cell receptors and internalization) [48,49]. For this reason, to present a more realistic behavior of the BGNPs in the biological environment (different protein concentrations can lead to different biomolecular corona compositions), [50] the nanostructures were exposed to an in vivo like protein concentration (50% v/v of serum), which will also be employed for in vitro testing [51].

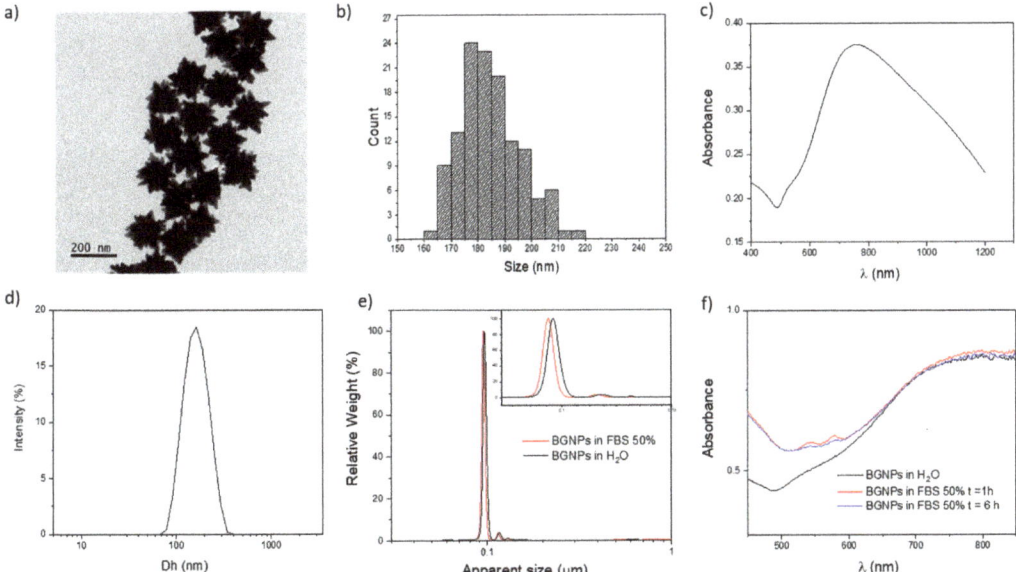

Figure 1. Characterization of BGNPs. (**a**) TEM micrograph. (**b**) TEM BGNP size distribution. (**c**) Vis–NIR absorption spectrum in H_2O. (**d**) DLS analysis (Dh = 164 nm, PDI = 0.06). (**e**) DCS analysis of BGNP in H_2O and cell culture media FBS 50% (apparent sizes of 100 nm and 97 nm respectively). (**f**) Absorption spectra related to the stability test of BGNPs in biological media: BGNPs were incubated in 50% FBS (in PBS) at 37 °C for different times (1 and 6 h). In the case of anisotropy, DLS and DCS do not represent the actual particle diameter. Consequently, representative particle distributions are reported rather than the actual sizes because of the incorrect geometrical assumption/approximation involved in the measurements.

3.2. Photothermal Performances of BGNPs in Phantom System

To explore the photothermal conversion efficiency of the BGNPs, we monitored the temperature of water solutions containing different concentrations of BGNPs during laser irradiation. The photothermal heating curves take the transferred heat from the BGNP to the medium into account. As such, the medium temperature only allows for an indirect view of the heat generated locally. In fact, the nanoparticles themselves may have much higher temperatures in their close proximity. Temperature differences of 70–90 °C were observed over distances of ~100 nm [52]. This aspect is crucial in biological experiments, where cells are sensitive to the local temperature of the nanoparticles, rather than medium temperature. The solutions were exposed to an 808-nm laser light source at a fixed power density (6.6 W cm^{-2}) for 90 s. The photothermal heating curves (Figure 2a), measured by an IR thermal camera (Figure 2b), showed a concentration-dependent photothermal effect, with the highest temperature increment of the solution with 0.25 mM Au^0 up to 65 °C (from 25 °C to 90 °C). The temperature increased proportionally with the increase of BGNPs concentration. In contrast, a negligible heating of only 2.2 °C was observed for water without BGNPs at the same exposure conditions. To provide a quantitative heating efficiency of our BGNPs comparing the results to similar gold nanoparticles presented in literature, the molar rate of heat transfer (Equation (1)) was calculated as proposed by Kuttner et al. [53].

$$\frac{\Delta Q}{c_{Au}} = \frac{(Q_{sample} - Q_{medium})}{c_{Au}} \quad (1)$$

The delivered thermal energy $\Delta Q = (Q_{sample} - Q_{medium})$ was calculated following the method described by Roper et al. [54] and Quintanilla et al. [55] (see Equations (S1)–(S4) and Figure S1 in Supplementary Materials), while the c_{Au} was calculated by inductively coupled plasma (ICP-OES) elemental analysis. The result of molar heat transfer rate is 0.53 W mM^{-1}, which is a value similar to suitable gold nanoparticles in PTT, such as gold nanorods [53].

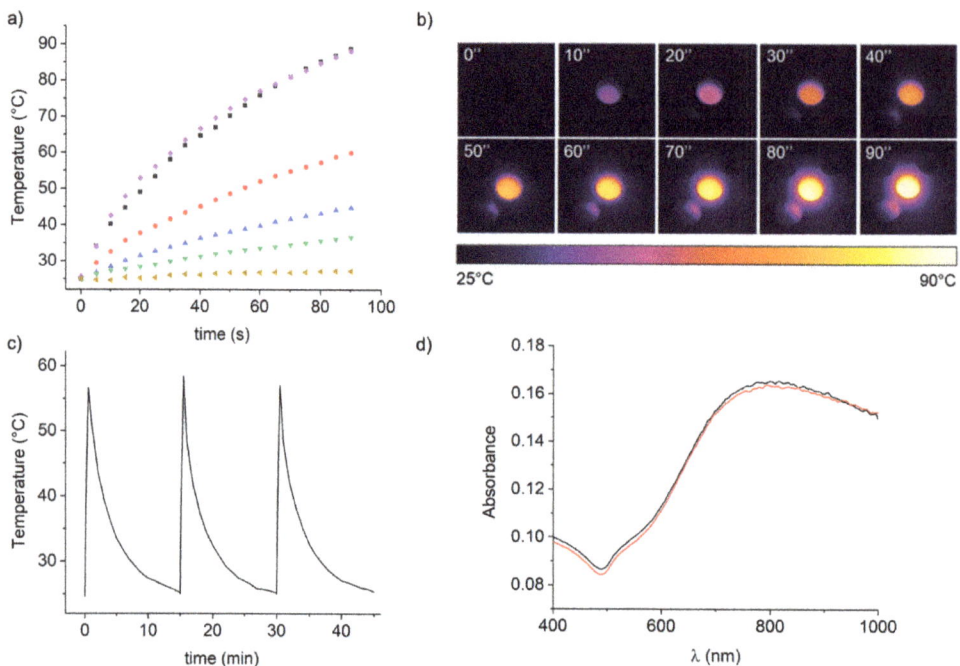

Figure 2. The photothermal effect of BGNPs in a phantom system. (**a**) Heating curves for different concentrations of BGNPs in water (0.25 mM Au^0 in violet, 0.1 mM Au^0 in red, 0.05 mM Au^0 in blue, 0.025 mM Au^0 in green, H$_2$O in yellow) and the BGNP biomolecular corona in water (0.25 mM Au^0 in black) during 808 nm NIR laser irradiation (6.6 W cm^{-2}). (**b**) Thermal imaging of the solution containing BGNPs (0.25 mM Au^0) for different times. (**c**) Temperature change of the solution containing BGNPs (0.25 mM Au^0), showing three laser on/off cycles of 808 NIR laser (6.6 W cm^{-2}). The sample was heated for 30 s, then the laser was switched off for 15 min and the solution was left to cool. (**d**) Vis–NIR spectra of the BGNPs before (black) and after (red) laser irradiation/heating.

The interaction with proteins may affect the photophysical properties of photosensitizers, [56–61] so we evaluated the BGNP performances in a physiological-like conditions, investigating the possible effects of the biomolecular corona during laser the irradiation/heating process [44]. We repeated the irradiation experiment for the FBS-dispersed BGNPs, using the highest concentration of BGNPs (0.25 mM Au^0 BGNPs). The results (Figure 2a, curves in violet and in black) are practically superimposable to the protein-free sample, indicating that the protein corona does not affect the photothermal behavior of the nanoparticles. It is known that some photothermal agents can degrade and eventually lose their photothermal properties during laser irradiation, in particular organic dyes such as cyanines and photobleach [62]. Other nanoparticles, like gold nanorods, are known to change their structure with laser absorption [63,64]. Thus, it is important to determine the photothermal stability of BGNPs to exclude heat-induced morphological changes and consequent LSPR shifts, which could prevent further cell death during in vitro laser treatment. As such, the BGNPs were subjected to multiple irradiation cycles (Figure 2c) and high-temperature treatment. A variation of 32 ± 1 °C (from 25 °C to 57 ± 1 °C) was obtained within 30 s and the light-to-heat conversion performances were maintained over the three cycles of heating and cooling performed, confirming the reproducibility of the photothermal response of the BGNPs (Figure 2c). To ensure the stability of the BGNPs after irradiation, the vis–NIR spectra were recorded before and after NIR laser irradiation (Figure 2d). The vis–NIR absorption spectrum of BGNPs remains unchanged after the three sequential cycles of heating and cooling, revealing that NIR irradiation does not affect the BGNPs colloidal stability and that there is no structural rearrangement of the gold nanoparticle due to laser irradiation/thermal heating. In fact, it is well-known that aggregation phenomena and the surface modification of BGNPs cause evident changes in their vis–NIR spectra. In addition, these results clearly confirm that BGNPs does not photodegrade during NIR treatment, as opposed to many organic dyes commonly used as photothermal agents. TEM analysis after irradiation were also performed (see Figure S2), confirming the thermostability of the nanostructures.

3.3. Uptake of BGNP in Colon Cancer Cells

A representative colon cancer cell line, DLD1, was used to study the uptake of BGNPs. To better take into account the potential influence of bio-nano interactions and biomolecular corona on the BGNP cell uptake (which are protein concentration-dependent), in vitro experiments were performed using culture media supplemented with 50% of the serum to get closer to an in vivo-like scenario with regards to the protein concentration. A large excess of protein can influence the nature of the biomolecular corona and the interactions of BGNPs with the cell [65]. In fact, binding competition of the free proteins crowds the media and commonly leads to reduced uptake, especially for large NPs [66]. BGNPs pre-dispersed with 50% FBS were incubated with DLD1 cells for 24 h, and then the cellular uptake of the BGNPs was studied by flow cytometry. BGNPs are phototheranostic platforms [60,67] that allow both therapy (PTT) and label-free imaging. In fact, BGNPs can be used for optical imaging because of their capacity to absorb and scatter light in the visible and NIR regions. In particular, the LSPR responsible for the photothermal effects of BGNPs, also provides large scattering cross sections, allowing for convenient detection of the BGNPs by scattering-based detection methods. Flow cytometry can measure quantitatively intracellular GNPs by collecting the light scattering from a large population of living cells through efficient single-cell analysis [33]. In flow cytometry, there are two modes of scattering measurements: side scattering and forward scattering. The side scattering channel (SSC) is commonly used as an indication of the cell's internal complexity or granularity. When nanoparticles are internalized by cells, the SSC intensity increases as a consequence of augmented intracellular complexity [33]. The (gated) side (SSC-A) and forward scatter (FSC-A) plots for DLD1 and DLD1 BGNPs-treated cells are reported in Figure 3A. Debris and death cells were excluded from the analysis based on morphology, thus gating the viable cells (R3) (Figure 3(Ac,Ad)). The cell granularity (SSC-A channel) of BGNPs-treated cells increased 1.74-fold compared to unexposed cells (Figure 3B,C), clearly indicating BGNP uptake. The same gating scheme was used for all the experiments.

To corroborate the BGNP cell internalization, reflectance confocal imaging [68] was performed in order to directly exploit the optical properties of the nanomaterials (label-free approach), avoiding potential problems related to dye leaching and conjugations, which inevitably alter the surface chemistry of the NPs and potentially also their biological interactions [69]. Performing a Z-stack across the whole cell body allowed the observation of the presence of BGNPs inside the cell cytoplasms (red spots) while in the close proximity of the nuclei (see Figure 4), where they are likely to be accumulated in the lysosomes [22,70].

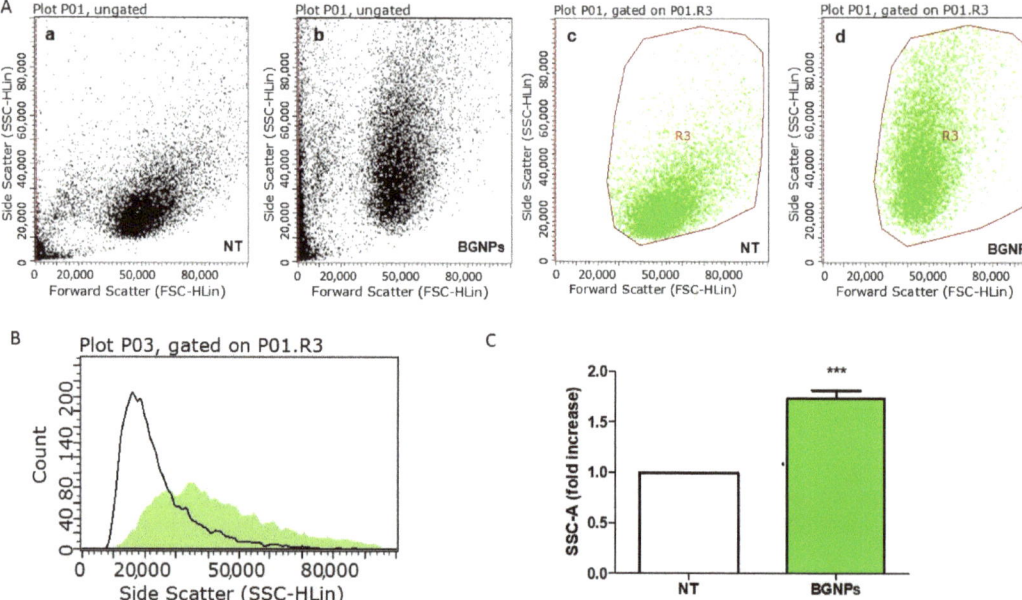

Figure 3. Flow-cytometric analysis of DLD1 after 24 h of BGNP exposure. (**A**) Representative gating plot of side scattering (SSC-A) versus forward scattering (FCS-A) of non-treated (NT) cells and BGNP-treated cells with all acquired events (**a,b**) and gated on living cells (R3) (**c,d**); (**B**) representative overlay of a side scattering histogram of cells exposed to BGNP compared to NT cells (dark line); (**C**) median relative fold-increase of SSC compared to NT cells of four independent experiments. *** $p < 0.001$ versus NT cells.

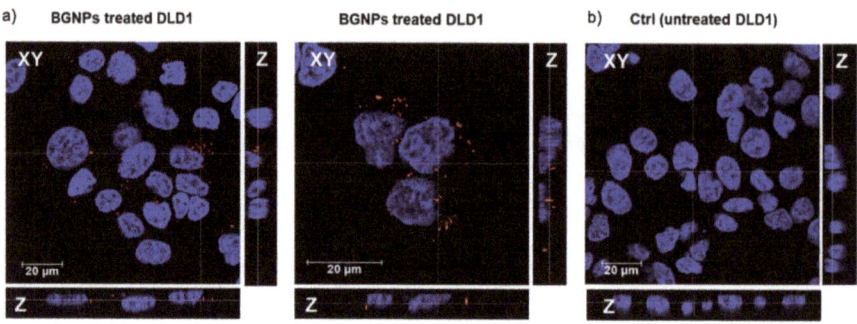

Figure 4. Confocal microscopy analysis. Representative images showing the XY planes and Z projections for (**a,b**) DLD1 cells after 24 h of BGNP exposure and (**b**) untreated DLD1 cell control. Nuclei are visualized by Hoechst staining (blue); BGNPs are visualized by reflected light (red). Bright filed XY transmission images are reported in Figure S3.

3.4. Efficacy of PTT Treatment in Colon Cancer Cells

To investigate the efficacy of BGNP-mediated PTT treatment on a cancer cell line, we incubated the DLD1 cells with 0.25 mM Au^0 BGNPs that were pre-dispersed in FBS for 24 h. After washing to remove the BGNPs that were not taken up, the DLD1 cells were irradiated with a NIR laser for different irradiance times and intensities. After 24 h from the irradiation, cell viability was measured using the MTT test. One of main concerns related to nanoparticle-based treatments is their potential intrinsic toxicity. Despite the well-known biocompatibility of GNPs, it is crucial to perform case-by-case studies to exclude size/shape-depended cytotoxicity against this particular cell line. Therefore, MTT assays were performed, to confirm the biocompatibility of BGNPs in the absence of laser irradiation (Figure 5a). No cytotoxic effect was observed on BGNPs treated DLD1 cells in dark conditions. On the opposite, a remarkable decrease in cell viability (4.76% viable cells, see Figure 5a) was observed after 3 min of irradiation at 6.6 W cm^{-2}. Interestingly, there was no cytotoxic effect when reducing the exposure time to 1 min or halving the laser irradiance to 3.3 W cm^{-2} while maintaining a period of 3 min of irradiation (Figure 5a).

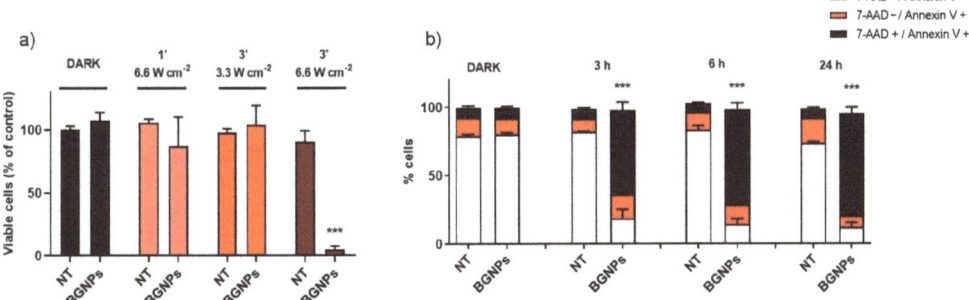

Figure 5. PTT treatment in colon cancer cells. (**a**) Percentage of viable cells (MTT) incubated with or without BGNPs, in dark condition or irradiated for different times and laser irradiance determined by MTT test. Percentage of viable cells is normalized on not treated (NT) cells in dark. (**b**) The percentage of living cells (white), cells undergoing programmed cell-death (red), and necrotic cells (black) after incubation or not with BGNPs in the dark or 3 h, 6 h, and 24 h after 3 min of irradiation at 6.6 W cm^{-2}. Data are the mean values of at least three independent experiments. *** $p < 0.001$ versus non-treated (NT) cells.

These results let us hypothesize the presence of a threshold for PTT to achieve cell death. The level of this threshold is paramount to reducing PTT side effects. For example, photosensitivity represents a major side effect of photodynamic therapy (PDT), in which a patient remains photosensitive for several weeks after cessation of the treatment, because sunlight or bright lights may activate a non-controlled generation of ROS, induced by the non-eliminated photosensitizer. In our case, BGNPs only generate heat/phototoxicity in the presence of a controllable source of laser light. Direct sunlight (~0.1 W cm^{-2}) or bright lights have irradiance intensities well below the threshold for BGNPs activation, thus they are not able to activate BGNP-dependent PTT. This aspect increases the control of the therapy such that PTT is activated only at the desired (localized) site of action, i.e., where the irradiation is focused, without collateral damage to surrounding tissues.

Typically, the application of PTT produces rapid temperature ramping, causing cellular death. Hyperthermia leads to cell membrane rupture, DNA damage and protein denaturation [13]. To discriminate the mechanisms of cell death, cells were counted for annexin V and 7-AAD staining in a flow cytometer, after 3 min of irradiation at 6.6 W cm^{-2}, with or without FBS-dispersed BGNPs. No significant increase in programmed cell death events was recorded, nor after short (3 h, 6 h) or long (24 h) post-treatment times. In contrast, a significant increase in the fraction of necrotic cells was observed already after 3 h after irradiation in BGNP-treated cells when compared to non-treated cells (62% versus 7%, respectively) (Figure 5b). Necrotic events reached the highest percentage 24 h after irradiation (75%) (Figure 5b). These results indicate that under laser irradiation, BGNPs induce cellular necrosis as the main cell death mechanism, conceivably due to the direct effect of the thermal stress on the cells. Our findings agree with several previous studies that identify necrosis as the main in vitro cellular response to PTT [13].

4. Conclusions

In this work, we have synthesized branched gold nanoparticles (BGNPs) as attractive agents for the photothermal eradication of colon cancer cells. The optical properties of the BGNPs were carefully tailored for effective absorbance in the first biological NIR window, a wavelength region of the light characterized by an optimal tissue penetration.

The FBS dispersed BGNPs were stable in physiological-like environments and were irradiated with an 808 nm laser source. They show an extremely efficient light-to-heat conversion capability. Sequential cycles of heating and cooling did not affect the BGNP stability.

Exploiting the intrinsic optical imaging offered by BGNPs, the uptake of BGNPs in colon cancer cells was confirmed using flow cytometry and confocal microscopy. In dark conditions BGNPs were fully biocompatible, while, when irradiated, BGNP-mediated PTT triggered rapid (3 h) cell death characterized by cell membrane rupturing, as evidenced by the high proportion of necrotic cells. These results agree with previous studies that identified necrosis as the main in vitro cellular response to PTT, leading to cell membrane rupture, DNA damage and protein denaturation. The passive accumulation of GNPs within cancer tissues, mediated by the enhanced permeability and retention effect, together with the possibility to easily functionalize the gold surfaces with targeting ligands [71], paves the way to providing robust double-targeting therapy approaches. The latter could exploit the recognition ability of conjugated targeting moieties with the possibility to focus the triggering light radiation at the desired site of action, lowering the collateral damage to healthy tissues, thus working towards a clinical need of crucial importance for the treatment of colon cancer.

Supplementary Materials: The following are available online at https://www.mdpi.com/article/10.3390/nano11061608/s1, Figure S1: Representative cooling curve of a dispersion of BGNPs with an exponential regression, Figure S2: Nanostructure thermal stability. TEM micrographs of BGNPs before and after laser irradiation, Figure S3: Confocal microscopy analysis of BGNPs uptake.

Author Contributions: For research articles with several authors, a short paragraph specifying their individual contributions must be provided. P.E.C., M.D.G., L.U., A.P., R.S.: Investigation, Data curation, Formal Analysis; C.F., P.P.P., A.D.: Supervision, Resources, Methodology. E.T., L.B.: Investigation, Data curation, Formal Analysis, Methodology. M.C.: Conceptualization, Methodology, Formal Analysis, Supervision, Resources, Funding acquisition. All authors: Writing—original draft preparation, Writing—review and editing. All authors have read and agreed to the published version of the manuscript.

Funding: M.D.G. was supported by a FIRC-AIRC fellowship for Italy (id. 22318). The research leading to these results has received funding from AIRC under MFAG 2019–ID. 22894 project-P.I. M.C.

Data Availability Statement: The data presented in this study are available on request from the corresponding authors.

Acknowledgments: The authors thank Alessandro Rossi and Valentina Alviani (Crisel Instruments) for assisting in the development of the instrumental setup for photothermal measurements. The paper is published with the contribution of the Department of Excellence program financed by the Minister of Education, University and Research (MIUR, L. 232 del 01/12/2016).

Conflicts of Interest: The authors declare no conflict of interest.

References

1. Rawla, P.; Sunkara, T.; Barsouk, A. Epidemiology of colorectal cancer: Incidence, mortality, survival, and risk factors. *Prz. Gastroenterol.* **2019**, *14*, 89–103. [CrossRef] [PubMed]
2. Taieb, J.; Gallois, C. Adjuvant chemotherapy for stage iii colon cancer. *Cancers* **2020**, *12*, 2679. [CrossRef]
3. Chen, J.; Zeng, Z.; Huang, L.; Luo, S.; Dong, J.; Zhou, F.H.; Zhou, K.; Wang, L.; Kang, L. Photothermal therapy technology of metastatic colorectal cancer. *Am. J. Transl. Res.* **2020**, *12*, 3089–3115.
4. Brace, C. Thermal tumor ablation in clinical use. *IEEE Pulse* **2011**, *2*, 28–38. [CrossRef]
5. Chu, K.F.; Dupuy, D.E. Thermal ablation of tumours: Biological mechanisms and advances in therapy. *Nat. Rev. Cancer* **2014**, *14*, 199–208. [CrossRef] [PubMed]

6. Vogl, T.J.; Eckert, R.; Naguib, N.N.N.; Beeres, M.; Gruber-Rouh, T.; Nour-Eldin, N.E.A. Thermal ablation of colorectal lung metastases: Retrospective comparison among laser-induced thermotherapy, radiofrequency ablation, and microwave ablation. *Am. J. Roentgenol.* **2016**, *207*, 1340–1349. [CrossRef] [PubMed]
7. Khot, M.I.; Andrew, H.; Svavarsdottir, H.S.; Armstrong, G.; Quyn, A.J.; Jayne, D.G. A Review on the Scope of Photothermal Therapy—Based Nanomedicines in Preclinical Models of Colorectal Cancer. *Clin. Colorectal Cancer* **2019**, *18*, e200–e209. [CrossRef]
8. Li, X.; Lovell, J.F.; Yoon, J.; Chen, X. Clinical development and potential of photothermal and photodynamic therapies for cancer. *Nat. Rev. Clin. Oncol.* **2020**, *17*, 657–674. [CrossRef]
9. Jaque, D.; Martínez Maestro, L.; Del Rosal, B.; Haro-Gonzalez, P.; Benayas, A.; Plaza, J.L.; Martín Rodríguez, E.; García Solé, J. Nanoparticles for photothermal therapies. *Nanoscale* **2014**, *6*, 9494–9530. [CrossRef] [PubMed]
10. Ali, M.R.K.; Wu, Y.; El-Sayed, M.A. Gold-Nanoparticle-Assisted Plasmonic Photothermal Therapy Advances toward Clinical Application. *J. Phys. Chem. C* **2019**, *123*, 15375–15393. [CrossRef]
11. Lal, S.; Clare, S.E.; Halas, N.J. Nanoshell-Enabled Photothermal Cancer Therapy: Impending Clinical Impact. *Acc. Chem. Res.* **2008**, *41*, 1842–1851. [CrossRef] [PubMed]
12. Huang, X.; Jain, P.K.; El-Sayed, I.H.; El-Sayed, M.A. Plasmonic photothermal therapy (PPTT) using gold nanoparticles. *Lasers Med. Sci.* **2008**, *23*, 217–228. [CrossRef] [PubMed]
13. Riley, R.S.; Day, E.S. Gold nanoparticle-mediated photothermal therapy: Applications and opportunities for multimodal cancer treatment. *Wiley Interdiscip. Rev. Nanomed. Nanobiotechnol.* **2017**, *9*, e1449. [CrossRef] [PubMed]
14. Vines, J.B.; Yoon, J.H.; Ryu, N.E.; Lim, D.J.; Park, H. Gold nanoparticles for photothermal cancer therapy. *Front. Chem.* **2019**, *7*, 167. [CrossRef]
15. Liu, X.; Atwater, M.; Wang, J.; Huo, Q. Extinction coefficient of gold nanoparticles with different sizes and different capping ligands. *Colloids Surf. B Biointerfaces* **2007**, *58*, 3–7. [CrossRef]
16. Haiss, W.; Thanh, N.T.K.; Aveyard, J.; Fernig, D.G. Determination of size and concentration of gold nanoparticles from UV-Vis spectra. *Anal. Chem.* **2007**, *79*, 4215–4221. [CrossRef]
17. Jung, H.S.; Verwilst, P.; Sharma, A.; Shin, J.; Sessler, J.L.; Kim, J.S. Organic molecule-based photothermal agents: An expanding photothermal therapy universe. *Chem. Soc. Rev.* **2018**, *47*, 2280–2297. [CrossRef]
18. Huang, X.; El-Sayed, I.H.; Qian, W.; El-Sayed, M.A. Cancer cell imaging and photothermal therapy in the near-infrared region by using gold nanorods. *J. Am. Chem. Soc.* **2006**, *128*, 2115–2120. [CrossRef] [PubMed]
19. Moros, M.; Lewinska, A.; Merola, F.; Ferraro, P.; Wnuk, M.; Tino, A.; Tortiglione, C. Gold Nanorods and Nanoprisms Mediate Different Photothermal Cell Death Mechanisms in Vitro and in Vivo. *ACS Appl. Mater. Interfaces* **2020**, *12*, 13718–13730. [CrossRef]
20. Ambrosone, A.; Del Pino, P.; Marchesano, V.; Parak, W.J.; De La Fuente, J.M.; Tortiglione, C. Gold nanoprisms for photothermal cell ablation in vivo. *Nanomedicine* **2014**, *9*, 1913–1922. [CrossRef]
21. Pérez-Hernández, M.; Del Pino, P.; Mitchell, S.G.; Moros, M.; Stepien, G.; Pelaz, B.; Parak, W.J.; Gálvez, E.M.; Pardo, J.; De La Fuente, J.M. Dissecting the molecular mechanism of apoptosis during photothermal therapy using gold nanoprisms. *ACS Nano* **2015**, *9*, 52–61. [CrossRef] [PubMed]
22. Espinosa, A.; Silva, A.K.A.; Sánchez-Iglesias, A.; Grzelczak, M.; Péchoux, C.; Desboeufs, K.; Liz-Marzán, L.M.; Wilhelm, C. Cancer Cell Internalization of Gold Nanostars Impacts Their Photothermal Efficiency In Vitro and In Vivo: Toward a Plasmonic Thermal Fingerprint in Tumoral Environment. *Adv. Healthc. Mater.* **2016**, *5*, 1040–1048. [CrossRef]
23. Van De Broek, B.; Devoogdt, N.; Dhollander, A.; Gijs, H.L.; Jans, K.; Lagae, L.; Muyldermans, S.; Maes, G.; Borghs, G. Specific cell targeting with nanobody conjugated branched gold nanoparticles for photothermal therapy. *ACS Nano* **2011**, *5*, 4319–4328. [CrossRef]
24. Yuan, H.; Fales, A.M.; Vo-Dinh, T. TAT peptide-functionalized gold nanostars: Enhanced intracellular delivery and efficient NIR photothermal therapy using ultralow irradiance. *J. Am. Chem. Soc.* **2012**, *134*, 11358–11361. [CrossRef]
25. Wang, S.; Huang, P.; Nie, L.; Xing, R.; Liu, D.; Wang, Z.; Lin, J.; Chen, S.; Niu, G.; Lu, G.; et al. Single continuous wave laser induced photodynamic/plasmonic photothermal therapy using photosensitizer-functionalized gold nanostars. *Adv. Mater.* **2013**, *25*, 3055–3061. [CrossRef]
26. Weissleder, R. A clearer vision for in vivo imaging. *Nat. Biotechnol.* **2001**, *19*, 316–317. [CrossRef] [PubMed]
27. Boselli, L.; Lopez, H.; Zhang, W.; Cai, Q.; Giannone, V.A.; Li, J.; Moura, A.; De Araujo, J.M.; Cookman, J.; Castagnola, V.; et al. Classification and biological identity of complex nano shapes. *Commun. Mater.* **2020**, *1*, 1–12. [CrossRef]
28. Donati, P.; Pomili, T.; Boselli, L.; Pompa, P.P. Colorimetric Nanoplasmonics to Spot Hyperglycemia From Saliva. *Front. Bioeng. Biotechnol.* **2020**, *8*, 1404. [CrossRef] [PubMed]
29. Maiorano, G.; Sabella, S.; Sorce, B.; Brunetti, V.; Malvindi, M.A.; Cingolani, R.; Pompa, P.P. Effects of cell culture media on the dynamic formation of protein-nanoparticle complexes and influence on the cellular response. *ACS Nano* **2010**, *4*, 7881–7891. [CrossRef] [PubMed]
30. Maiorano, G.; Rizzello, L.; Malvindi, M.A.; Shankar, S.S.; Martiradonna, L.; Falqui, A.; Cingolani, R.; Pompa, P.P. Monodispersed and size-controlled multibranched gold nanoparticles with nanoscale tuning of surface morphology. *Nanoscale* **2011**, *3*, 2227–2232. [CrossRef]
31. Potenza, M.A.C.; Krpetić, Ž.; Sanvito, T.; Cai, Q.; Monopoli, M.; De Araújo, J.M.; Cella, C.; Boselli, L.; Castagnola, V.; Milani, P.; et al. Detecting the shape of anisotropic gold nanoparticles in dispersion with single particle extinction and scattering. *Nanoscale* **2017**, *9*, 2778–2784. [CrossRef]

32. Li, J.; Wu, J.; Zhang, X.; Liu, Y.; Zhou, D.; Sun, H.; Zhang, H.; Yang, B. Controllable synthesis of stable urchin-like gold nanoparticles using hydroquinone to tune the reactivity of gold chloride. *J. Phys. Chem. C* **2011**, *115*, 3630–3637. [CrossRef]
33. Wu, Y.; Ali, M.R.K.; Dansby, K.; El-Sayed, M.A. Improving the Flow Cytometry-based Detection of the Cellular Uptake of Gold Nanoparticles. *Anal. Chem.* **2019**, *14261–14267*. [CrossRef] [PubMed]
34. Klingberg, H.; Oddershede, L.B.; Loeschner, K.; Larsen, E.H.; Loft, S.; Møller, P. Uptake of gold nanoparticles in primary human endothelial cells. *Toxicol. Res.* **2015**, *4*, 655–666. [CrossRef]
35. Grzelczak, M.; Pérez-Juste, J.; Mulvaney, P.; Liz-Marzán, L.M. Shape control in gold nanoparticle synthesis. *Chem. Soc. Rev.* **2008**, *37*, 1783–1791. [CrossRef]
36. Personick, M.L.; Mirkin, C.A. Making sense of the mayhem behind shape control in the synthesis of gold nanoparticles. *J. Am. Chem. Soc.* **2013**, *135*, 18238–18247. [CrossRef] [PubMed]
37. Castagnola, V.; Cookman, J.; De Araújo, J.M.; Polo, E.; Cai, Q.; Silveira, C.P.; Krpetić; Yan, Y.; Boselli, L.; Dawson, K.A. Towards a classification strategy for complex nanostructures. *Nanoscale Horiz.* **2017**, *2*, 187–198. [CrossRef] [PubMed]
38. Calvaresi, M. The route towards nanoparticle shape metrology. *Nat. Nanotechnol.* **2020**, *15*, 512–513. [CrossRef]
39. Wang, J.; Chen, H.J.; Hang, T.; Yu, Y.; Liu, G.; He, G.; Xiao, S.; Yang, B.R.; Yang, C.; Liu, F.; et al. Physical activation of innate immunity by spiky particles. *Nat. Nanotechnol.* **2018**, *13*, 1078–1086. [CrossRef] [PubMed]
40. Talamini, L.; Violatto, M.B.; Cai, Q.; Monopoli, M.P.; Kantner, K.; Krpetić, Ž.; Perez-Potti, A.; Cookman, J.; Garry, D.; Silveira, C.P.; et al. Influence of Size and Shape on the Anatomical Distribution of Endotoxin-Free Gold Nanoparticles. *ACS Nano* **2017**, *11*, 5519–5529. [CrossRef] [PubMed]
41. Centi, S.; Cavigli, L.; Borri, C.; Milanesi, A.; Milanesi, A.; Banchelli, M.; Chioccioli, S.; Khlebtsov, B.N.; Khlebtsov, N.G.; Khlebtsov, N.G.; et al. Small Thiols Stabilize the Shape of Gold Nanorods. *J. Phys. Chem. C* **2020**, *124*, 11132–11140. [CrossRef]
42. Pelaz, B.; Del Pino, P.; Maffre, P.; Hartmann, R.; Gallego, M.; Rivera-Fernández, S.; De La Fuente, J.M.; Nienhaus, G.U.; Parak, W.J. Surface Functionalization of Nanoparticles with Polyethylene Glycol: Effects on Protein Adsorption and Cellular Uptake. *ACS Nano* **2015**, *9*, 6996–7008. [CrossRef]
43. Dai, Q.; Walkey, C.; Chan, W.C.W. Polyethylene glycol backfilling mitigates the negative impact of the protein corona on nanoparticle cell targeting. *Angew. Chem. Int. Ed.* **2014**, *53*, 5093–5096.
44. Polo, E.; Araban, V.; Pelaz, B.; Alvarez, A.; Taboada, P.; Mahmoudi, M.; del Pino, P. Photothermal effects on protein adsorption dynamics of PEGylated gold nanorods. *Appl. Mater. Today* **2019**, *15*, 599–604. [CrossRef]
45. Perez-Potti, A.; Lopez, H.; Pelaz, B.; Abdelmonem, A.; Soliman, M.G.; Schoen, I.; Kelly, P.M.; Dawson, K.A.; Parak, W.J.; Krpetic, Z.; et al. In depth characterisation of the biomolecular coronas of polymer coated inorganic nanoparticles with differential centrifugal sedimentation. *Sci. Rep.* **2021**, *11*, 1–12.
46. Tebbe, M.; Kuttner, C.; Männel, M.; Fery, A.; Chanana, M. Colloidally Stable and Surfactant-Free Protein-Coated Gold Nanorods in Biological Media. *ACS Appl. Mater. Interfaces* **2015**, *7*, 5984–5991. [CrossRef] [PubMed]
47. Di Giosia, M.; Valle, F.; Cantelli, A.; Bottoni, A.; Zerbetto, F.; Fasoli, E.; Calvaresi, M. High-throughput virtual screening to rationally design protein—Carbon nanotube interactions. Identification and preparation of stable water dispersions of protein —Carbon nanotube hybrids and efficient design of new functional materials. *Carbon* **2019**, *147*, 70–82. [CrossRef]
48. Castagnola, V.; Zhao, W.; Boselli, L.; Lo Giudice, M.C.; Meder, F.; Polo, E.; Paton, K.R.; Backes, C.; Coleman, J.N.; Dawson, K.A. Biological recognition of graphene nanoflakes. *Nat. Commun.* **2018**, *9*, 1–9. [CrossRef] [PubMed]
49. Dawson, K.A.; Yan, Y. Current understanding of biological identity at the nanoscale and future prospects. *Nat. Nanotechnol.* **2021**, *16*, 229–242. [CrossRef]
50. Monopoli, M.P.; Walczyk, D.; Campbell, A.; Elia, G.; Lynch, I.; Baldelli Bombelli, F.; Dawson, K.A. Physical-Chemical aspects of protein corona: Relevance to in vitro and in vivo biological impacts of nanoparticles. *J. Am. Chem. Soc.* **2011**, *133*, 2525–2534. [CrossRef]
51. Monopoli, M.P.; Åberg, C.; Salvati, A.; Dawson, K.A. Biomolecular coronas provide the biological identity of nanosized materials. *Nat. Nanotechnol.* **2012**, *7*, 779–786. [CrossRef] [PubMed]
52. Maity, S.; Wu, W.C.; Xu, C.; Tracy, J.B.; Gundogdu, K.; Bochinski, J.R.; Clarke, L.I. Spatial temperature mapping within polymer nanocomposites undergoing ultrafast photothermal heating via gold nanorods. *Nanoscale* **2014**, *6*, 15236–15247. [CrossRef]
53. Kuttner, C.; Höller, R.P.M.; Quintanilla, M.; Schnepf, M.J.; Dulle, M.; Fery, A.; Liz-Marzán, L.M. SERS and plasmonic heating efficiency from anisotropic core/satellite superstructures. *Nanoscale* **2019**, *11*, 17655–17663. [CrossRef] [PubMed]
54. Roper, D.K.; Ahn, W.; Hoepfner, M. Microscale heat transfer transduced by surface plasmon resonant gold nanoparticles. *J. Phys. Chem. C* **2007**, *111*, 3636–3641. [CrossRef]
55. Quintanilla, M.; Kuttner, C.; Smith, J.D.; Seifert, A.; Skrabalak, S.E.; Liz-Marzán, L.M. Heat generation by branched Au/Pd nanocrystals: Influence of morphology and composition. *Nanoscale* **2019**, *11*, 19561–19570. [CrossRef]
56. Di Giosia, M.; Bomans, P.H.H.; Bottoni, A.; Cantelli, A.; Falini, G.; Franchi, P.; Guarracino, G.; Friedrich, H.; Lucarini, M.; Paolucci, F.; et al. Proteins as supramolecular hosts for C60: A true solution of C60 in water. *Nanoscale* **2018**, *10*, 9908–9916. [CrossRef]
57. Di Giosia, M.; Nicolini, F.; Ferrazzano, L.; Soldà, A.; Valle, F.; Cantelli, A.; Marforio, T.D.; Bottoni, A.; Zerbetto, F.; Montalti, M.; et al. Stable and Biocompatible Monodispersion of C 60 in Water by Peptides. *Bioconjug. Chem.* **2019**, *30*, 808–814. [CrossRef] [PubMed]
58. Soldà, A.; Cantelli, A.; Di Giosia, M.; Montalti, M.; Zerbetto, F.; Rapino, S.; Calvaresi, M. C60@lysozyme: A new photosensitizing agent for photodynamic therapy. *J. Mater. Chem. B* **2017**, *5*, 6608–6615. [CrossRef]

59. Cantelli, A.; Piro, F.; Pecchini, P.; Di Giosia, M.; Danielli, A.; Calvaresi, M. Concanavalin A-Rose Bengal bioconjugate for targeted Gram-negative antimicrobial photodynamic therapy. *J. Photochem. Photobiol. B Biol.* **2020**, *206*, 111852. [CrossRef]
60. Di Giosia, M.; Soldà, A.; Seeger, M.; Cantelli, A.; Arnesano, F.; Nardella, M.I.; Mangini, V.; Valle, F.; Montalti, M.; Zerbetto, F.; et al. A Bio-Conjugated Fullerene as a Subcellular-Targeted and Multifaceted Phototheranostic Agent. *Adv. Funct. Mater.* **2021**, *31*, 2101527. [CrossRef]
61. Di Giosia, M.; Zerbetto, F.; Calvaresi, M. Incorporation of Molecular Nanoparticles Inside Proteins: The Trojan Horse Approach in Theranostics. *Acc. Mater. Res.* **2021**. [CrossRef]
62. Zhao, Y.; He, Z.; Zhang, Q.; Wang, J.; Jia, W.; Jin, L.; Zhao, L.; Lu, Y. 880 Nm Nir-Triggered Organic Small Molecular-Based Nanoparticles for Photothermal Therapy of Tumor. *Nanomaterials* **2021**, *11*, 773. [CrossRef] [PubMed]
63. Link, S.; Burda, C.; Nikoobakht, B.; El-Sayed, M.A. Laser-induced shape changes of colloidal gold nanorods using femtosecond and nanosecond laser pulses. *J. Phys. Chem. B* **2000**, *104*, 6152–6163. [CrossRef]
64. Takahashi, H.; Niidome, T.; Nariai, A.; Niidome, Y.; Yamada, S. Photothermal reshaping of gold nanorods prevents further cell death. *Nanotechnology* **2006**, *17*, 4431–4435. [CrossRef]
65. Spedalieri, C.; Gergo, P.; Werner, S.; Guttmann, P. Probing the Intracellular Bio-Nano Interface in Different Cell Lines with Gold Nanostars. *Nanomaterials* **2021**, *11*, 1183. [CrossRef] [PubMed]
66. Muraca, F.; Boselli, L.; Castagnola, V.; Dawson, K.A.; Dawson, K.A. Ultrasmall Gold Nanoparticle Cellular Uptake: Influence of Transient Bionano Interactions. *ACS Appl. Bio Mater.* **2020**, *3*, 3800–3808. [CrossRef]
67. D'Hollander, A.; Vande Velde, G.; Jans, H.; Vanspauwen, B.; Vermeersch, E.; Jose, J.; Struys, T.; Stakenborg, T.; Lagae, L.; Himmelreich, U. Assessment of the theranostic potential of gold nanostars-a multimodal imaging and photothermal treatment study. *Nanomaterials* **2020**, *10*, 2112. [CrossRef]
68. Guggenheim, E.J.; Rappoport, J.Z. *Reflectance Imaging for Visualization of Unlabelled Structures Using Nikon A1 and N-SIM*; Application Note; Nikon Instruments Inc.: Tokyo, Japan, 2018.
69. Klein, S.; Petersen, S.; Taylor, U.; Rath, D.; Barcikowski, S. Quantitative visualization of colloidal and intracellular gold nanoparticles by confocal microscopy. *J. Biomed. Opt.* **2010**, *15*, 036015. [CrossRef]
70. Ma, X.; Wu, Y.; Jin, S.; Tian, Y.; Zhang, X.; Zhao, Y.; Yu, L.; Liang, X.J. Gold nanoparticles induce autophagosome accumulation through size-dependent nanoparticle uptake and lysosome impairment. *ACS Nano* **2011**, *5*, 8629–8639. [CrossRef]
71. Knights, O.; Freear, S.; McLaughlan, J.R. Improving plasmonic photothermal therapy of lung cancer cells with anti-EGFR targeted gold nanorods. *Nanomaterials* **2020**, *10*, 1307. [CrossRef]

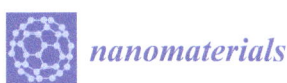

Article

880 nm NIR-Triggered Organic Small Molecular-Based Nanoparticles for Photothermal Therapy of Tumor

Yunying Zhao [1,†], Zheng He [1,†], Qiang Zhang [1], Jing Wang [1], Wenying Jia [1], Long Jin [1], Linlin Zhao [1,2,*] and Yan Lu [1]

[1] School of Materials Science & Engineering, Tianjin Key Laboratory for Photoelectric Materials and Devices, Key Laboratory of Display Materials & Photoelectric Devices, Ministry of Education, Tianjin University of Technology, Tianjin 300384, China; 17853483674@163.com (Y.Z.); 13752723282@163.com (Z.H.); zhangqiang@email.tjut.edu.cn (Q.Z.); wangjing@iccas.ac.cn (J.W.); jia15249238411@163.com (W.J.); KimYong0205@163.com (L.J.); luyan@tjut.edu.cn (Y.L.)
[2] State Key Laboratory of Molecular Engineering of Polymers, Fudan University, Shanghai 200433, China
* Correspondence: linlinzhao@email.tjut.edu.cn
† These authors contributed equally to this work.

Abstract: Photothermal therapy (PTT) has received constant attention as an efficient cancer therapy method due to locally selective treatment, which is not affected by the tumor microenvironment. In this study, a novel 880 nm near-infrared (NIR) laser-triggered photothermal agent (PTA), 3TT-IC-4Cl, was used for PTT of a tumor in deep tissue. Folic acid (FA) conjugated amphiphilic block copolymer (folic acid-polyethylene glycol-poly (β-benzyl-L-aspartate)$_{10}$, FA-PEG-PBLA$_{10}$) was employed to encapsulate 3TT-IC-4Cl by nano-precipitation to form stable nanoparticles (TNPs), and TNPs exhibit excellent photothermal stability and photothermal conversion efficiency. Furthermore, the in vitro results showed TNPs display excellent biocompatibility and significant phototoxicity. These results suggest that 880 nm triggered TNPs have great potential as effective PTAs for photothermal therapy of tumors in deep tissue.

Keywords: photothermal therapy; NIR-triggered; photothermal agent; deep tissue; nanoparticles

1. Introduction

Phototherapy has attracted extensive attention in recent years as a powerful cancer treatment method due to characteristics such as convenience, noninvasiveness, locally selective treatment, negligible drug resistance and minimized adverse side effects [1]. Photodynamic therapy (PDT) and photothermal therapy (PTT) are two typical phototherapy approaches, PTT is based on the photothermal agents (PTA), which are preferentially taken up and retained by diseased tissue; then after excitation by appropriate wavelength laser, the PTA convert light to heat to induce cancer cell apoptosis or necrosis. Compared to PDT, PTT is not affected by the tumor microenvironment, such as the local oxygen level, so PTT has received increasing attention and developed rapidly in recent years.

PTAs are one of the most important factors determining the efficiency of PTT, and many kinds of PTA have been developed in recent years. Current PTAs can be classified as inorganic and organic materials, and compared to inorganic PTAs, the organic PTAs with easy chemical structure tuning, good biocompatibility, low-toxicity and an easy metabolism in the biological system are more desirable for clinical photo-theranostics [2–7], such as cyanine dyes [8–13], diketopyrrolopyrrole derivatives [14,15], croconaine-based agents [16,17], porphyrin-based agents [18–21], conjugated polymers [22–29], squaraine derivatives [30,31], boron dipyrromethane (BODIPY) dyes [32] and so on. In organic PTAs, the polymeric PTA was limited due to its complicated fabrication processes, indistinct biodegradation and potential biosafety [21]. Therefore, the small organic molecules have received increasing attention as potential alternatives to nanomaterials in the area of PTT recently.

In addition, another main challenge for phototherapy is to efficiently treat cancers at a deep tissue level. Near-infrared (NIR) light is referred to as the "optical window" of the biological tissues due to the minimal light absorption and scattering. Compared with the UV or visible light, NIR shows larger penetration distance in tissue, lower photodamage effect and higher signal-to-noise ratio [33,34]. The organic molecules with extended π-conjugation usually show strong NIR absorbance, which is beneficial for deep tumor tissue diagnosis and phototherapy [35–37]. The well-designed, conjugated small molecules of organic PTA, especially the recently reported acceptor-donor-acceptor (A-D-A) structure PTA, would open a new gate for efficient PTT of tumor in deep tissues [38–40].

However, a problem limiting the use of conjugated small molecules of organic PTA is their low water solubility; the hydrophobic PTAs are difficult to use to prepare pharmaceutical formulations and cannot be directly injected intravenously. To overcome these problems, various strategies have been employed to prepare water-soluble and stable formulations of hydrophobic organic PTA, such as conjugate to water-soluble polymers [11], loaded into mesoporous materials [19] or carbon materials [41–43], encapsulate in colloidal carriers such as liposomes [18] and polymer nanoparticles [9,10,14,15,20–24,32,44,45].

In this study, an A-D-A structure non-fullerene molecule, 3TT-IC-4Cl, which includes three fused thieno[3,2-b]thiophene as the central core and difluoro-substituted indanone as the end group was selected as PTA for PTT. Similarly to other A-D-A structure non-fullerene molecules, 3TT-IC-4Cl exhibits both broad absorption and effectively suppressed fluorescence [39], and especially, 3TT-IC-4Cl exhibits strong and broad absorption in the 800–900 nm region after forming nanoparticles, and it is indicated that the 3TT-IC-4Cl has the potential as PTA for NIR-triggered PTT of cancer in deep tissue. In order to effectively utilize 3TT-IC-4Cl for PTT, herein, our previous reported folic acid (FA) conjugated amphiphilic block copolymer (folic acid-polyethylene glycol-poly (β-benzyl-L-aspartate)$_{10}$, FA-PEG-PBLA$_{10}$) was employed to encapsulate 3TT-IC-4Cl by nano-precipitation and dialysis process to form stable nanoparticles (TNPs) and improve 3TT-IC-4Cl solubility in aqueous solution. In the TNPs system, the 3TT-IC-4Cl and PBLA segment of the copolymer was an inner core for 3TT-IC-4Cl storage, 3TT-IC-4Cl was the heat source and the PEG segment was the outer shell to improve solubility, stability and biocompatibility of this system, and the active targeting ligand FA was introduced to the surface of nanoparticles to enhance the selectivity of nanoparticles.

Recently, the NIR-triggered organic small molecular based PTT systems have been developed [9,10,14,15,19,24,32,46]; however, few systems of A-D-A type small molecular organic PTA-based and 880 nm-triggered PTT have been reported.

2. Materials and Methods

2.1. Materials

Folic Acid (FA), PEG-bis(amine) (Mn: 3.4 kDa), β-benzyl-L-aspartate (BLA), Triethylamine (TEA), Thiazolyl Blue Tetrazolium Bromide (MTT), Phosphate Buffered Saline (PBS), and Sodium Bicarbonate were purchased from Sigma Chemical Co. (St. Louis, MO, USA). Triphosgene was purchased from Aldrich Chemical Co. (Milwaukee, WI, USA). N-hydroxysuccinimide (NHS) and N,N'-dicyclohexylcarbodiimide were purchased from Fluka (Buchs, Switzerland). Then, 3TT-IC-4Cl was provided by Zhongsheng Huateng Technology Co., Ltd. (Beijing, China) according to a previously reported method [47]. Indocyanine Green (ICG) was purchased from Adamas (Shanghai, China). CHCl$_3$ was purchased from Sinopharm Chemical Reagent Co., Ltd. (Shanghai, China). Dimethyl sulfoxide (DMSO) was purchased from Fuchen Chemical Reagent Co., Ltd. (Tianjin, China). Chloroform-d was purchased from Tenglong Weibo Technology Co., Ltd. (Qingdao, China). DMSO-d$_6$ was purchased from Ningbo Cuiying Chemical Technology Co., Ltd. (Ningbo, China). Dulbecco's modified Eagle's medium (DMEM), Fetal Bovine Serum (FBS), Penicillin and Streptomycin were purchased from Gibco BRL (Invitrogen Corp., Carlsbad, CA, USA). All other chemicals were of an analytical grade and used as received without further purification.

2.2. Characterization

The chemical structure was determined by 400 MHz ^{1}H NMR (AVANCE III HD 400 MHz, Bruker, Fällanden, Switzerland) using CHCl$_3$-d and DMSO-d$_6$ as the solvent. The photophysical properties of samples in aqueous solution were confirmed by UV-visible spectrophotometry (UV-2550, Shimadzu, Tokyo, Japan) and fluorescence spectrophotometer (F-4600, Hitachi, Tokyo, Japan). The morphologies, sizes and size distributions of nanoparticles were determined by transmission electron microscopes (TEM) (TECNAI G2 Spirit TWIN, FEI, Hillsboro, FL, USA) and dynamic light scattering (DLS) (Zetasizer Nano ZS90, Malvern Instruments Co, Malvern, UK) at 25 °C using a He-Ne laser (633 nm) as a light source. The temperature was monitored by IR thermal camera (TiS65, Fluke, Everett, WA, USA). The NIR laser (880 nm) used in this study was purchased from Beijing Laserwave Optoelectronics Technology Co., Ltd. (LWIRL880-20W-F, Laserwave, Beijing, China).

2.3. Preparation of TNPs

In order to prepare TNPs, first, the amphiphilic block copolymer FA-PEG-PBLA$_{10}$ used for 3TT-IC-4Cl encapsulation was synthesized by ring-opening polymerization as our previous reported [48]. The chemical structure of FA-PEG-PBLA$_{10}$ was confirmed by ^{1}H NMR (400 MHz, DMSO). Then, the TNPs were prepared by the nanoprecipitation method. Briefly, 5 mg 3TT-IC-4Cl was dissolved in 1 mL THF; then, the 3TT-IC-4Cl solution was added into to 50 mL FA-PEG-PBLA$_{10}$ solution (0.5 mg/mL in DMSO) dropwise, and then the mixture was transfered to dialysis tubs (Cut-off 3.5 K Mw) to remove THF and DMSO, followed by freeze drying, after which the TNPs were obtained.

2.4. Photothermal Effect

To confirm the PTT application potential, the photothermal property of TNPs was investigated, and a series of concentrations of TNPs (0, 30, 90, 180 and 250 µg/mL) in water were irradiated by 880 nm laser (0.7 W/cm^2, where, the power densities (W/cm^2) = laser beam power/laser beam area) for 720 s, the temperature of TNPs solution was recorded by an IR thermal camera every 30 s. In addition, the constant concentration (180 µg/mL) of TNPs were irradiated by an 880 nm laser for 720 s with various power densities (0.3, 0.5, 0.8 and 1.5 W/cm^2) was investigated by the same method.

2.5. Stability of TNPs

In order to investigated the stability of TNPs, TNPs (180 µg/mL, 30 µg/mL free 3TT-IC-4Cl equiv.) and free ICG (30 µg/mL) were irradiated with an 880 nm laser (0.7 W/cm^2) for 5 min; then the laser was turned off and the sample was cooled to the room temperature naturally, and the temperature of samples was recorded using the IR thermal camera every 30 s. Subsequently, the procedures were repeated four times.

2.6. In Vitro Phototoxicity and Biocompatibility of TNPs

HeLa cells (provided by Dingguo Biology Technology Co., Ltd., 1×10^4 cells/well) were seeded onto 96-well plates in 200 µL DMEM and allowed to attach for 24 h. After cell attachment, the medium was replaced with 100 µL of fresh medium containing FA-PEG-PBLA$_{10}$ (the polymer dispersed in aqueous medium) and TNPs with a series of concentration (0, 30, 60, 90, 120, 180 and 250 µg/mL), and then incubated for 4 h. The cells were washed with PBS and replace with fresh DMEM. The samples were irradiated with a laser (880 nm, 0.7 mW/cm^2) for 5 min. Then, irradiated cells were incubated at 37 °C for 24 h and cell viability was evaluated by MTT assay. Data presented are averaged results of quadruplicate experiments. For biocompatibility, HeLa cells (1×10^4 cells/well) were seeded onto 96-well plates in 200 µL DMEM and allowed to attach for 24 h. After cell attachment, the medium was replaced with 100 µL of fresh medium containing FA-PEG-PBLA$_{10}$ and TNPs with a series of concentration (0, 30, 60, 90, 120, 180 and 250 µg/mL), and then they were incubated for 24 h. The cell viability was evaluated by an MTT assay. Data presented are averaged results of quadruplicate experiments.

3. Results and Discussion

3.1. Synthesis and Characterization of TNPs

A novel PTA with an 880 nm-triggered A-D-A structure non-fullerene molecule, 3TT-IC-4Cl, which included three fused thieno[3,2-b]thiophene as the central core and difluoro substituted indanone as the end group [47] was selected for PTT. In order to effectively utilize 3TT-IC-4Cl for tumor therapy. An amphiphilic block copolymer (FA-PEG-PBLA$_{10}$) was synthesized as in our previous reported method [48] and used for 3TT-IC-4Cl encapsulation, 3TT-IC-4Cl was encapsulated in FA-PEG-PBLA$_{10}$ by nano-precipitation and a dialysis process to form stable nanoparticles (TNPs), as shown in Figure 1, the PBLA segment of the copolymer was used as a reservoir for 3TT-IC-4Cl storage in the inner core, the PEG segment was used as the outer shell to improve solubility, stability and biocompatibility of TNPs, the active targeting ligand FA was introduced to the surface of nanoparticles to enhance selectivity of nanoparticles, the chemical structure was confirmed by ^{1}H NMR, as shown in Figure 2A, and the characteristic peaks a and b are belong to FA-PEG-PBLA$_{10}$, and the characteristic peaks c, d, e, f, g and h attribute to 3TT-IC-4Cl, respectively. It indicated that the 3TT-IC-4Cl was encapsulated in FA-PEG-PBLA$_{10}$ successfully, the encapsulation rate (93.5%) was calculated by the relative intensity ratio of the methylene proton of PEG at 3.5 ppm and the proton of the alkane chain of in 3TT-IC-4Cl at about 1 ppm.

For nanomedicine used in cancer therapy, size, morphology and stability are the key properties that influence in vivo performance. These factors affect the bio-distribution and circulation time of the drug carriers. Stable and suitable-sized particles have reduced uptake by the reticuloendothelial systems (RES) and provide efficient passive tumor targeting ability via an enhanced permeation and retention (EPR) effect [49]. The incomplete tumor vasculature results in leaky vessels with gap sizes of 100 nm to 2 μm depending on the tumor type, and some studies have shown that particles with diameters of <200 nm are more effective [49,50]. The morphology of TNPs was evaluated by TEM, as shown in Figure 3. The TNPs were submicron in size and uniform and nearly spherical with no aggregation between nanoparticles observed due to the polymer modification, the average diameter was 150 nm. DLS measurements showed average hydrodynamic diameters of TNPs were about 200 nm (Figure 3, inset), a suitable size for passive targeting ability through the EPR effect. The size distribution of TNPs maintained a narrow and monodisperse unimodal pattern. Zeta potential of TNPs was measured as shown in Figure S1. It was shown that TNPs have negative surface charges, and zeta potential is about −13.2 mV. The zeta potential of TNPs showed that it would more stable against aggregation. Furthermore, the size of TNPs in DMEM remains almost same within 60 days (Figure S2).

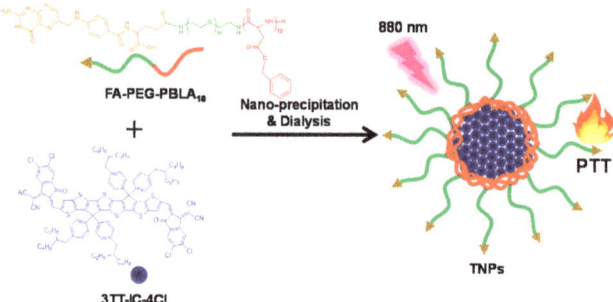

Figure 1. Schematic illustration demonstrating of stable nanoparticles (TNPs) formation and photothermal therapy (PTT) effect.

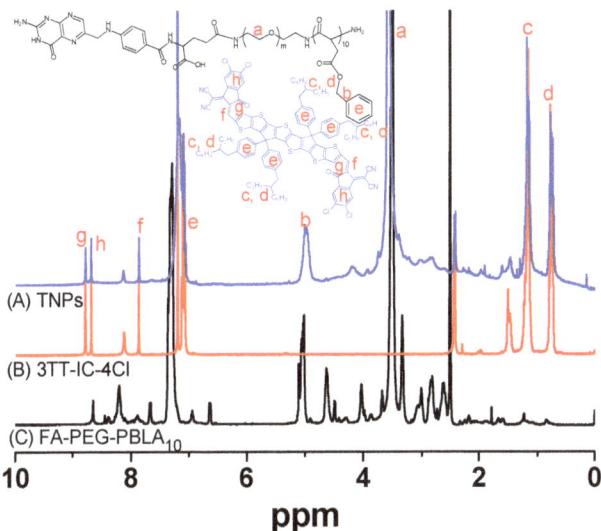

Figure 2. ¹H NMR spectra of (**A**) TNPs, (**B**) 3TT-IC-4Cl, and (**C**) FA-PEG-PBLA$_{10}$.

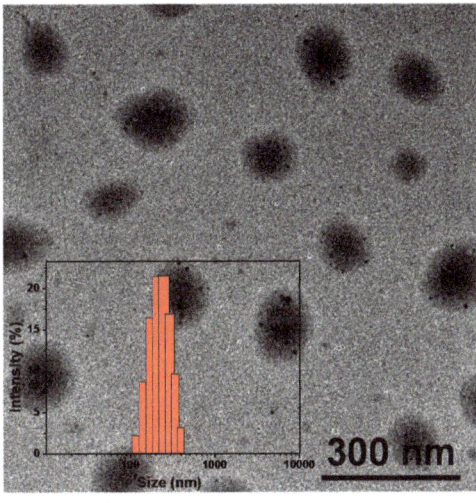

Figure 3. TEM image of TNPs and typical size distributions of TNPs (insert).

3.2. Optical Properties of TNPs

The optical properties of TNPs were investigated by UV-vis absorption spectra and fluorescence spectra (Figure 4A,B), for free 3TT-IC-4Cl in CHCl$_3$ solution, and it shows strong absorption at 772 nm and a maximal fluorescence at about 840 nm. However, after the formation of nanoparticles, the TNPs aqueous solution exhibits strong absorption at 874 nm, the significant red shift was due to the π-π stacking of 3TT-IC-4Cl during the nanoparticles formation and this result would be conducive to trigger TNPs by an 880 nm NIR light source for the phototherapy of the tumor in deep tissue. On the other hand, compared to free 3TT-IC-4Cl in CHCl$_3$ solution, in the TNPs aqueous solution, nearly no fluorescence signal was observed due to the 3TT-IC-4Cl aggregation during the nanoparticle formation, which would significantly increase non-radiative heat generation and enhance PTT efficiency [20,51].

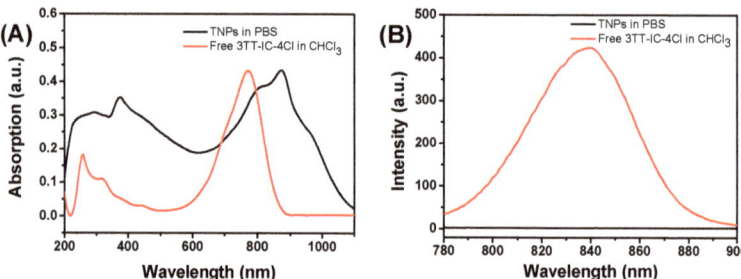

Figure 4. (**A**) UV–Vis absorption spectra of free 3TT-IC-4Cl (red) and TNPs (black), and (**B**) Fluorescence spectra of free 3TT-IC-4Cl (red) and TNPs (black).

3.3. Photothermal Properties of TNPs In Vitro

To investigate the photothermal conversion property of the TNPs, the temperature of TNP aqueous solution with a series of concentrations (from 0 to 250 µg/mL) under the 880 nm laser irradiation (0.7 W/cm^2) for 15 min was monitored (Figure 5A), and the related infrared (IR) thermal images of TNPs aqueous solution were showed in Figure 5C. As shown in the Figures, the temperature increased significantly as TNP concentration increased. It is noted that the TNPs at 90 µg/mL exhibit effective hyperthermia (>50 °C), which is sufficient to induce apoptosis or necrosis of cancer cells [52]. The relationship between temperature of TNPs aqueous solution (180 µg/mL) and different laser power (from 0.3 to 1.5 W/cm^2) was future measured, as shown in Figure 5B, and the temperature of the TNPs aqueous solution depends on the laser power. The related infrared (IR) thermal images of TNP aqueous solution were showed in Figure 5D. On the other hand, we also investigated the photothermal conversion efficiency of TNPs through a cycle of heat-up and cooling using the previously reported method (Figure S3) [53]. The photothermal conversion efficiency of the TNPs was 31.5%, which is higher than other PTAs such as cyanine dyes (e.g., ≈26.6%) and gold nanorods (e.g., ≈21.0%) [24,54,55]. The strong absorption and high photothermal conversion efficiency of TNPs in the NIR region provided the potential of photothermal treatment of cancer.

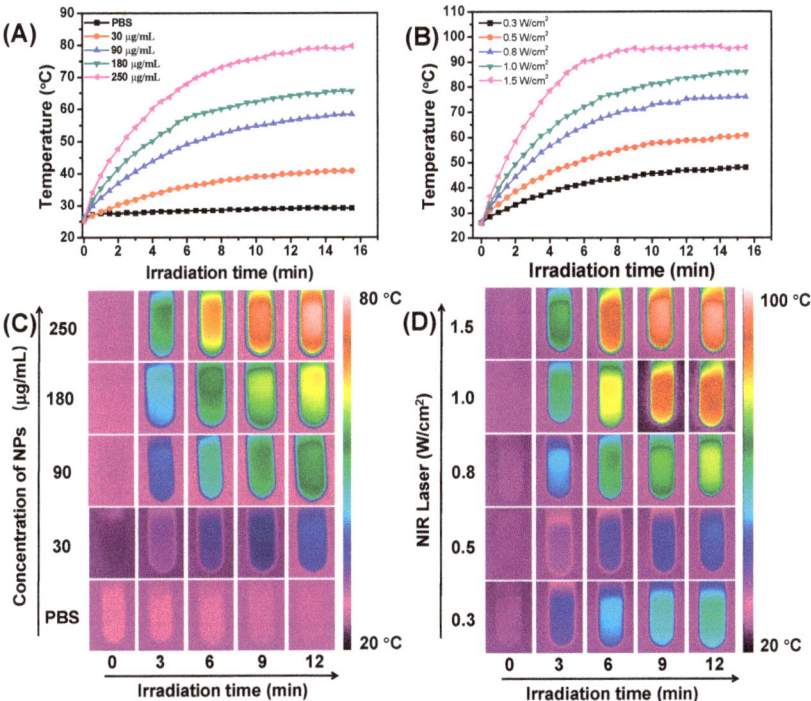

Figure 5. (**A**) Photothermal conversion behavior of TNPs at different concentrations (0–250 μg/mL) under 880 nm irradiation at 0.7 W/cm^2, (**B**) Photothermal conversion behavior of TNPs at different laser power (0.3–1.5 W/cm^2) under 880 nm irradiation at 0.7 W/cm^2, and (**C**) IR thermal images of TNPs at different concentrations (0–250 μg/mL) under 880 nm irradiation at 0.7 W/cm^2, and (**D**) IR thermal images of TNPs at different laser power (0.3–1.5 W/cm^2) under 880 nm irradiation at 0.7 W/cm^2.

3.4. Photothermal Stability of TNPs

The photothermal stability is an important parameter of photothermal drugs for PTT applications, and it would be crucial for clinical applications and therapeutic efficiency. The photothermal stability of TNPs was evaluated by monitoring its ability to maintain the temperature elevation. As shown in Figure 6A, the TNPs were irradiated at 0.7 W/cm^2 for 5 min, then the laser was turned off, the following samples were cooled down to room temperature, the temperature was recorded by IR thermal camera throughout the process, this irradiation/cooling procedures were repeated five times, as Figure 6A shows, and TNPs displayed negligible change in their temperature elevation after five irradiation/cooling cycles. However, the temperature elevation of free ICG decreased significantly after one irradiation/cooling cycle. On the other hand, we also observed the changes in the color of the samples, as shown in Figure 6B, and after 5 min irradiation the color of free ICG solution changed observably, but the TNPs exhibit no change after 30 min irradiation. These results indicated the TNPs exhibit excellent photothermal stability.

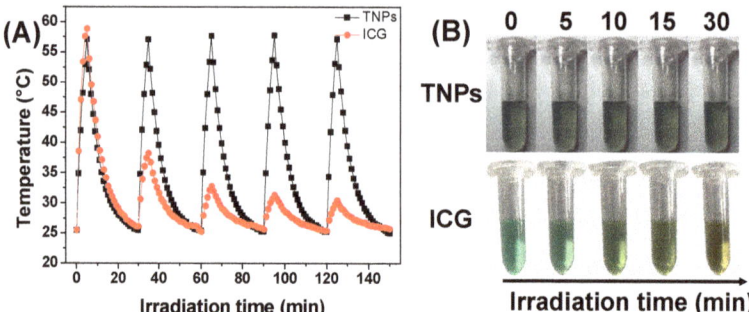

Figure 6. (**A**) Temperature elevation of TNPs, and free ICG under five irradiation/cooling cycles (under 880 nm irradiation at 0.7 W/cm^2 for 5 min), (**B**) Photographs of the TNPs, and free ICG in PBS solutions after 880 nm light irradiation for different time.

3.5. In Vitro Cell Test

In order to investigate the feasibility of TNPs as nano photothermal agents for PTT, in vitro cytotoxicity of TNPs was investigated by MTT assay and the average cell viability was monitored. For a biocompatibility test, the dark toxicity of TNPs was investigated. As shown in Figure 7A, both FA-PEG-PBLA$_{10}$ and TNPs exhibited no significant dark toxicity. As the concentration increased, the average cell viability was greater than 90% even when cells were treated with 250 µg/mL of TNPs. For the phototoxicity test, we investigated the concentration dependent (0, 30, 60, 90, 120, 180 and 250 µg/mL) cytotoxicity of TNPs with 880 nm laser irradiation. As shown in Figure 7B, after irradiation at 0.7 W/cm^2 for 5 min, the cell viability gradually decreased as the TNPs concentration increased. Taken together, these results indicate that the TNPs could considerably enhance the efficiency of PTT for tumor in deep tissue, even at low concentrations.

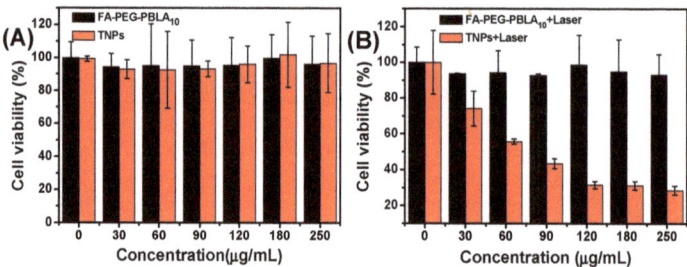

Figure 7. In vitro cytotoxicity test using FA-PEG-PBLA$_{10}$ and TNPs against HeLa cells (**A**) dark toxicity depending on the nanoparticles concentration and (**B**) phototoxicity depending on nanoparticles concentration.

4. Conclusions

In summary, an 880 nm NIR laser that triggered TNPs as PTA for photothermal therapy of a tumor in deep tissue was developed. In this work, a novel PTA, 3TT-IC-4Cl, was selected and used for PTT; it included three fused thieno[3,2-b]thiophene as the central core and difluoro-substituted indanone as the end group. After encapsulation by the FA-PEG-PBLA$_{10}$ block copolymer and forming nanoparticles, the TNP aqueous solution exhibited strong absorption at 880 nm due to the π-π stacking. DLS and TEM measurements showed that the TNPs have a spherical shape and narrow size distribution with a mean diameter of 150 nm. TNPs exhibit excellent photothermal stability and high photothermal conversion efficiency after 880 nm laser irradiation. In the in vitro test, TNPs display excellent biocompatibility and significant phototoxicity. Therefore, the 880 nm-triggered TNPs have great potential as an effective PTA for the photothermal therapy of tumor in deep tissue.

Supplementary Materials: The following are available online at https://www.mdpi.com/2079-4991/11/3/773/s1, Figure S1: Zeta potential of TNPs in water, Figure S2: Changes of hydrodynamic diameters of TNPs in DMEM with time, [TNPs] = 180 μg/mL, Figure S3: (A) Temperature elevation of TNPs (180 μg/mL) under 880 nm irradiation at 0.7 W/cm^2 for 5 min, followed by subsequent cooling to room temperature and (B) Linear time data versus-Ln (θ) obtained from the cooling period of NIR la-ser off.

Author Contributions: Conceptualization, L.Z.; Data curation, Y.Z., Z.H., J.W., W.J. and L.J.; Formal analysis, Y.Z. and Z.H.; Funding acquisition, L.Z. and Y.L.; Methodology, Q.Z.; Writing—original draft, L.Z.; Writing—review & editing, L.Z. and Y.L. All authors have read and agreed to the published version of the manuscript.

Funding: This research was supported by the National Natural Science Foundation of China (Grant Nos. 51703163), the Natural Science Foundation of Tianjin (18JCZDJC34600 and 18JCYBJC86700) and the Program for Prominent Young College Teachers of Tianjin Educational Committee.

Conflicts of Interest: The authors declare no conflict of interest.

References

1. Li, J.; Pu, K. Development of organic semiconducting materials for deep-tissue optical imaging, phototherapy and photoactivation. *Chem. Soc. Rev.* **2019**, *48*, 38–71. [CrossRef] [PubMed]
2. Li, Y.; Lin, T.Y.; Luo, Y.; Liu, Q.; Xiao, W.; Guo, W.; Lac, D.; Zhang, H.; Feng, C.; Wachs-mann-Hogiu, S.; et al. A smart and versatile theranostic nanomedicine platform based on nanoporphyrin. *Nat. Commun.* **2014**, *5*, 4712. [CrossRef] [PubMed]
3. Antaris, A.L.; Chen, H.; Cheng, K.; Sun, Y.; Hong, G.; Qu, C.; Diao, S.; Deng, Z.; Hu, X.; Zhang, B.; et al. A small-molecule dye for NIR-II imaging. *Nat. Mater.* **2015**, *15*, 235. [CrossRef] [PubMed]
4. Zhang, Y.; Jeon, M.; Rich, L.J.; Hong, H.; Geng, J.; Zhang, Y.; Shi, S.; Barnhart, T.E.; Alexan-dridis, P.; Huizinga, J.D.; et al. Non-invasive multimodal functional imaging of the intestine with frozen micellar naphthalocyanines. *Nat. Nanotechnol.* **2014**, *9*, 631. [CrossRef] [PubMed]
5. Abuteen, A.; Zanganeh, S.; Akhigbe, J.; Samankumara, L.P.; Aguirre, A.; Biswal, N.; Braune, M.; Vollertsen, A.; Röder, B.; Brückner, C.; et al. The evaluation of NIR-absorbing porphyrin derivatives as contrast agents in photoacoustic imaging. *Phys. Chem. Chem. Phys.* **2013**, *15*, 18502–18509. [CrossRef]
6. Song, X.; Chen, Q.; Liu, Z. Recent advances in the development of organic photothermal nano-agents. *Nano Res.* **2015**, *8*, 340–354. [CrossRef]
7. Jung, H.S.; Verwilst, P.; Sharma, A.; Shin, J.; Sessler, J.L.; Kim, J.S. Organic molecule-based photothermal agents: An expanding photothermal therapy universe. *Chem. Soc. Rev.* **2018**, *47*, 2280–2297. [CrossRef]
8. Wang, H.; Chang, J.; Shi, M.; Pan, W.; Li, N.; Tang, B. A Dual-targeted organic photothermal agent for enhanced photothermal therapy. *Angew. Chem. Int. Ed.* **2019**, *58*, 1057–1061. [CrossRef]
9. Asadian-Birjand, M.; Bergueiro, J.; Wedepohl, S.; Calderón, M. Near Infrared dye conjugated nanogels for combined photodynamic and photothermal therapies. *Macromol. Biosci.* **2016**, *16*, 1432–1441. [CrossRef]
10. Luo, S.; Tan, X.; Fang, S.; Wang, Y.; Liu, T.; Wang, X.; Yuan, Y.; Sun, H.; Qi, Q.; Shi, C. Mito-chondria-targeted small-molecule fluorophores for dual modal cancer phototherapy. *Adv. Funct. Mater.* **2016**, *26*, 2826–2835. [CrossRef]
11. Yang, W.; Noh, J.; Park, H.; Gwon, S.; Singh, B.; Song, C.; Lee, D. Near infrared dye-conjugated oxidative stress amplifying polymer micelles for dual imaging and synergistic anticancer phototherapy. *Biomaterials* **2018**, *154*, 48–59. [CrossRef] [PubMed]
12. Heshmati Aghda, N.; Abdulsahib, S.M.; Severson, C.; Lara, E.J.; Torres Hurtado, S.; Yildiz, T. Induction of immunogenic cell death of cancer cells through nanoparticle-mediated dual chemotherapy and photothermal therapy. *Int. J. Pharm.* **2020**, *589*, 119787. [CrossRef] [PubMed]
13. Liu, X.; He, Z.; Chen, Y.; Zhou, C.; Wang, C.; Liu, Y. Dual drug delivery system of photothermal-sensitive carboxymethyl chitosan nanosphere for photothermal-chemotherapy. *Int. J. Biol. Macromol.* **2020**, *163*, 156–166. [CrossRef] [PubMed]
14. Cai, Y.; Liang, P.; Tang, Q.; Yang, X.; Si, W.; Huang, W.; Zhang, Q.; Dong, X. Diketo-pyrrolopyrrole–triphenylamine organic nanoparticles as multifunctional reagents for photoacoustic imaging-guided photodynamic/photothermal synergistic tumor therapy. *ACS Nano* **2017**, *11*, 1054–1063. [CrossRef] [PubMed]
15. Wang, Q.; Dai, Y.; Xu, J.; Cai, J.; Niu, X.; Zhang, L.; Chen, R.; Shen, Q.; Huang, W.; Fan, Q. All-in-one phototheranostics: Single laser triggers NIR-II fluorescence/photoacoustic imaging guided photothermal/photodynamic/chemo combination therapy. *Adv. Funct. Mater.* **2019**, *29*, 1901480. [CrossRef]
16. Spence, G.T.; Hartland, G.V.; Smith, B.D. Activated photothermal heating using croconaine dyes. *Chem. Sci.* **2013**, *4*, 4240–4244. [CrossRef]

17. Spence, G.T.; Lo, S.S.; Ke, C.; Destecroix, H.; Davis, A.P.; Hartland, G.V.; Smith, B.D. Near-infrared croconaine rotaxanes and doped nanoparticles for enhanced aqueous photothermal heating. *Chem. Eur. J.* **2014**, *20*, 12628–12635. [CrossRef]
18. Lovell, J.F.; Jin, C.S.; Huynh, E.; Jin, H.; Kim, C.; Rubinstein, J.L.; Chan, W.C.W.; Cao, W.; Wang, L.V.; Zheng, G. Porphysome nanovesicles generated by porphyrin bilayers for use as multi-modal biophotonic contrast agents. *Nat. Mater.* **2011**, *10*, 324. [CrossRef]
19. Peng, J.; Zhao, L.; Zhu, X.; Sun, Y.; Feng, W.; Gao, Y.; Wang, L.; Li, F. Hollow silica nanoparticles loaded with hydrophobic phthalocyanine for near-infrared photodynamic and photothermal combination therapy. *Biomaterials* **2013**, *34*, 7905–7912. [CrossRef]
20. Zhang, J.; Yang, C.; Zhang, R.; Chen, R.; Zhang, Z.; Zhang, W.; Peng, S.H.; Chen, X.; Liu, G.; Hsu, C.S.; et al. Biocompatible D–A semiconducting polymer nanoparticle with light-harvesting unit for highly effective photoacoustic imaging guided photothermal therapy. *Adv. Funct. Mater.* **2017**, *27*, 1605094. [CrossRef]
21. Zou, Q.; Abbas, M.; Zhao, L.; Li, S.; Shen, G.; Yan, X. Biological photothermal nanodots based on self-assembly of peptide–porphyrin conjugates for antitumor therapy. *J. Am. Chem. Soc.* **2017**, *139*, 1921–1927. [CrossRef] [PubMed]
22. Chen, P.; Ma, Y.; Zheng, Z.; Wu, C.; Wang, Y.; Liang, G. Facile syntheses of conjugated polymers for photothermal tumour therapy. *Nat. Commun.* **2019**, *10*, 1192. [CrossRef] [PubMed]
23. Guo, B.; Sheng, Z.; Hu, D.; Li, A.; Xu, S.; Manghnani, P.N.; Liu, C.; Guo, L.; Zheng, H.; Liu, B. Molecular engineering of conjugated polymers for biocompatible organic nanoparticles with highly efficient photoacoustic and photothermal performance in cancer theranostics. *ACS Nano* **2017**, *11*, 10124–10134. [CrossRef]
24. Yang, T.; Liu, L.; Deng, Y.; Guo, Z.; Zhang, G.; Ge, Z.; Ke, H.; Chen, H. Ultrastable near-infrared conjugated-polymer nanoparticles for dually photoactive tumor inhibition. *Adv. Mater.* **2017**, *29*, 1700487. [CrossRef]
25. Zhang, W.; Li, Y.; Xu, L.; Wang, D.; Long, J.; Zhang, M. Near-Infrared-absorbing conjugated polymer nanoparticles loaded with doxorubicin for combinatorial photothermal-chemotherapy of cancer. *ACS Appl. Polym. Mater.* **2020**, *2*, 4180–4187. [CrossRef]
26. Wang, Y.; Zhang, H.; Wang, Z.; Feng, L. Photothermal conjugated polymers and their biological applications in imaging and therapy. *ACS Appl. Polym. Mater.* **2020**, *2*, 4222–4240. [CrossRef]
27. Wang, Y.; Meng, H.M.; Song, G.; Li, Z.; Zhang, X.B. Conjugated-polymer-based nanomaterials for photothermal therapy. *ACS Appl. Polym. Mater.* **2020**, *2*, 4258–4272. [CrossRef]
28. Huff, M.E.; Gökmen, F.Ö.; Barrera, J.S.; Lara, E.J.; Tunnell, J.; Irvin, J. Induction of immunogenic cell death in breast cancer by conductive polymer nanoparticle-mediated photothermal therapy. *ACS Appl. Polym. Mater.* **2020**, *2*, 5602–5620. [CrossRef]
29. Lu, K.Y.; Jheng, P.R.; Lu, L.S.; Rethi, L.; Mi, F.L.; Chuang, E.Y. Enhanced anticancer effect of ROS-boosted photothermal therapy by using fucoidan-coated polypyrrole nanoparticles. *Int. J. Biol. Macromol.* **2021**, *166*, 98–107. [CrossRef]
30. Prostota, Y.; Kachkovsky, O.D.; Reis, L.V.; Santos, P.F. New unsymmetrical squaraine dyes derived from imidazo[1,5-a]pyridine. *Dye. Pigment.* **2013**, *96*, 554–562. [CrossRef]
31. Gao, F.P.; Lin, Y.X.; Li, L.L.; Liu, Y.; Mayerhöffer, U.; Spenst, P.; Su, J.G.; Li, J.Y.; Würthner, F.; Wang, H. Supramolecular adducts of squaraine and protein for noninvasive tumor imaging and photothermal therapy in vivo. *Biomaterials* **2014**, *35*, 1004–1014. [CrossRef]
32. Guo, Z.; Zou, Y.; He, H.; Rao, J.; Ji, S.; Cui, X.; Ke, H.; Deng, Y.; Yang, H.; Chen, C.; et al. Bifunctional platinated nanoparticles for photoinduced tumor ablation. *Adv. Mater.* **2016**, *28*, 10155–10164. [CrossRef] [PubMed]
33. Du, Y.; Xu, B.; Fu, T.; Cai, M.; Li, F.; Zhang, Y.; Wang, Q. Near-infrared photoluminescent Ag_2S quantum dots from a single source precursor. *J. Am. Chem. Soc.* **2010**, *132*, 1470–1471. [CrossRef] [PubMed]
34. Zhou, J.; Yu, M.; Sun, Y.; Zhang, X.; Zhu, X.; Wu, Z.; Wu, D.; Li, F. Fluorine-18-labeled $Gd^{3+}/Yb^{3+}/Er^{3+}$ codoped $NaYF_4$ nanophosphors for multimodality PET/MR/UCL imaging. *Biomaterials* **2011**, *32*, 1148–1156. [CrossRef] [PubMed]
35. Atilgan, S.; Ekmekci, Z.; Dogan, A.L.; Guc, D.; Akkaya, E.U. Water soluble distyryl-boradiazaindacenes as efficient photosensitizers for photodynamic therapy. *Chem. Commun.* **2006**, 4398–4400. [CrossRef] [PubMed]
36. Tian, J.; Zhou, J.; Shen, Z.; Ding, L.; Yu, J.S.; Ju, H. A pH-activatable and aniline-substituted photosensitizer for near-infrared cancer theranostics. *Chem. Sci.* **2015**, *6*, 5969–5977. [CrossRef]
37. Drogat, N.; Gady, C.; Granet, R.; Sol, V. Design and synthesis of water-soluble polyaminated chlorins and bacteriochlorins with near-infrared absorption. *Dye. Pigment.* **2013**, *98*, 609–614. [CrossRef]
38. Li, X.; Liu, L.; Li, S.; Wan, Y.; Chen, J.X.; Tian, S.; Huang, Z.; Xiao, Y.F.; Cui, X.; Xiang, C.; et al. Biodegradable π-conjugated oligomer nano-particles with high photothermal conversion efficiency for cancer theranostics. *ACS Nano* **2019**, *13*, 12901–12911. [CrossRef]
39. He, Z.; Zhao, L.; Zhang, Q.; Chang, M.; Li, C.; Zhang, H.; Lu, Y.; Chen, Y. An acceptor–donor–acceptor structured small molecule for effective nir triggered dual phototherapy of cancer. *Adv. Funct. Mater.* **2020**, *30*, 1910301. [CrossRef]
40. Cai, Y.; Wei, Z.; Song, C.; Tang, C.; Huang, X.; Hu, Q.; Dong, X.; Han, W. Novel acceptor–donor–acceptor structured small molecule-based nanoparticles for highly efficient photothermal therapy. *Chem. Commun.* **2019**, *55*, 8967–8970. [CrossRef] [PubMed]
41. Tian, B.; Wang, C.; Zhang, S.; Feng, L.; Liu, Z. Photothermally enhanced photodynamic therapy delivered by nano-graphene oxide. *ACS Nano* **2011**, *5*, 7000–7009. [CrossRef]
42. Yan, H.; Wu, H.; Li, K.; Wang, Y.; Tao, X.; Yang, H.; Li, A.; Cheng, R. Influence of the surface structure of graphene oxide on the adsorption of aromatic organic compounds from water. *ACS Appl. Mater. Interfaces* **2015**, *7*, 6690–6697. [CrossRef] [PubMed]

43. Liang, X.; Shang, W.; Chi, C.; Zeng, C.; Wang, K.; Fang, C.; Chen, Q.; Liu, H.; Fan, Y.; Tian, J. Dye-conjugated single-walled carbon nanotubes induce photothermal therapy under the guidance of near-infrared imaging. *Cancer Lett.* **2016**, *383*, 243–249. [CrossRef] [PubMed]
44. Qi, J.; Fang, Y.; Kwok, R.T.K.; Zhang, X.; Hu, X.; Lam, J.W.Y.; Ding, D.; Tang, B.Z. Highly stable organic small molecular nanoparticles as an advanced and biocompatible phototheranostic agent of tumor in living mice. *ACS Nano* **2017**, *11*, 7177–7188. [CrossRef] [PubMed]
45. Zhang, S.; Guo, W.; Wei, J.; Li, C.; Liang, X.J.; Yin, M. Terrylenediimide-based intrinsic theranostic nanomedicines with high photothermal conversion efficiency for photoacoustic imaging-guided cancer therapy. *ACS Nano* **2017**, *11*, 3797–3805. [CrossRef] [PubMed]
46. Jang, B.; Park, J.Y.; Tung, C.H.; Kim, I.H.; Choi, Y. Gold nanorod–photosensitizer complex for near-infrared fluorescence imaging and photodynamic/photothermal therapy in vivo. *ACS Nano* **2011**, *5*, 1086–1094. [CrossRef]
47. Gao, H.H.; Sun, Y.; Wan, X.; Ke, X.; Feng, H.; Kan, B.; Wang, Y.; Zhang, Y.; Li, C.; Chen, Y. A new nonfullerene acceptor with near infrared absorption for high performance ternary-blend organic solar cells with efficiency over 13%. *Adv. Sci.* **2018**, *5*, 1800307. [CrossRef]
48. Zhao, L.; Kim, T.H.; Huh, K.M.; Kim, H.W.; Kim, S.Y. Self-assembled photosensitizer-conjugated nanoparticles for targeted photodynamic therapy. *J. Biomater. Appl.* **2013**, *28*, 434–447. [CrossRef]
49. Byrne, J.D.; Betancourt, T.; Brannon-Peppas, L. Active targeting schemes for nanoparticle systems in cancer therapeutics. *Adv. Drug Deliv. Rev.* **2008**, *60*, 1615–1626. [CrossRef]
50. Peer, D.; Karp, J.M.; Hong, S.; Farokhzad, O.C.; Margali, R.; Langer, R. Nanocarriers as an emerging platform for cancer therapy. *Nat. Nanotechnol.* **2007**, *2*, 751–760. [CrossRef]
51. Lyu, Y.; Fang, Y.; Miao, Q.; Zhen, X.; Ding, D.; Pu, K. Intraparticle molecular orbital engineering of semiconducting polymer nanoparticles as amplified theranostics for in vivo photoacoustic imaging and photothermal therapy. *ACS Nano* **2016**, *10*, 4472–4481. [CrossRef] [PubMed]
52. Hahn, G.M.; Braun, J.; Har-Kedar, I. Thermo/chemotherapy: Synergism between hyperthermia (42–43 degrees) and adriamycin (of bleomycin) in mammalian cell inactivation. *Proc. Natl. Acad. Sci. USA* **1975**, *72*, 937–940. [CrossRef] [PubMed]
53. Liu, Y.; Ai, K.; Liu, J.; Deng, M.; He, Y.; Lu, L. Dopamine-melanin colloidal nanospheres: An efficient near-infrared photothermal therapeutic agent for in vivo cancer therapy. *Adv. Mater.* **2013**, *25*, 1353–1359. [CrossRef] [PubMed]
54. Deng, Y.; Huang, L.; Yang, H.; Ke, H.; He, H.; Guo, Z.; Yang, T.; Zhu, A.; Wu, H.; Chen, H. Cyanine-anchored silica nanochannels for light-driven synergistic thermo-chemotherapy. *Small* **2017**, *13*, 1602747. [CrossRef] [PubMed]
55. Sun, Z.; Xie, H.; Tang, S.; Yu, X.F.; Guo, Z.; Shao, J.; Zhang, H.; Huang, H.; Wang, H.; Chu, P.K. Ultrasmall black phosphorus quantum dots: Synthesis and use as photothermal agents. *Angew. Chem. Int. Ed.* **2015**, *54*, 11526–11530. [CrossRef] [PubMed]

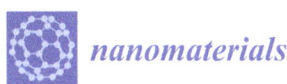

Article

Improving Plasmonic Photothermal Therapy of Lung Cancer Cells with Anti-EGFR Targeted Gold Nanorods

Oscar Knights [1], Steven Freear [1] and James R. McLaughlan [1,2,]

[1] School of Electronic and Electrical Engineering, University of Leeds, Leeds LS2 9JT, UK; O.B.Knights@leeds.ac.uk (O.K.); s.freear@leeds.ac.uk (S.F.)
[2] Leeds Institute of Medical Research, St James' University Hospital, University of Leeds, Leeds LS9 7TF, UK
* Correspondence: j.r.mclaughlan@leeds.ac.uk

Received: 12 June 2020; Accepted: 1 July 2020; Published: 3 July 2020

Abstract: Lung cancer is a particularly difficult form of cancer to diagnose and treat, due largely to the inaccessibility of tumours and the limited available treatment options. The development of plasmonic gold nanoparticles has led to their potential use in a large range of disciplines, and they have shown promise for applications in this area. The ability to functionalise these nanoparticles to target to specific cancer types, when combined with minimally invasive therapies such as photothermal therapy, could improve long-term outcomes for lung cancer patients. Conventionally, continuous wave lasers are used to generate bulk heating enhanced by gold nanorods that have accumulated in the target region. However, there are potential negative side-effects of heat-induced cell death, such as the risk of damage to healthy tissue due to heat conducting to the surrounding environment, and the development of heat and drug resistance. In this study, the use of pulsed lasers for photothermal therapy was investigated and compared with continuous wave lasers for gold nanorods with a surface plasmon resonance at 850 nm, which were functionalised with anti-EGFR antibodies. Photothermal therapy was performed with both laser systems, on lung cancer cells (A549) in vitro populations incubated with untargeted and targeted nanorods. It was shown that the combination of pulse wave laser illumination of targeted nanoparticles produced a reduction of 93% $\pm$ 13% in the cell viability compared with control exposures, which demonstrates a possible application for minimally invasive therapies for lung cancer.

Keywords: nanoparticles; gold nanorods; cancer therapy; photothermal therapy; photoacoustic imaging; lung cancer; EGFR-targeting

1. Introduction

Cancer is a leading cause of death worldwide with approximately 70% of deaths occurring in low- and middle-income countries [1]. Lung cancer is the most prevalent and deadly form of cancer since there exists very few options for diagnosis or treatment. Plasmonic photothermal therapy (PPTT) is a therapeutic modality, when combined with AuNRs could provide a highly selective, minimally invasive treatment option for cancer. It would be beneficial if PPTT could be administered with a pulsed-wave (PW) laser since it would reduce the potential damage to surrounding tissues by eliminating the bulk heating effect caused by continuous wave (CW) lasers. The photothermal effect relies heavily on a light source that can deliver sufficient of energy to a localised region, and thus a laser is often used [2]. Laser ablation (LA), a common clinical therapeutic technique that relies on lasers, is predominantly used to compliment additional therapies by reducing tumour volume [3]. It is mostly used for treating superficial and lung cancers where laser access and light delivery is feasible [4]. Continuous wave (CW) lasers with high powers (around 5 W) are employed to induce bulk heating and irreversible thermal damage in the target tissue; however, pulsed wave (PW) lasers have also shown potential for photothermal applications [5]. Depending on the type of laser system employed—either PW or CW—there will be significant differences in the observed outcomes. CW lasers can induce either apoptosis or necrosis, depending on laser intensity and AuNR distribution, whereas PW lasers can only induce necrosis [6]. These two pathways for cell death have their own advantages and disadvantages. For example, an apoptotic pathway can lead to cells developing drug and thermal resistance but does not cause immunogenic or inflammatory responses, while the opposite is true for a necrotic pathway [7]. PW lasers create a highly-localised rapid temperature increase in the target AuNRs [8], and this almost-instantaneous and high temperature increase causes large mechanical stresses (peak pressures of 10–100 MPa [9]) that can induce necrotic cell death depending on particle location and laser energy. There are very few reports on pulsed wave plasmonic photothermal therapy (PW-PPTT), also known as photoacoustic plasmonic photothermal therapy (PA-PPTT), and the majority predominately use either high energy laser pulses, ultra-short laser pulses (femtosecond), or alternative photoabsorbers, with little in the way of low-energy, nanosecond pulses that utilise AuNRs as the absorbing agent. Moreover, there are few reports addressing how the size of the AuNRs may affect the treatment efficacy of both PW-PPTT and conventional PPTT at equivalent concentrations. The optimisation of both the optical absorbers and laser parameters is crucial to the success of this technique. If PW lasers can be used to destroy target regions of tissue successfully and efficiently, with similar or superior outcomes to that of CW lasers, then new and combined diagnostic and therapeutic techniques may be possible.

The functionalisation of AuNRs to molecularly target specific binding sites, such as epidermal growth factor receptors (EGFR), is increasingly seen as an essential aspect of using AuNRs for biomedical purposes. This is largely due to the need for high numbers of AuNRs to be localised in a tumour region for a sufficient PA or PPTT effect to be observed. Furthermore, relying solely on the enhanced permeability and retention (EPR) effect to accumulate AuNRs in target tissue may not be sufficient [10,11]. If the target ligand is known, then the AuNRs can be functionalised with monoclonal antibodies (for example anti-EGFR) that will enable monovalent affinity. This is a highly desirable characteristic that can result in a much larger accumulation of AuNRs at a site. It is known that many forms of cancer express EGFR-positive ligands and it has therefore become a common method for molecular targeting for a range of imaging techniques such as photoacoustic imaging PAI [12]. The aim of this study was to investigate the effects that AuNR targeting to EGFR positive lung cancer cells has on both CW and PW laser treatment.

2. Materials and Methods

To determine the EGFR expression of lung cancer cells, immunofluorescence (IF) staining was performed using a standard IF protocol. Briefly, the A549 cells were grown in a 6-well plate on microscope coverslips. Once 70% confluence was reached, the media was removed and the cell monolayer was washed with Dulbecco's Phosphate-Buffered Saline (DPBS, Thermo Fisher Scientific, Waltham, MA USA). To fix the cells to the coverslips, 4% PFA (Paraformaldehyde, Thermo Fisher Scientific, Waltham, MA USA) was added and left for 15 min at room temperature. The coverslips were then washed twice with DPBS before being permeabilised with a solution of DPBS and 0.3% Triton X-100. The coverslips were then washed twice in DPBS, followed by sample blocking in 10% FBS (fetal bovine serum, Thermo Fisher Scientific, Waltham, MA USA) for 1 h. The blocking buffer was removed and Alexa Flour 488-conjugated anti-EGFR antibodies, diluted in 5% FBS, was added to the coverslips and incubated for 2 h at room temperature. Finally, the coverslips were washed 3 times in DPBS and mounted on microscope slides using DAPI (4′,6-diamidino-2-phenylindole, Thermo Fisher Scientific, Waltham, MA USA) reagent (ProLong Gold Antifade Mountant). The same protocol was repeated to form a control group without adding the conjugated antibodies. The level of EGFR expression (as determined from the IF images in Figure 1) in A549 cells was not as high as expected. Nevertheless,

EGFR expression was observed during the IF staining and therefore it was decided that the effect of targeting AuNRs to the EGFR receptors would be investigated.

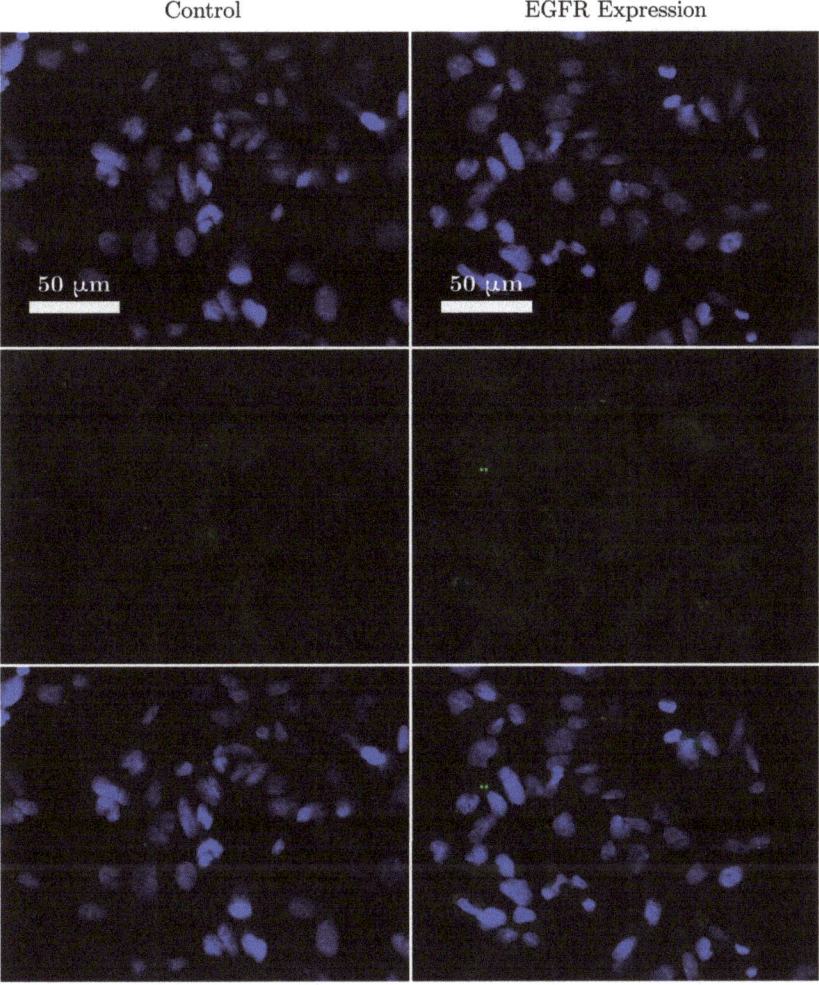

Figure 1. A fluorescence image of lung cancer cells (A549) showing the expression of anti-epidermal growth factor receptors receptors. Blue represents the staining of the cell nucleus and green shows the expression of EGFR.

AuNR-targeting was considered using dark-field microscopy. Highly concentrated Streptavidin-conjugated AuNRs were purchased (Table 1) from Nanopartz—a company that is able to synthesis AuNRs on a large scale with repeatable characteristics—to enable them to be easily functionalised with an anti-EGFR targeting ligand (Figure 2). A protocol was designed to enable the comparison of cellular uptake for targeted versus untargeted S-Au40-849s at three different time-points: 4 h, 8 h, and 24 h. These were chosen to provide an indication of the timescales required for wide-spread affinity of the targeted AuNRs to the lung cancer cells. We previously observed high levels of uptake after 4 h incubation [13]. The biotinylated antibody used in this study was a mouse monoclonal antibody (ab24293, abcam) and the amount required to facilitate the conjugation with the AuNRs was explored along-side the targeting efficiency. A series of 21 microscope coverslips were soaked in ethanol overnight before being allowed to dry completely and were then placed inside a separate well of six 6-well plates. For each time-point there was enough cover-slips to allow for: one blank (3), two untargeted (6), two targeted with 10 µL biotinylated antibody (6), and two targeted with 20 µL biotinylated antibody (6). A human non-small cell lung epithelial carcinoma cell line (A549, ATCC, Middlesex, UK) was cultured in DMEM (Dulbecco's Modified Eagle Medium) media supplemented with 10% FBS (Fetal Bovine Serum). When the cells reached 80% confluency, the 6-well plates were seeded with 4×10^3 cells per well and incubated for 48 h. Before the AuNRs were added to the wells, a functionalising protocol was followed (Figure 3). The stock S-Au40-849s (concentration = 13.2 mg mL^{-1}) were first sonicated for 15 min to minimise aggregation and then 45 µL of the stock S-Au40-849s was split between three sterile Eppendorfs (i.e., 15 µL per Eppendorf). The first Eppendorf (named 'UT') was reserved for untargeted AuNRs, 10 µL of the biotinylated antibody was added to the second Eppendorf (named 'T10'), and 20 µL of the biotinylated antibody was added to the final Eppendorf (named 'T20'). All of the Eppendorfs were then topped up with Dulbecco's phosphate-buffered saline (DPBS, 14190-094, Thermo Fisher Scientific, Waltham, MA USA) to a total volume of 40 µL (i.e., 25 µL DPBS in Eppendorf UT, 15 µL DPBS in Eppendorf T10, and 5 µL DPBS in Eppendorf T20). All three Eppendorfs were then sonicated for 10 min before being placed on a vortex for 30 min to facilitate the conjugation of the AuNRs and antibodies. The AuNRs were then purified by centrifuging for 10 min at a relative centrifugal force (r.c.f.) of 5900, followed by the removal of the supernatant and addition of 40 µL DPBS, and then further mixing was performed with the vortex for 2 min followed by sonication for 10 min. After repeating the purification process twice, the supernatant was replaced with 100 µL DMEM media before being added to separate 15 mL falcon tubes filled with DMEM media to a total volume of 6 mL. Finally, each falcon tube was vortexed for 2 min and sonicated for 10 min before the media-AuNR solutions were added to the 6-well plates at a total volume of 2 mL per well, giving a final AuNR concentration of 30 µg mL^{-1}. The plates were then incubated for different lengths of time (4 h, 8 h, and 24 h) before a standard protocol for preparing microscope slides for dark-field imaging was followed. A549 cells were plated onto 22 × 22 mm glass cover-slips in a 6-well plate at a density of 1×10^5 well^{-1} and allowed to grow for two days. The AuNR-media was removed from each well and the cell monolayer on the cover-slip was twice-rinsed with DPBS, fixed in 4% paraformaldehyde/DPBS for 10 min at room temperature and rinsed with DPBS five times. The fixed coverslips were then mounted and sealed onto glass slides. Bright and dark-field microscopy imaging was performed with an inverted microscope (Nikon Eclipse Ti-E, Nikon UK Ltd., Kingston upon Thames, Surrey, UK) using an oil coupled 100x objective (CFI Plan Fluor, Nikon UK Ltd., Kingston upon Thames, Surrey, UK). Images were recorded with a 5 Megapixel colour camera (DS-Fi1, Nikon UK Ltd., Kingston upon Thames, Surrey, UK) and saved using the NIS-Elements D software (Nikon UK Ltd., Kingston upon Thames, Surrey, UK). The height of objectives focal plane was monitored to establish that images were acquired within the cells. Open-source software package ImageJ [14] was used to crop and enhance the contrast of saved images. To ensure valid comparisons could be made, all of the images were enhanced in the same way.

Table 1. Certified dimensions and measured surface plasmon resonance of all AuNRs used in study.

AuNR Name	Width (nm)	Length (nm)	Aspect Ratio	SPR (nm)
S-Au40-849	40	148	3.7	849

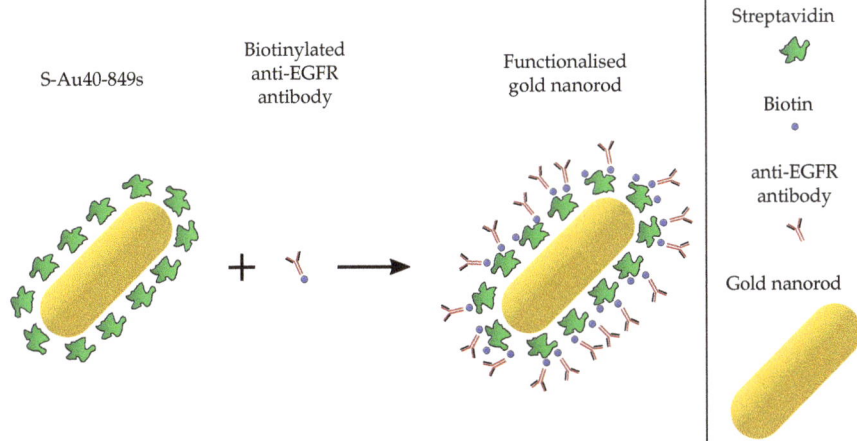

Figure 2. The biotinylated anti-EGFR antibodies exhibit high affinity to the streptavidin proteins that are already conjugated to the AuNR.

For the photothermal therapy experiments, targeting was achieved using the same methodology (Figure 3) for conjugating the S-Au40-849s to anti-EGFR monoclonal antibodies was followed as described. However, the 6-well plates were replaced with two 96-well plates and were seeded with A549 cells at a concentration of 1×10^5 cells per well. The experimental procedure was similar to that previously described [13], with untargeted (UT) AuNRs were add to one plate and targeted (T10) AuNRs were added to the other—both at a concentration of $30\,\mu\text{g}\,\text{mL}^{-1}$—and left to incubate for either 4 h or 24 h. Immediately prior to laser exposure, the media in the wells of the 96-well plate was removed, the cell monolayer washed once with DPBS, and then 100 µL of fresh media was added. This washing step was performed to minimise the number of AuNRs remaining in the wells that were not bound to the cell surface receptors or taken up by the cells. The laser systems used were a pulsed tuneable laser (Surelite, OPO Plus, Continuum, San Jose, CA, USA) operating at a pulse repetition frequency of 10 Hz with a pulse duration of 7 ns, spot size of 9 mm (at the bottom of the 96-well plate) and radiant exposure of $25\,\text{mJ}\,\text{cm}^{-2}$, and a continuous wave diode laser (B4-852-1500-15C, Sheaumann Laser, Marlborough, MA, USA) operating at 1.5 W across a spot size of 9 mm with a fixed wavelength at 854 nm. The pulsed laser system was tuned to the same wavelength as the CW laser (854 nm) to ensure an accurate comparison could be made between the two laser types, by facilitating an equivalent optical absorption by the AuNRs. This wavelength was confirmed using a direct measurement of the beam with a UV-VIS-NIR spectrometer (HR4000, Ocean Optics, Orlando, FL, USA). Output from either laser was coupled directly into broadband optical fibres that were mounted onto a 3-axis motorised translation stage [13] to enable the scanning of the fibre tips across the 96-well plates. The wells that were targeted with the lasers were alternated to reduce any effects from the laser heating of neighbouring wells, and each well was exposed for a total of 5 min.

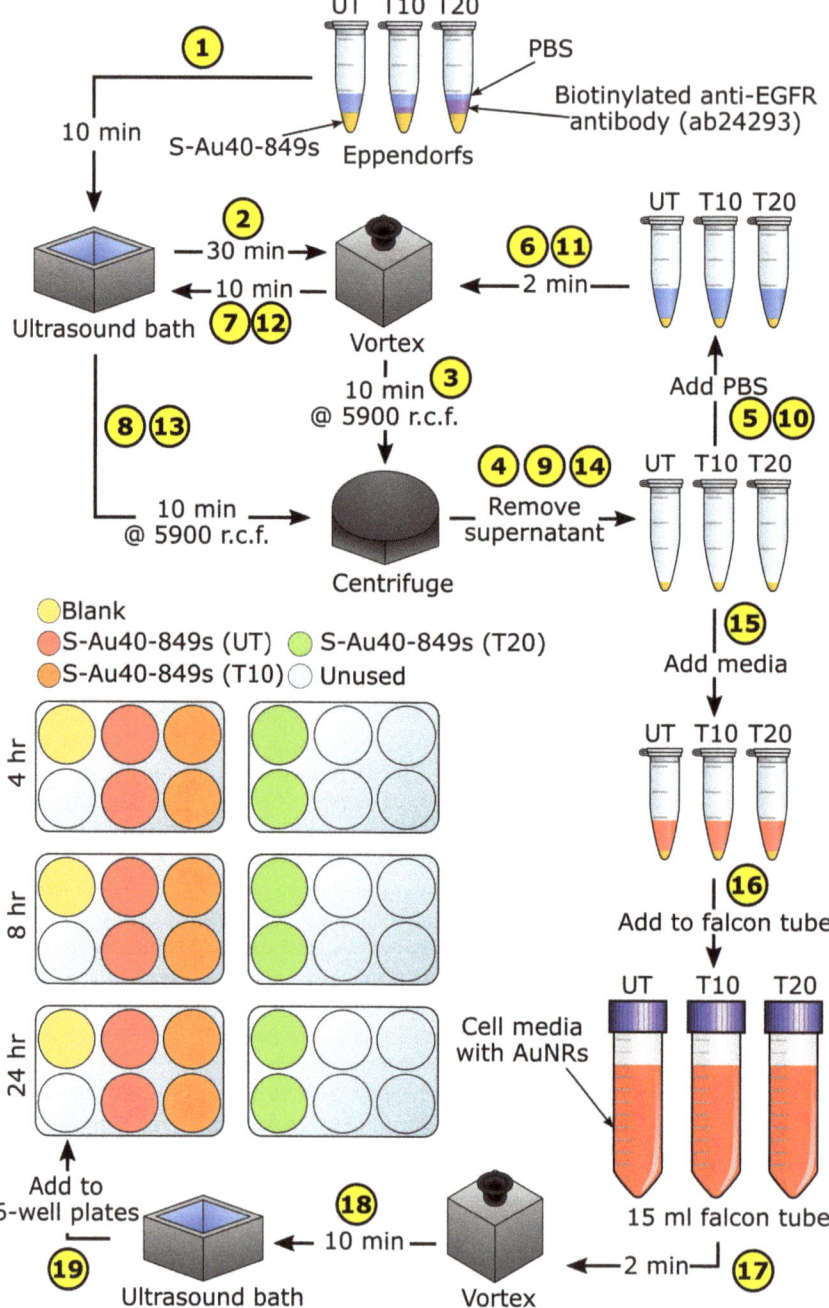

Figure 3. A schematic depicting the functionalisation process for the S-Au40-849s. UT = untargeted AuNRs, T10 = targeted AuNRs (10 µL antibody), T20 = targeted AuNRs (20 µL antibody).

To measure cell viability, a standard MTT (3-[4,5-dimethylthiazol-2-yl]-2,5 diphenyl tetrazolium bromide) colorimetric assay protocol was followed [15] to establish the level of cell death between the two laser types. This metabolic assay provides an indication of cell viability by measuring the enzymatic activity of cellular mitochondria [16]. After laser irradiation, the media from each well of the 96-well plate was replaced with fresh media and the plate was placed in the incubator. 24 h later, the media was removed from each well and a solution of media containing MTT (500 µg mL^{-1}) was added. After a further 3.5 h incubation the media containing MTT was removed from each well and the 96-well plate was wrapped in foil and stored at approximately 4 °C ready for absorbance measurements. Before measuring the plates with a plate reader (Mithras LB 940, Berthold Technologies, Bad Wildbad, Germany), 100 µL DMSO was added to each well. The divided sections of the plate were averaged to obtain a single absorbance value for each AuNR concentration, and the background absorbance level was subtracted from each of the other values. The cell viability was finally calculated by the ratio of mean absorbance of the sample with respect to mean absorbance of the control group (cells with media and no laser or AuNR exposure).

3. Results

Bright and dark-field imaging was used to assess the targeting of AuNR clusters to the lung cancer cells. Several images (N = 248) were acquired by scanning pseudo-randomly across the microscope slides to cover the majority of the sample and ensure a representative illustration of the cellular uptake was observed. Figure 4 shows a selection of those images to demonstrate the typical distribution observed. The volume of biotinylated antibodies (10 µL or 20 µL) that was used in the conjugation process appeared to affect the aggregation of AuNRs. As can be seen from Figure 5, large aggregates formed when 20 µL biotinylated antibodies was used in the conjugation process. The AuNR aggregates did appear to be bound to the surface of the A549 cells, however the large number of AuNRs making up the aggregates lead to a decrease in the distribution of AuNRs across the cell sample. When 10 µL was used, a reduction in AuNR aggregates was seen and the overall distribution of AuNRs throughout the cell population was more uniform.

Figures 6 and 7 show the cell viability data of the A549 cells after incubation with both untargeted and targeted S-Au40-849s for 4 h and 24 h, respectively. After a 4 h incubation period, there was no discernible reduction in cell viability induced from the AuNRs, either on their own or following laser irradiation. The lack of photothermal ablation can be attributed to an insufficient number of AuNRs remaining in the absorbing region after washing. This is in agreement with the cellular uptake data (Figure 4) where a 4 h incubation period resulted in minimal uptake of both untargeted and targeted S-Au40-849s. Conversely, after 24 h incubation with S-Au40-849s (Figure 7), reduced cell viability was observed in some cases. The AuNRs that received no laser exposure did not reduce the viability of the lung cancer cells, independent of whether they had been functionalised with the anti-EGFR ligands.

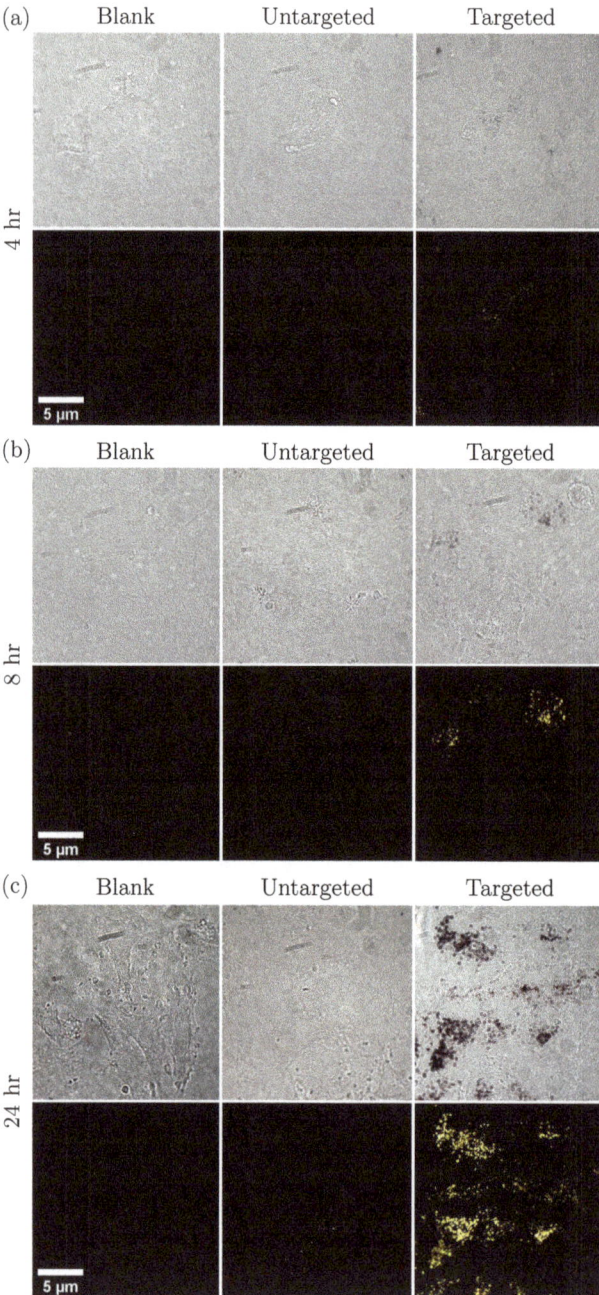

Figure 4. Bright- and dark-field images of lung cancer cells (A549) incubated with untargeted versus targeted (10 μL antibody) S-Au40-849s for (**a**) 4 h, (**b**) 8 h, and (**c**) 24 h.

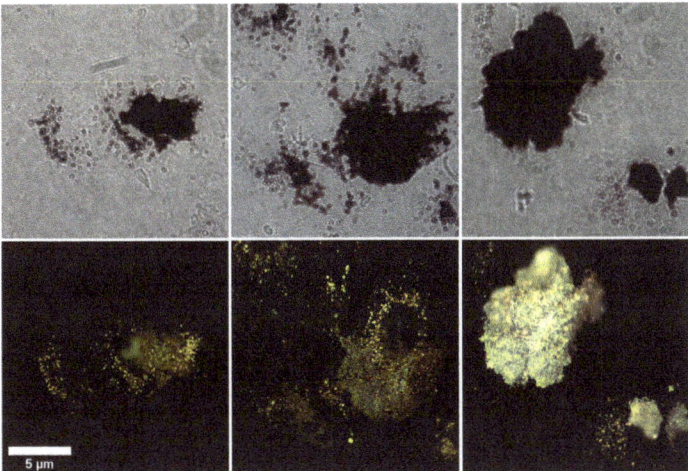

Figure 5. Large AuNR aggregates were apparent when a high volume (20 µL) of biotinylated anti-EGFR antibodies were used in the conjugation process of the S-Au40-849s, after 24 h of incubation.

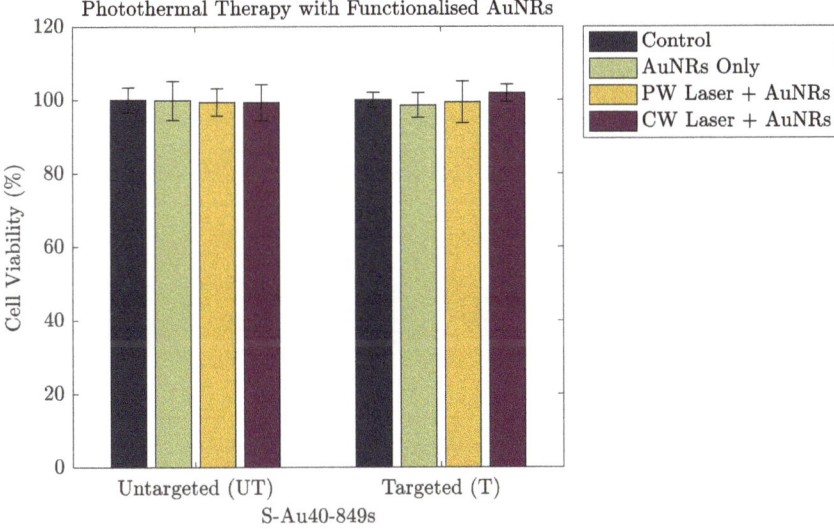

Figure 6. The cell viability of a lung cancer cell line after 4 h incubation with either untargeted S-Au40-849s or targeted S-Au40-849s.

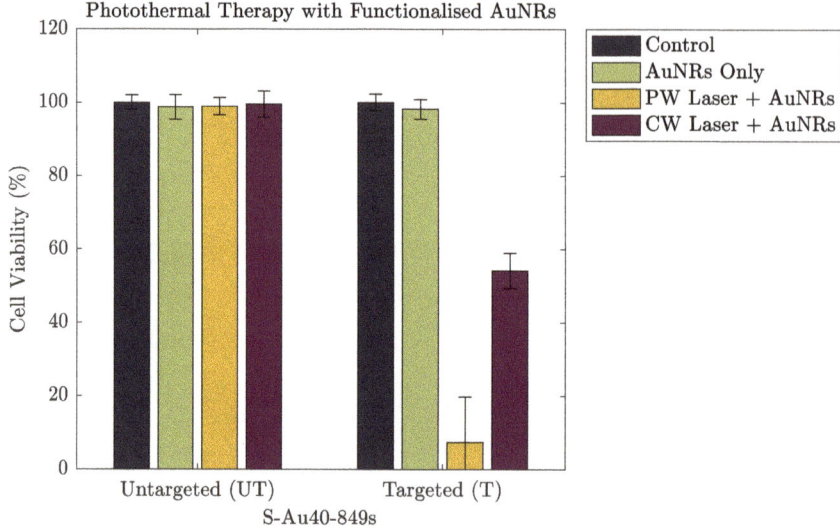

Figure 7. The cell viability of a lung cancer cell line after 24 h incubation with either untargeted S-Au40-849s or targeted S-Au40-849s.

4. Discussion

The untargeted S-Au40-849s displayed little cellular uptake across all of the time points, which was surprising since it might be expected that after 24 h incubation, much higher levels of uptake would be seen compared to that which was observed here. In comparison with the dark-field images taken of the citrate-capped AuNRs used in [13,17], there was considerably less cellular uptake of the untargeted S-Au40-849s. This was likely due to the streptavidin ligands that were already conjugated to the surface of the AuNRs, limiting the penetration of the S-Au40-849s into the lung cancer cells, since streptavidin has a relatively large molecular weight (approximately 60 kDa) and has been shown to restrict cellular uptake [18]. Furthermore, the potentially reduced biocompatibility of untargeted S-Au40-849s may negatively affect cellular uptake. Conversely, the targeted S-Au40-849s significantly enhanced AuNR uptake by the lung cancer cells after 8 h and 24 h (potentially via affinity to EGFR receptors) and while minimal uptake was observed after 4 h incubation with the A549 cells, there was an increase in overall uptake compared with their untargeted counterparts. The conjugation of the S-Au40-849 AuNRs with the anti-EGFR monoclonal antibodies had a considerable effect on the overall uptake when incubated with the lung cancer cells for longer than 4 h and the results provide a compelling argument to use molecularly targeted AuNRs for the selective delivery of high concentrations of AuNRs to malignant tissues. This was in contrast to a previous study [13] where a small but notable reduction in cell viability (approximately 20%) was observed. Differences between these studies can be attributed to the differences in the surface chemistry of the AuNRs used. In this study, the AuNRs were either surrounded by streptavidin proteins—which reduce cellular uptake (Figure 4) and therefore reduce toxic effects—or were conjugated with anti-EGFR ligands and were bound to the surface receptors on the cell membrane, limiting penetration into the cells. The cells that experienced a combination of untargeted S-Au40-849s and either CW or PW laser irradiation, also did not display a reduction in cell viability after the 5 min laser exposure. As discussed previously, the untargeted AuNRs had limited penetration into the cell membranes due to the large streptavidin molecules bound to the surface of the AuNRs and so were likely almost entirely removed during the washing stage.

Perhaps the most significant result was that the PW laser reduced the viability of 93% ± 12% of the population of lung cancer cells when combined with anti-EGFR targeting S-Au40-849s (after 24 h incubation), in comparison to the CW which destroyed almost half (46%) of the cells. A direct comparison of the energy/power density of these two laser systems is difficult due to their different modes of operation (see Supplementary Materials for further discussion), but by just taking average power, gives an $P_{ave} = 160$ mW for the PW laser and 950 mW or the CW laser. There are likely multiple contributing factors to the enhanced PPTT efficacy of the PW laser. The first reason may be that the efficacy of the CW laser for inducing cell-death is at its highest when there are a large number of AuNRs in the absorbing region and the light can be efficiently converted into wide-spread, bulk heating. The washing of the cell monolayer removed any AuNRs that were not bound to the cell surface and the number remaining in the path of the laser will not have been high enough to induce hyperthermia. The AuNRs that did persist would still have absorbed the incoming laser-light and converted it into heat, causing damage to the cells, however the overall heat generated from the exposure was not enough to provide a broad destruction of cells. The second reason may be due to an enhanced optical absorption and bubble-formation around the AuNRs under PW exposure due to AuNR clustering. It has been shown that the accumulation of antibody conjugated AuNRs on the surface of a cell membrane can further facilitate the self-assembly of the AuNRs into nanoclusters [19]. This in turn leads to an enhancement of the bubble formation around the AuNRs under high intensity laser pulses and subsequently an increase in damage to the cellular membrane. Zharov et al. (2005) concluded that pulsed lasers were more effective at inducing cell death when AuNRs formed nanoclusters on the cell membrane, and this agrees with our findings. Highly localised bubble formation due to the presence of nanoparticles can have other benefits for both therapeutic and imaging applications [20,21].

5. Conclusions

CW lasers induce bulk temperature changes in an absorbing medium whereas localised heating occurs when PW lasers are used. This suggests that PW lasers are only able to destroy cancer cells via a necrotic pathway, which reduces the risk of the cells developing drug or heat resistance but can cause immunogenic or inflammatory responses due to the immediate expulsion of the cells internals. Conversely, depending on the laser exposure parameters, CW lasers have been shown in the literature to induce cell death via either apoptosis or necrosis (although this aspect was not addressed in this study). Understanding these important distinctions between the two laser types is imperative for guiding therapy design. The relevant temperatures required to initiate the destruction of cells and the inducement of hyperthermia is in excess of 42 °C, which is only approximately 5 °C above internal body temperature. The length of time the cells remain at elevated temperatures influences the therapeutic efficiency and a clinically relevant parameter known as the thermal isoeffective dose (TID) is often used to compare thermal treatments. There is a large range of TID threshold values in the literature for determining when complete destruction of tissue is achieved, and this is due to the differences between the cellular compositions of different tissues. If TID values are to be used as a clinical measure of therapy, it is necessary to determine a TID threshold for the specific tissue that is being treated, otherwise it may be difficult to ensure maximum therapeutic effect.

Further to the consideration of AuNR size on photothermal efficacy, the effect of targeting AuNRs to the lung cancer cells was demonstrated. AuNRs with a similar size and aspect ratio to those used previously were purchased with streptavidin proteins conjugated to the surface, enabling the AuNRs to be easily functionalised with anti-EGFR targeting ligands. Lung cancer cells (along with many other malignant tissues, [22]) have been shown to overexpress anti-EGFR receptors and provide a potential method for increasing AuNR delivery efficiency to the cells—a critical aspect to the success of this therapy. The cellular uptake of untargeted S-Au40-849s was compared with that of targeted ones, and the results demonstrated the importance of molecularly targeting AuNRs for increased uptake. The untargeted AuNRs showed minimal uptake across the cell samples after the longest incubation time studied (24 h), however the accumulation and uptake of targeted AuNRs was evident.

Under laser irradiation, targeting also provided a significant advantage over untargeted AuNRs, when the incubation time was long enough (24 h). After 4 h there was no observed reduction in cell viability for any of the parameters studied, which agreed with the uptake study. However, a 24 h incubation resulted in an observable reduction in cell viability in some cases. The untargeted AuNRs were not able to reduce cell viability under any laser exposure parameters. In the case for targeted AuNRs, the PW laser was the most efficient laser system, destroying almost 93% of the total population of lung cancer cells, compared with almost half for the CW laser. This reversal in photothermal efficacy between the laser types may be due to the AuNRs forming nanoclusters, facilitated by the anti-EGFR targeting ligands, and increasing the mechanical stresses induced by the PW laser. In terms of the therapeutic efficacy of different sized un-targeted AuNRs, it appears that smaller AuNRs (width = 10 nm) are most suited as photoabsorbers under both CW and PW laser illumination, whereas AuNRs with a width of 25 nm were the least suited. The location of AuNRs was a critical aspect for therapeutic efficacy and targeting them to bind specifically to cell-receptors, such as EGFR, can improve cellular uptake and overall therapeutic outcome. Furthermore, if the eventual goal is to use AuNRs as clinical therapeutic agents then it is crucial that the production of AuNRs with consistent and uniform dimensions, properties and coatings, can be scaled-up to a level that ensures the practicality and safety of wide-spread clinical use.

Supplementary Materials: The following are available online at http://www.mdpi.com/2079-4991/10/7/1307/s1, Figure S1: A schematic representation of the differences between pulsed and continuous wave illumination.

Author Contributions: O.K. and J.R.M. conceived and designed the experiments, and analyzed the data; O.K. performed the experiments and wrote the manuscript with input from J.R.M., S.F. provided editorial input on the manuscript. All authors have read and agreed to the published version of the manuscript.

Funding: This research was funded by the UKRI (EP/S001069/1), and the Royal Society grant number (RG 170324).

Acknowledgments: Oscar B. Knights would like to acknowledge the EPSRC for supporting his Ph.D. through the Doctoral Training Grant Studentship. James R. McLaughlan would like to acknowledge support from an UKRI Innovation Fellowship.

Conflicts of Interest: The authors declare no conflict of interest.

Abbreviations

The following abbreviations are used in this manuscript:

AuNR	Gold Nanorod
EGFR	Epidermal growth factor receptor
EPR	Enhanced Permeability and Retention
PA	Photoacoustic
PPTT	Plasmonic Photothermal Therapy
PTT	Photothermal Therapy
TID	Thermal Iso-effective dose
rcf	Relative Centrifugal Force

References

1. World Health Organisation (WHO). *Cancer Fact Sheet No. 297*; World Health Organisation: Geneva, Switzerland, 2018.
2. El-Sayed, I.H.; Huang, X.; El-Sayed, M.A. Selective laser photo-thermal therapy of epithelial carcinoma using anti-EGFR antibody conjugated gold nanoparticles. *Cancer Lett.* **2006**, *239*, 129–135. [CrossRef] [PubMed]
3. Oto, A.; Sethi, I.; Karczmar, G.; McNichols, R.; Ivancevic, M.K.; Stadler, W.M.; Watson, S.; Eggener, S. MR imaging–guided focal laser ablation for prostate cancer: phase I trial. *Radiology* **2013**, *267*, 932–940. [CrossRef] [PubMed]
4. Zhao, Q.; Tian, G.; Chen, F.; Zhong, L.; Jiang, T. CT-guided percutaneous laser ablation of metastatic lung cancer: Three cases report and literature review. *Oncotarget* **2017**, *8*, 2187. [CrossRef] [PubMed]

5. Huang, X.; Qian, W.; El-Sayed, I.H.; El-Sayed, M.A. The potential use of the enhanced nonlinear properties of gold nanospheres in photothermal cancer therapy. *Lasers Surg. Med. Off. J. Am. Soc. Laser Med. Surg.* **2007**, *39*, 747–753. [CrossRef] [PubMed]
6. Yang, W.; Liang, H.; Ma, S.; Wang, D.; Huang, J. Gold nanoparticle based photothermal therapy: Development and application for effective cancer treatment. *Sustain. Mater. Technol.* **2019**, *22*, e00109. [CrossRef]
7. Pérez-Hernández, M.; del Pino, P.; Mitchell, S.G.; Moros, M.; Stepien, G.; Pelaz, B.; Parak, W.J.; Gálvez, E.M.; Pardo, J.; de la Fuente, J.M. Dissecting the molecular mechanism of apoptosis during photothermal therapy using gold nanoprisms. *ACS Nano* **2014**, *9*, 52–61. [CrossRef] [PubMed]
8. Qin, Z.; Bischof, J.C. Thermophysical and biological responses of gold nanoparticle laser heating. *Chem. Soc. Rev.* **2012**, *41*, 1191–1217. [CrossRef] [PubMed]
9. Zhong, J.; Yang, S.; Zheng, X.; Zhou, T.; Xing, D. In vivo photoacoustic therapy with cancer-targeted indocyanine green-containing nanoparticles. *Nanomedicine* **2013**, *8*, 903–919. [CrossRef] [PubMed]
10. Danhier, F. To exploit the tumor microenvironment: Since the EPR effect fails in the clinic, what is the future of nanomedicine? *J. Control. Release* **2016**, *244*, 108–121. [CrossRef] [PubMed]
11. Sindhwani, S.; Syed, A.M.; Ngai, J.; Kingston, B.R.; Maiorino, L.; Rothschild, J.; MacMillan, P.; Zhang, Y.; Rajesh, N.U.; Hoang, T.; et al. The entry of nanoparticles into solid tumours. *Nat. Mater.* **2020**, *19*, 1–10. [CrossRef] [PubMed]
12. Weber, J.; Beard, P.C.; Bohndiek, S.E. Contrast agents for molecular photoacoustic imaging. *Nat. Methods* **2016**, *13*, 639. [CrossRef]
13. Knights, O.; McLaughlan, J. Gold Nanorods for Light-Based Lung Cancer Theranostics. *Int. J. Mol. Sci.* **2018**, *19*, 3318. [CrossRef] [PubMed]
14. Schneider, C.A.; Rasband, W.S.; Eliceiri, K.W. NIH Image to ImageJ: 25 years of image analysis. *Nat. Methods* **2012**, *9*, 671–675. [CrossRef] [PubMed]
15. Van Meerloo, J.; Kaspers, G.J.; Cloos, J. Cell sensitivity assays: the MTT assay. In *Cancer Cell Culture*; Springer: Berlin, Germany, 2011; pp. 237–245.
16. Alkilany, A.M.; Murphy, C.J. Toxicity and cellular uptake of gold nanoparticles: What we have learned so far? *J. Nanopart. Res.* **2010**, *12*, 2313–2333. [CrossRef] [PubMed]
17. Knights, O.B.; Ye, S.; Ingram, N.; Freear, S.; McLaughlan, J.R. Optimising gold nanorods for photoacoustic imaging in vitro. *Nanosc. Adv.* **2019**, *1*, 1472–1481. [CrossRef]
18. Ahmed, W.; Elhissi, A.; Dhanak, V.; Subramani, K. Carbon nanotubes: Applications in cancer therapy and drug delivery research. In *Emerging Nanotechnologies in Dentistry*; Elsevier: Amsterdam, The Netherlands, 2018; pp. 371–389.
19. Zharov, V.; Letfullin, R.; Galitovskaya, E. Microbubbles-overlapping mode for laser killing of cancer cells with absorbing nanoparticle clusters. *J. Phys. D Appl. Phys.* **2005**, *38*, 2571. [CrossRef]
20. Cavigli, L.; Centi, S.; Borri, C.; Tortoli, P.; Panettieri, I.; Streit, I.; Ciofini, D.; Magni, G.; Rossi, F.; Siano, S.; et al. 1064-nm-resonant gold nanorods for photoacoustic theranostics within permissible exposure limits. *J. Biophoton.* **2019**, *12*, e201900082. [CrossRef] [PubMed]
21. McLaughlan, J.R.; Roy, R.A.; Ju, H.; Murray, T.W. Ultrasonic enhancement of photoacoustic emissions by nanoparticle-targeted cavitation. *Opt. Lett.* **2010**, *35*, 2127–2129. [CrossRef] [PubMed]
22. Nicholson, R.; Gee, J.; Harper, M.. EGFR and cancer prognosis. *Eur. J. Cancer* **2001**, *37*, 9–15. [CrossRef]

© 2020 by the authors. Licensee MDPI, Basel, Switzerland. This article is an open access article distributed under the terms and conditions of the Creative Commons Attribution (CC BY) license (http://creativecommons.org/licenses/by/4.0/).

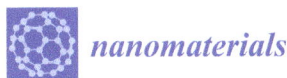

Article

Single-Step Photochemical Formation of Near-Infrared-Absorbing Gold Nanomosaic within PNIPAm Microgels: Candidates for Photothermal Drug Delivery

Sreekar B. Marpu [1,*], Brian Leon Kamras [1,†], Nooshin MirzaNasiri [1,†], Oussama Elbjeirami [1,‡], Denise Perry Simmons [2], Zhibing Hu [3,‡] and Mohammad A. Omary [1,*]

1. Department of Chemistry, University of North Texas, Denton, TX 76203, USA; briankamras@my.unt.edu (B.L.K.); nooshinmirzanasiri@my.unt.edu (N.M.); elbjeirami@unt.edu (O.E.)
2. Department of Mechanical and Energy Engineering, University of North Texas, Denton, TX 76203, USA; denise.simmons@unthsc.edu
3. Department of Physics, University of North Texas, Denton, TX 76203, USA; Zhibing.Hu@unt.edu
* Correspondence: sreekarbabu.marpu@unt.edu (S.B.M.); mohammad.omary@unt.edu (M.A.O.)
† These authors contribute equally to this work.
‡ Deceased.

Received: 18 May 2020; Accepted: 18 June 2020; Published: 28 June 2020

Abstract: This work demonstrates the dynamic potential for tailoring the surface plasmon resonance (SPR), size, and shapes of gold nanoparticles (AuNPs) starting from an Au(I) precursor, chloro(dimethyl sulfide)gold (I) (Au(Me$_2$S)Cl), in lieu of the conventional Au(III) precursor hydrogen tetrachloroaurate (III) hydrate (HAuCl$_4$). Our approach presents a one-step method that permits regulation of an Au(I) precursor to form either visible-absorbing gold nanospheres or near-infrared-window (NIRW)-absorbing anisotropic AuNPs. A collection of shapes is obtained for the NIR-absorbing AuNPs herein, giving rise to spontaneously formed nanomosaic (NIR-absorbing anisotropic gold nanomosaic, NIRAuNM) without a dominant geometry for the tesserae elements that comprise the mosaic. Nonetheless, NIRAuNM exhibited high stability; one test sample remains stable with the same SPR absorption profile 7 *years post-synthesis thus far*. These NIRAuNM are generated within thermoresponsive poly(*N*-isopropylacrylamide) (PNIPAm) microgels, without the addition of any growth-assisting surfactants or reducing agents. Our directed-selection methodology is based on the photochemical reduction of a light-, heat-, and water-sensitive Au(I) precursor via a disproportionation mechanism. The NIRAuNM stabilized within the thermoresponsive microgels demonstrates a light-activated size decrease of the microgels. On irradiation with a NIR lamp source, the percent decrease in the size of the microgels loaded with NIRAuNM is at least five times greater compared to the control microgels. The concept of photothermal shrinkage of hybrid microgels is further demonstrated by the release of a model luminescent dye, as a drug release model. The absorbance and emission of the model dye released from the hybrid microgels are over an order of magnitude higher compared to the absorbance and emission of the dye released from the unloaded-control microgels.

Keywords: nanoparticles; anisotropy; plasmonic photothermal therapy; surface plasmon resonance; light scattering; cancer treatment; drug release; microgels

1. Introduction

Stimuli-responsive polymers, hydrogels, and microgels are appealing to biomedical researchers as potential drug delivery candidates, based upon their ability to undergo phase transitions in response to various environmental factors (e.g., temperature, light, pH, and/or ionic strength). High water content, hydrophilicity, softness, flexibility, biocompatibility, and properties similar to biological tissues render such polymer hydrogel materials as suitable platforms for various biomedical applications [1–7]. To extend their functionality, numerous investigations have demonstrated the loading and/or stabilization of different nanomaterials such as metallic nanoparticles and quantum dots within these microgels [8]. Poly(N-isopropylacrylamide) (PNIPAm) is often used because of its thermoresponsiveness results in "smart gel" materials. PNIPAm, which has a lower critical solution temperature (LCST)–32 °C, can be tuned by varying its composition and crosslinking density [9]. In a related area, AuNPs are frequently studied for their structural, optical, electronic, and catalytic properties. Among those, AuNPs with anisotropic shapes (e.g., rods, triangles, cubes, truncated octahedra, shells, stars, etc.) with surface plasmon resonances (SPR) that extend beyond the visible region are desirable for sensing and plasmonic photothermal therapy (PPTT) applications [10–12].

1.1. Overview of Anisotropic AuNPs Usage

By regulating the size and shape of a given anisotropic gold nanoparticle, the NIR SPR resonance band can be tuned to lie within the "near-infrared window" (NIRW) that lies within 700–1300 nm [13]. Due to their strong NIR absorption and high extinction coefficient [12,14,15], anisotropic AuNPs are highly appealing candidates for plasmonic photothermal therapy (PPTT) [15]. Usually, researchers exploiting the plasmonic photothermal properties or localized sensitive properties of Near infrared gold nanoparticles (NIRAuNPs) use gold nanorods (AuNRs) stabilized in the highly cytotoxic (vide infra) surfactant reagent cetyltrimethylammonium bromide (CTAB) made using the classic seed-mediated method, developed by the Murphy group and later modified by El-Sayed et al. [16]. In addition to the classic seed-mediated method, there are also seedless and polyol processes developed by numerous researchers [17]. For example, Huang et al. produced gold nanorods (AuNRs) with high aspect ratios by employing silver bromide (AgBr) as a capping agent, CTAB as the growth-directing surfactant, and HCl to modulate pH [17]. Wang et al. used 5-Bromosalicylic acid as a templating factor in addition to the typical CTAB surfactant and silver nitrate as a capping agent, which produced rods at a practically quantitative yield [18]. In addition to AuNRs, other anisotropic shapes including nanoplates, nanotriangles, nanocubes, and nanostars with sharp edges and NIR SPR features are equally attractive candidates for biosensing and surface-enhanced Raman scattering (SERS) applications [19]. These anisotropic particles are mainly synthesized using protocols resembling the AuNR synthesis [6,20].

1.2. Toxicity Challenges

The abovementioned methods involve surfactants such as CTAB or silver ions, which are both reported to be toxic by various research groups [21]. Even without CTAB, overcoming the inherent toxicity of silver ions is still challenging [21]. The toxicity of CTAB and the role of CTAB in AuNRs synthesis have been detailed by many groups [22,23]. In 2017, Bandyopadhyay illustrated that the positive surface charge of CTAB induces cytotoxicity and hinders the adsorption of serum proteins onto the particle surface, which can alter the process of endocytosis [24]. The role of CTAB in complicating the biomedical applications of AuNRs was explained by Kohanloo et al., who determined the critical CTAB:nanorod concentration ratio to be approximately 740,000:1 to attain nanorods stability upon the formation of a CTAB double-layer, whereas experimentally, an even larger excess of CTAB is added [25]. Additionally, Choi et al. demonstrated the necessity of replacing or removing CTAB for in vivo application of AuNRs. Currently, CTAB toxicity is circumvented by ligand exchange using thiolated polyethylene glycol (PEG-SH) because of the latter's water solubility, biocompatibility, and relatively higher binding affinity for Au than CTAB [26]. Although gold nanoparticle cores alone are shown to be nontoxic in numerous in vitro studies, the stabilizing ligand can be toxic. Therefore, differentiating the toxicity due to the stabilizing ligands versus the gold core itself is critical. These potential problems and risks are high with anisotropic AuNPs due to their highly exposed surfaces and defects compared to spherical AuNPs [21].

1.3. Nontoxic Tuning Methods

Among the few methodologies that do not use surfactants or CTAB, Guo and coworkers have shown success using a seed-mediated growth approach to create size-tunable AuNPs in the range of 5 to 200 nm by reduction of Au(III) with sodium borohydride (NaBH$_4$) and hydroxylamine hydrochloride (NH$_2$OH·HCl) [27]. Alternatively, some research groups have explored "green" synthesis methods to overcome cytotoxicity issues and the tedious ligand exchange processes inherent to conventional syntheses of various NIRAuNPs [26]. Biological extracts are known to be employed as reducing/stabilizing substances for making both spherical and anisotropic AuNPs. Among them, the biological synthesis of triangular gold nanoprisms, stabilized in lemongrass by Sastry et al., has attracted immense interest [28]. Sakthivel and coworkers have used *Coleus amboinicus* extracts as reducing and stabilizing agents for producing different sizes of spherical, polydispersed AuNPs [29]. Kitching et al. described the advantages of fungal biosynthesis of gold nanoparticles and have also explained the complications involved in understanding the biosynthetic mechanism of AuNPs formation within biological media [30]. In 2014, the Menon group successfully synthesized NIR-absorbing anisotropic AuNPs using a cocoa extract and explained the challenges involved in making AuNPs with NIRW-absorbing features within these biological [31].

1.4. Photochemical Formation of AuNPs

Numerous literature examples have demonstrated the photochemical formation of silver nanoparticles, but an extension of this methodology to AuNPs is still limited. This is likely due to easy access to the light-sensitive silver precursors, which contrast with the relative stability of the hydrogen tetrachloroaurate (III) hydrate (HAuCl$_4$) precursor. However, there are a few examples of spherical and anisotropic AuNPs made from HAuCl$_4$ precursors by employing photochemistry. The Zhao group demonstrated the formation of small, spherical AuNPs by irradiation of HAuCl$_4$ with a 300 nm wavelength light source [32]. In 2005, the El-Sayed group demonstrated the formation of Au(0) with continuous excitation of HAuCl$_4$ in the presence of ethylene glycol and polyvinylpyrrolidone (PVP) using a 250–400 nm light source [33]. Pal has demonstrated the photochemical formation of spherical AuNPs in the presence of sodium dodecyl sulfate (SDS) and dopamine hydrochloride [34]. There are even fewer literature examples illustrating the photochemical formation of anisotropic AuNPs. Among them, the photochemical synthesis of gold nanorods by Kim et al. is notable for tuning the aspect ratio of AuNRs by using photochemistry in the presence of CTAB and silver ions [35]. Zhu et al. have shown the photochemical formation of a mixture of anisotropic AuNPs within room-temperature ionic liquids (RTILs) [36]. In 2016, Wei et al. demonstrated a plasmon-driven synthesis of Au nanoprisms within PVP [37]. Analyzing the growth of AuNRs by photochemical means, some researchers have also analyzed the role of CTAB, silver ions, and photoinitiators [38]. Pignatelli et al. found that varying the irradiation time, wavelength, and intensity can tune the absorption and aspect ratio of AuNRs [39].

1.5. Stabilization of AuNPs within PNIPAm Hydrogels/Microgels

Several groups have modified AuNPs, postsynthesis, by binding PNIPAm or surface-functionalized PNIPAm to the AuNPs surface and found that the resulting hybrid material exhibits a thermoreversible phase shift and corresponding color-absorption shift [40]. Despite the synergistic properties of temperature sensitivity and heat-generating ability, only a handful of demonstrations exist that incorporate AuNRs or NIR-absorbing AuNPs within PNIPAm microgels or hydrogels. Zhao et al. loaded CTAB-stabilized AuNRs into a triblock copolymer of randomly arranged acrylamide, acrylonitrile, and dimethylacrylamide to exploit the polymers' upper critical solution temperature (UCST); such methods afforded a temperature-responsive, "switchable" composite material [41]. This composite, when irradiated with visible light, resulted in the release of an adsorbed protein from within the pores of the composite. Liz-Marzan et al. found that CTAB-stabilized AuNRs adsorbed within PNIPAm microgel spheres undergo a phase-transition, which red-shifts the rod's SPR when irradiated with NIR light [42]. Kawano et al. have demonstrated photothermal heating using CTAB stabilized, silica-coated AuNRs within PNIPAm nanogels [43]. In 2010, Jiang et al. demonstrated the formation of PNIPAm-AuNR composites by using the seed-mediated growth method; they reasoned that such PNIPAm composites have great advantages in surface-enhanced Raman scattering (SERS) as these composites combine the thermoresponsive behavior of microgels and the SERS effect of AuNRs [44]. In 2015, F.-Lopez et al. have demonstrated reversible plasmon coupling from AuNRs with differing aspect ratios doped within PNIPAm [45]. However, most or all of these methods, to the best of our knowledge, are based on loading or tethering premade anisotropic AuNPs or AuNRs to PNIPAm polymers or hydrogels [40–45].

1.6. Formation of AuNPs from Au(I) Precursor

Our literature search found a handful of studies investigating Au(I) species as AuNP precursors. In 1988, Vogler et al. formed AuNPs by reducing gold azide complexes via photolysis [46]. In 2004, Lee et al. demonstrated the formation of spherical AuNPs from Au(I)-SC18–alkane thiolates by electron beam irradiation [47]. Another important demonstration of using Au(I) compounds for the synthesis of gold nanostructures comes from the 2008 report by the Xia group, using Au(I) halides including AuCl and AuBr to make AuNPs in chloroform in the presence of alkylamines with heating at 60 °C. The method demonstrated that the relatively low stability of Au(I) halides resulted in AuNP formation in the absence of any reducing agents [48]. Included in this handful of reports, our group demonstrated for the first time, the aurophilicity and ligand π-acceptance ability to sensitize the photoreactivity of Au(I) complexes. In 2007, we reported our findings on the propensity of Au(I) isonitriles to form AuNPs by photolysis in the presence of polyamidoamine (PAMAM) dendrimers in organic media [49]. These findings led to the discovery of Au(I) isonitriles transition through an Au(0) intermediate and present a possible mechanism for the formation of AuNPs. We continue to build upon our findings, and to the best of our knowledge, we report herein, the very first photochemical synthesis method for selectively making strong NIRW-absorbing AuNPs comprising a mixture of anisotropic shapes. Our method uses an Au(I) precursor within PNIPAm-*co*-allylamine microgels medium in the complete absence of any synergetic reducing agents or surfactants. To evaluate the wide range potential of this methodology, our work involves the formation of different sizes of spherical AuNPs, ranging from 5 to 50 nm, within different types of stabilizing media, again in the complete absence of any additional (potentially toxic) chemicals. The stabilizing media types included: agarose, alginic acid, chitosan, hydroxypropyl cellulose (HPC), polyvinyl alcohol (PVA), polyacrylic acid (PAA), PNIPAm microgels, and sodium dodecyl sulfate (SDS).

2. Materials and Methods

N-isopropylacrylamide (NIPA) monomer, allylamine, acrylic acid, *N*,*N*'-Methylenebis(acrylamide) (BIS), potassium persulfate (KPS), and sodium dodecyl sulfate (SDS) were purchased from Polysciences Inc., Warrington, PA, USA). Ethanol (99.5%), diethyl ether, dimethyl sulfide (Me_2S), 85% deacetylated medium-molecular-weight chitosan, 50,000 Mw 30% polyacrylic acid, 100,000 Mw alginic acid sodium salt, 80,000 Mw hydroxypropyl cellulose, 90,000 Mw poly(vinyl alcohol), 96% bovine serum albumin (BSA), and wide-range agarose were bought from Sigma-Aldrich (St. Louis, MO, USA). Dialysis tubing (10 k MWCO) was purchased from California Biological (Burlington, NC, USA). All chemicals are used as received. For all experiments, 18.2 MΩ-cm (at 25 °C) ultrapure water (MilliporeSigma, Burlington, MA, USA)) was used. All glassware were cleaned in a bath of freshly prepared aqua regia, and were then rinsed thoroughly with ultrapure water. There were multiple samples made throughout the years using the same synthesis protocol and likewise for the experimental measurements below–all of which have attained high reproducibility.

2.1. Physical Measurements

A 450-W medium-pressure immersion mercury vapor lamp (Ace Glass) was placed into a photochemistry chamber equipped with a magnetic stirrer and a variable-temperature hot plate was used for all photochemical reactions. Based upon the manufacturer's specifications of the total output energy from the mercury lamp, approximately 40–48% is in the ultraviolet region, 40–43% is in the visible region, and the remainder is in the infrared region. Regular borosilicate (BS) and quartz (SQ) silica glass were selectively utilized for the different syntheses. The same lamp source setup was employed for the synthesis of both spherical and anisotropic gold nanoparticle compositions. Absorption spectra were acquired using a Perkin-Elmer Lambda 900 double-beam UV/VIS-NIR spectrophotometer. The size, morphology, dispersity, and elemental analysis of different gold nanoparticle samples were determined using a high-resolution analytical transmission electron microscope (TEM). Specifically, a FEI Co. Tecnai G2 F20 S-TWIN 200 keV field-emission scanning transmission electron microscope (STEM) was used. A 1-nm STEM probe allowed for an imaging resolution of 0.19 nm, and a high angle annular dark field detector (HAADF) allowed for Z-contrast imaging in STEM mode at high resolution. High-resolution analytical capabilities were provided on the F20 STEM, which was equipped with an energy-dispersive X-ray spectrometer (EDS, also known as EDX), and a Gatan Tridiem parallel electron energy loss spectrometer (EELS) with a 2k × 2k CCD for energy-filtered imaging and high-rate spectrum imaging EELS. Unless otherwise mentioned, all images were collected in a bright field mode. Scanning electron microscopy (SEM) images were collected using an FEI Nova 200 NanoLab, which is a dual column ultrahigh resolution field emission scanning electron microscope. The nanoscale chemical analysis was performed with an EDS system with spectrum imaging control.

2.2. Syntheses of Gold(I) Precursor

The chloro(dimethyl sulfide)gold(I) complex (Au(Me$_2$S)Cl) was synthesized by slightly modifying our earlier-established procedure described elsewhere [50]. Tetrahydrothiophene (THT) was replaced with dimethyl sulfide (Me$_2$S) in the procedure. Before use, the glassware was oven-dried overnight at 150 °C. All manipulations were carried out under an atmosphere of purified nitrogen using the standard Schlenk technique. Briefly, the procedure involved 2 steps. In the first step, 1.8 g of gold (from the gold coin) was dissolved in 12 mL of aqua regia (9 mL of HCl and 3 mL of HNO$_3$) in a 100 mL Schlenk flask. The reaction mixture was heated at 70 °C with continuous stirring to dissolve the solid gold. After dissolving the gold, heating was continued for an additional 30 min, followed by the addition of 3 mL of HCl. At this stage, heating was discontinued, and 30 mL of ethanol and 20 mL of water were added. The reaction was allowed to reach ambient temperature. At this stage, a yellow-orange colored solution was obtained. In the second step, the drop-wise addition of 2 mL of Me$_2$S ligand resulted in the formation of a white precipitate. The reaction flask was then cooled in an ice bath, and the precipitate (product) was collected by sequential filtration with cold ethanol, followed by cold ether. The product was then dried overnight under vacuum. It should be noted that this heat-, light-, and water-sensitive Au(I) complex is always stored refrigerated and in the dark (foil wrap) away from the refrigerator's light source.

2.3. Syntheses of PNIPAm Microgels

The hydrogel nanoparticles were made using the free radical precipitation method [50–54]. Precisely, 3.814 g of N-isopropylacrylamide monomer, 0.2 g of either allylamine or acrylic acid (for PNIPAm-co-allylamine and PNIPAm-co-acrylic acid, respectively), 0.066 g of BIS, and 0.08 g of SDS were dissolved in 245 g of ultrapure water. The solution was stirred under an N$_2$ atmosphere for 40 min at 60 °C, and then, 5.0 mL of KPS (0.166 g) was added to initiate radical polymerization. Heating was continued for 5 h under a nitrogen atmosphere at 60 °C. The resulting PNIPAm-co-allylamine and PNIPAm-co-acrylic acid colloidal particles were transferred to 10,000 MWCO dialysis tubing and dialyzed against deionized (DI) water for 1 week at ambient temperature, followed by further purification via ultracentrifugation. The hydrodynamic radius (R_h) of the microgels with and without AuNPs is measured by the dynamic light-scattering (DLS) technique. A commercial laser light-scattering (LLS) spectrometer (ALV/DLS/SLS-5000, Langen, Germany) equipped with an ALV-5000 Digital Time Correlator was used with a He–Ne laser (Uniphase 1145P, output power = 22 mW, and λ = 632.8 nm) as the light source. All size measurements were performed at a scattering angle of 90°. The volume shrinkage studies were conducted by controlling the temperature of the samples by a circulating water bath (Brinkmann Lauda Super RM-6, American Laboratory Trading, East Lyme, CT, USA) to within 0.02 °C. The samples for all the dynamic light scattering analysis were prepared by homogenization followed by dilution with Millipore water. Each sample was measured three times, and the mean radius was reported. The zeta potential was measured on a Zetasizer Nano ZS (Malvern Instruments, Westborough MA, USA) by loading samples into maintenance-free cells. Figure S1 shows the initial size of the PNIPAm microgels with and without AuNPs.

2.4. Syntheses of Spherical AuNPs within PNIPAm Microgels

In a typical procedure, a particular weight percent concentration of PNIPAm solution (2.0% w/v) is initially diluted to 0.2% w/v with ultrapure water and homogenized by stirring at ambient temperature (22 °C). Au(Me$_2$S)Cl (5.0 mg, 1.68 µmol) is directly added to the PNIPAm microgel solution and stirred at ambient temperature for 5–10 min until all the Au(I) powder is homogeneously dispersed in the microgel medium. The freshly prepared PNIPAm-Au dispersion is immediately transferred into an SQ glass vial followed by irradiation in the photochemistry chamber equipped with a medium-pressure immersion mercury lamp as described in methods. All PNIPAm microgel samples containing the Au(I) complex are irradiated at ambient temperature. The temperature of the photochemistry chamber is maintained at 22 °C during the entire course of irradiation. For testing the effect of ambient conditions (room light and ambient temperature), the initial microgel solution containing the Au(I) precursor was transferred into a BS glass vial and then subjected to stirring at ambient temperature and ambient light. In all cases, AuNPs formation within the PNIPAm microgels was monitored by sampling the reaction solution over time and observing the recorded changes in absorption spectra. Depending upon the reaction conditions and the nature of the PNIPAm microgels (co-allylamine or co-acrylic acid), the total reaction time varied from 30 to 180 min. The absorption spectra were collected after placing the samples into 1-cm path length quartz cuvettes. For calculating the photochemical quantum yield of AuNPs within PNIPAm microgels, the changes in absorption of the samples with respect to time were analyzed.

2.5. Synthesis of Spherical AuNPs within Different Media

In a typical procedure, 1.0% *w/v* of a stabilizing media (alginic acid, chitosan, poly(acrylic acid), poly (vinyl alcohol), hydroxypropyl cellulose, sodium dodecyl sulfate, and bovine serum albumin) is dissolved in ultrapure water and homogenized for 10 min. Au(Me$_2$S)Cl (5.0 mg, 1.68 µmol), is added to each of the abovementioned media, and the solution is subjected to photoirradiation in an SQ or BS glass container or heated at 37 °C. The reaction time varied for each solution depending upon the stabilizer used. Each reaction was stopped when the absorbance of AuNPs on the UV/VIS–NIR spectrophotometer ranged from 1.0 to 1.5 units (an arbitrary but consistent scale).

2.6. Synthesis of Anisotropic AuNPs (NIRAuNM) within PNIPAm-Co-allylamine Microgels

In a typical procedure, a particular weight percent concentration of the PNIPAm-*co*-allylamine solution (2.0% *w/v*) was initially diluted to 0.5% w/v with ultrapure water and homogenized by stirring at ambient temperature. The pH of the diluted microgel solution was adjusted to 4.0 by the dropwise addition of 0.1 M acetic acid (0.5 mL). Au(Me$_2$S)Cl (3.0–9.0 mg, 1.02–3.02 µmol) was then added to the PNIPAm microgel solution and stirred at room temperature for 5–10 min until all the Au(I) powder is homogeneously dispersed in the microgels medium. The freshly prepared PNIPAm-Au solution was immediately transferred into a (BS) glass container followed by irradiation in the photochemistry chamber equipped with a medium-pressure immersion mercury lamp. For photoirradiated samples, the temperature was maintained between 0 and 5 °C throughout the reaction. For samples prepared by thermolysis, the PNIPAm microgel solution containing Au(Me$_2$S)Cl was initially heated in a water bath at 37 °C for 10 to 15 min. After the initial color change, the reaction beaker was immediately transferred into an ice-water bath, and the temperature maintained between 0 and 5 °C throughout the remainder of the reaction time. NIRAuNM formation within the PNIPAm-co-allylamine microgel media was monitored by observing the recorded changes in absorption spectra as a function of time. Depending on reaction conditions, the total reaction time varied from 45 to 90 min. The absorption spectra were collected by collecting the samples into 1-cm path length quartz cuvettes. In all cases, the size, shape, distribution, and morphology of the AuNPs were determined using a field-emission scanning electron microscopy (FE-SEM, an FEI Co, Hillsboro, OR, USA.) and transmission electron microscopy (TEM, an EFI Co, Hillsboro, OR, USA). The samples were prepared by the drop-cast method on respective grids. The elemental composition of AuNPs was determined from EDS measurements.

2.7. Preparation of Samples for Electron Microscopy

For SEM, the microgel samples loaded with AuNPs were directly deposited on to SEM stubs and dried overnight inside a vacuum chamber. The samples were diluted with DI water as required for better microscopy results. For TEM, diluted hybrid microgel samples were added drop-wise on to the formvar carbon support copper grids and dried in a vacuum chamber for an hour. All samples for microscopy were stored strictly inside closed boxes to prevent any contamination. The SEM and TEM grids were obtained from Ted Pella, Redding, CA, USA.

3. Results and Discussion

3.1. Potential of Au(I) Precursor as an Alternative Precursor to Au(III) Salts for Making AuNPs

The schematics representing the in situ formation of both visible absorbing spherical AuNPs and NIR-absorbing anisotropic AuNPs within PNIPAm microgels are shown in Scheme 1. The one-electron photoreduction of Au(I) to Au(0) proceeds rapidly and spontaneously at ambient temperature in aqueous media. Compared to conventional Au(III) systems, the photochemical reduction of Au(Me$_2$S)Cl in water was so spontaneous that it resulted in aggregated or decomposed Au(0) within a few minutes of irradiation (Figure 1A)– indicating its sensitivity to light. The broad SPR peak spreads across 550–900 nm, the faint red color of the Au(I)-water solution at 0 min irradiation, and the aggregation of Au(0) as revealed from the changes in absorption spectra (Figure 1A) within 2 min of irradiation all indicated both water and light sensitivity of Au(Me$_2$S)Cl. After 2 min of irradiation, the absorption spectrum indicated the aggregation of Au(0) in absence of any stabilizer, shown by the high absorption baseline and disappearance of the broad SPR peak (Figure 1A). The TEM images collected from the unstable Au(I)-water system showed the expected aggregation of Au(0) nanostructures (Figure 1A"). UV/VIS–NIR absorption spectra, daylight images, and TEM images of Au(I) in aqueous media confirmed that the Au(Me$_2$S)Cl can undergo photochemical reduction to form metallic gold(0) without any external reducing agents. The evidence in Figure 1, supported our hypothesis for the rest of the manuscript. We deduced this hypothesis based on both the literature as well as our earlier AuNP work, which revealed that dimethyl sulfide (Me$_2$S) is an ideal ligand for making nontoxic [55] gold nanoparticles, because of its inherent low toxicity and high volatility (e.g., it is responsible for the foul smell upon boiling cabbage). The literature notes that AuNP formation from Au(I) precursors is rarely explored in organic media [49] and completely unexplored in aqueous media, possibly because Au(I) compounds are known to undergo spontaneous decomposition in aqueous media even at ambient temperature, as confirmed in our current body of work in Figure 1.

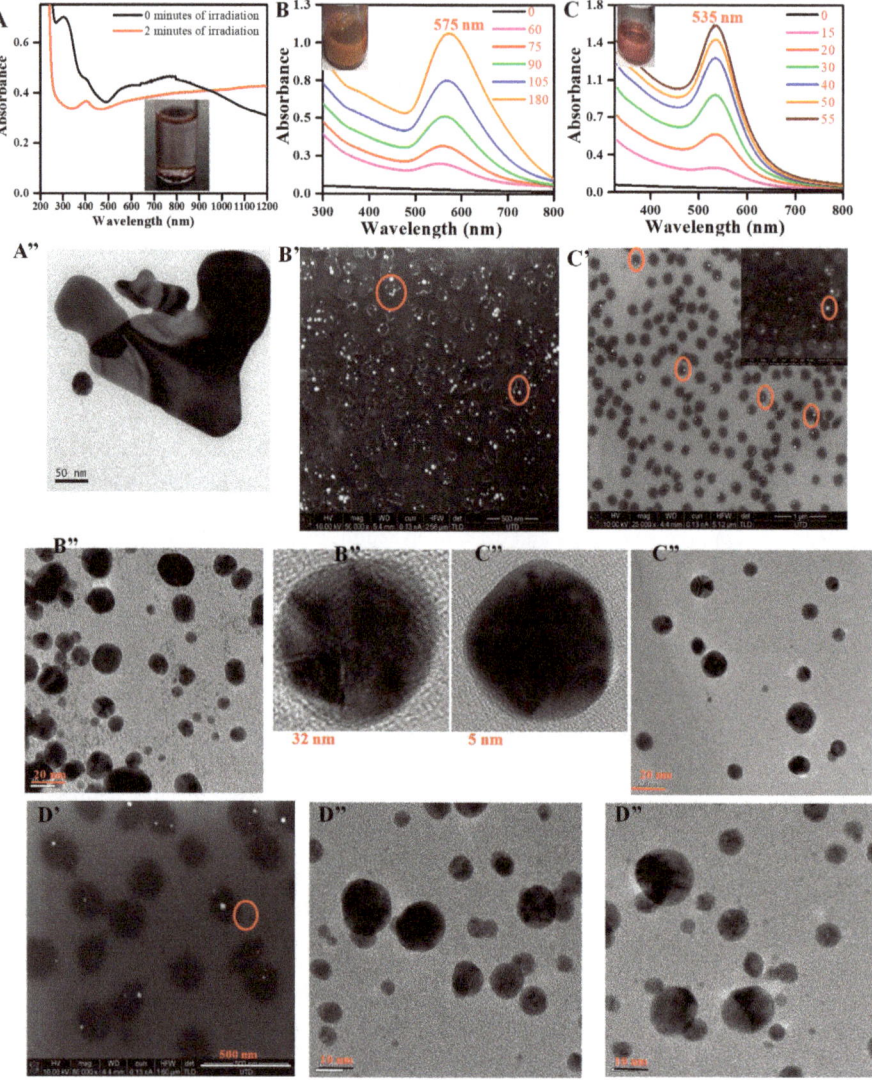

Figure 1. Absorption spectra and electron microscopy images of spherical gold nanoparticles (AuNPs) formed using chloro(dimethyl sulfide)gold (I) (Au(Me$_2$S)Cl) precursor under different irradiation conditions within deionized (DI) water and poly(N-isopropylacrylamide) (PNIPAm) microgels. Traces (**A,A″**) illustrate absorption spectra and TEM images of decomposed Au(I) in DI water. Traces (**B,B′,B″**) depict absorption changes vs. time (minutes), SEM and TEM images for AuNPs formed under ambient light within PNIPAm-co-allylamine microgels. Traces (**C,C′,C″**) represent absorption changes vs. time (minutes), SEM, and TEM images for AuNPs formed by photoirradiation within PNIPAm-co-allylamine microgels. Traces (**D′,D″**) show SEM and TEM images of AuNPs formed by photoirradiation within PNIPAm-co-acrylic acid microgels. Refer to Figure S3 for the corresponding absorption spectra of sample (**D′,D″**).

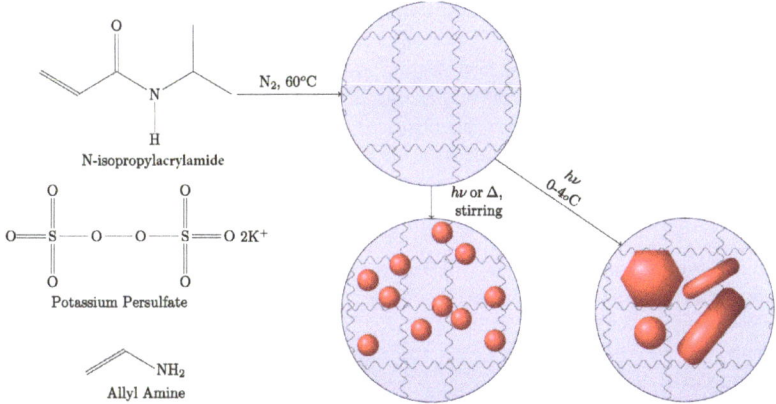

Scheme 1. Synthesis of poly(N-isopropylacrylamide) (PNIPAm)-co-allylamine microgels, followed by the formation of spherical and anisotropic gold nanoparticles (AuNPs) within the microgels (hυ and Δ represent light and heat, respectively). The heating is performed at 37 °C for 10–15 min. The irradiation times are included in the actual data figures.

3.2. In Situ Formation of Spherical Gold Nanoparticles within PNIPAm Microgels

To start with, the formation of spherical AuNPs was investigated under ambient and photoirradiation conditions within the PNIPAm-co-allylamine microgels (Figure 1B,C and Figure S2). Except for PNIPAm microgels, no additional or assisting reducing agents were employed during the reaction. AuNPs formed under photoirradiation exhibited smaller size, narrower size distribution, and higher photochemical quantum yield compared to those prepared under ambient conditions (Figure 1B vs. Figure 1C). Under both conditions, a typical PNIPAm-co-allylamine microgel sample containing Au(I) changes from colorless to pink color as evidenced by the evolution of an SPR peak around 575 nm (ambient conditions) or 530 nm (photoirradiation conditions) during the first 60 or 15 min of the reaction, respectively (Figure 1B,C). Under otherwise identical reaction conditions, the photoirradiated sample attained an arbitrary absorbance of 1.0 unit in less than 40 min, whereas the sample under ambient conditions required over 105 min to attain the same absorbance. The SPR peak maxima and full-width-half-max (FWHM) of the AuNPs spectra show that the AuNPs in the photoirradiated sample were monodispersed and smaller than those produced in ambient light (12.1 ± 4 nm or 862 cm^{-1} for λ_{max} = 530 nm vs. 21.0 ± 6 nm or 1270 cm^{-1} for λ_{max} = 575 nm, respectively). Additionally, FE-SEM images from both samples show visible differentiation of AuNPs and polymer microgel boundaries, with single to multiple AuNPs within a single microgel particle. Aggregated gold cores were more prevalent in the sample prepared using ambient light, as expected from the comparatively broad SPR peak. FE-SEM images indicate that in both cases, the microgels acted as host matrices which stabilized the AuNPs. Note that microgels containing multiple gold cores were more prevalent in the sample prepared under ambient conditions. PNIPAm microgels copolymerized with acrylic acid were synthesized separately to investigate the effect of surface charge of microgels during the formation of AuNPs. The surface charge of control PNIPAm-co-allylamine and PNIPAm-co-acrylic acid microgels were confirmed to be + 30 ±4.5 and − 25 ± 3.8 mV, respectively, as determined via zeta potential measurements. Except for a few minor variations, similar size, spherical AuNPs were obtained by utilizing negatively charged PNIPAm-co-acrylic acid gels, as shown in Figure 1D and Figure S3. Under similar experimental conditions, the acid-containing microgels attained 1.0 unit of arbitrary absorbance in less than 10 min, compared to 30 min for positively charged microgels (Figure 1C and Figure S3). The data from Table 1 showed that negatively charged microgels are preferable for making spherical AuNPs compared to positively charged PNIPAm microgels. The reason for this is likely due to the stronger electrostatic interactions between the negatively charged stabilizing surface and the

Au$^+$ atomic cations that potentially cover the surface of the AuNP; even in absence of such cations, the electrophilic nature of even neutral Au or other metal atoms is conducive to greater affinity to negatively charged stabilizers. The data from Figure 1 demonstrated the formation of spherical AuNPs within both positively charged and negatively charged PNIPAm hydrogel microspheres under similar experimental conditions. During these reactions, we have noticed that, under similar experimental conditions, usage of HAuCl$_4$ does not result in the formation of AuNPs. No change in color or evolution of SPR was noticed even after 1 h of irradiation, emphasizing the significance of Au(I) precursor as a preferential replacement for HAuCl$_4$ as the gold precursor in this study.

Table 1. Correlating absorption spectra (SPR) with a TEM-determined particle size (average diameter, d_{avg}) of gold nanoparticles (AuNPs) obtained from different compositions of poly(N-isopropylacrylamide) (PNIPAm) microgels.

Stabilizing Media	Experimental Condition	SPR λ_{max} (nm)	FWHM * (nm)	FWHM * (cm^{-1})	TEM d_{avg} (nm)	PQY *
PNIPAm-co-allylamine microgels	Ambient light	575	676	5825	21.0 ± 6.0	NA
PNIPAm-co-allylamine microgels	Photoirradiation	535	591	4584	12.1 ± 4.0	0.07
PNIPAm-co-acrylic acid microgels	Photoirradiation	533	595	4932	10.6 ± 3.7	0.1

* PQY = photochemical quantum yield; FWHM = full-width-half-max (nanometers (nm) and wavenumbers (cm^{-1})).

3.3. Hybrid Crystalline PNIPAm Microgels Containing Gold Nanoparticles

Spherical PNIPAm microgel nanoparticles are well-known for their ability to form environmentally sensitive colloidal crystals. When microgels containing AuNPs were concentrated (2–3 wt%) and centrifuged, followed by heating above their LCST and slow cooling, lustrous colloidal crystals were formed (Figure 2). Turbidity measurements of these hybrid colloidal crystals showed two characteristic peaks: a Bragg's diffraction peak due to the orderly arrangement of PNIPAm colloidal crystals [4] and a second peak from the AuNPs' SPR. The presence of the Bragg's diffraction peak and SPR peak in the hybrid colloidal array signifies the retention of characteristic traits of both AuNPs and an orderly arrangement of PNIPAm crystalline microgels. Consistent with our investigation, there are reports of AuNPs formation within PNIPAm microgels and also demonstrations of color tunability within environmentally sensitive hydrogels and polymers [44]; however, the formation of hybrid PNIPAm colloidal crystals is demonstrated herein for the first time, to our knowledge. We believe that the additional environmentally sensitive SPR trait of these hybrid colloidal crystals will further benefit their photonic applications.

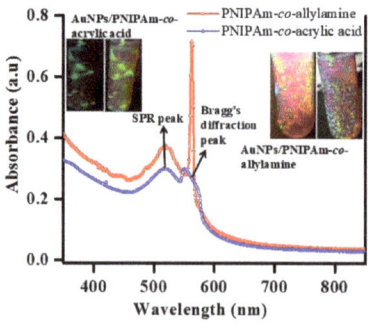

Figure 2. UV/VIS absorption spectra of hybrid poly(N-isopropylacrylamide) (PNIPAm) colloidal microgel crystals. The absorption spectra show the characteristic surface plasmon resonance (SPR) of spherical AuNPs and Bragg's diffraction peak of orderly arranged PNIPAm colloidal crystals.

3.4. In Situ Formation of NIR-Absorbing Anisotropic Gold Nanomosaic (NIRAuNM) within PNIPAm-Co-Allylamine Microgels

After investigating the formation of spherical AuNPs, our focus shifted towards the formation of more challenging and intriguing anisotropic and/or NIR-absorbing AuNPs. Particles which absorb in the NIR region open a new range of applications, most importantly plasmonic photothermal therapy. The photothermal heating of nanoparticles is shown to exhibit cell death through membrane blebbing [56]. Currently, there are scant literature examples of single-step methods for making NIR-absorbing anisotropic AuNPs and no literature methods that have demonstrated the formation of NIRAuNPs from Au(I) systems. Based on spherical AuNPs results, the light was selected as the energy source for exploring the formation of NIRAuNPs within PNIPAm-co-allylamine microgels. The entire procedure is performed using only two reagents: Au(Me$_2$S)Cl and dialyzed PNIPAM-co-allylamine microgels. In a typical reaction, the formation of anisotropic AuNPs can be followed by observing the changes in time-dependent UV/VIS–NIR spectra (Figure 3). At the beginning of the irradiation, no NIR peaks were observed from the reaction mixture. The relatively high baseline in the UV region was attributed to microgels scattering. After 15–20 min of irradiation, the evolution of a broad SPR peak at 550 nm indicated the slow generation of spherical AuNPs. As the irradiation continued, the absorption band at 550 nm remained unchanged, whereas the evolution of a broad SPR peak in the NIR region with a peak maximum > 750 nm was observed. Upon further irradiation, the absorbance of the broad NIR peak (>750 nm) increased, accompanied by a blue shift in the peak maximum. After 70 min of continuous irradiation, the growth of the NIR peak halted with a peak maximum stabilizing at 715 nm. The time-dependent absorption spectrum (Figure 3) indicated that small particles bearing an SPR peak 550 nm were formed first, and we assumed eventual coalesce into anisotropic structures upon further irradiation. This was indicated by the evolution and continuous growth of the NIR peak but not the 550 nm peak. These data suggested a fusion growth pattern, where small particles congealed to form larger particles. To understand if the formation of these particles is only short-lived, TEM images were collected from the samples 1 week after synthesis. The absorption spectra obtained before the collection of TEM images showed no change in absorption spectra 1 week after synthesis, indicating the stability of the anisotropic nanoparticles. The mixture of different sizes and shapes of anisotropic particles observed in the TEM images were congruent with the broad NIR SPR peak. The mixture of shapes included rods, triangles/prisms, and other polygonal structures along with some large spherical/semispherical nanostructures, somewhat akin to the construction of a mosaic from individual tesserae blocks that need not be of a uniform shape. Hence, we coin the phrase "nanomosaic" for this type of particle in general; indeed, when we highlight the plasmonic absorption properties we will be using the more specific term "NIR-absorbing anisotropic gold nanomosaic" abbreviated henceforth as "NIRAuNM." A closer observation reveals that the longitudinal length of these anisotropic nanostructures, especially rods and triangles, was over 50 nm, which was consistent with both their NIR SPR peak (λ_{max} > 700 nm) and published literature [31,37,57]. We believe that the blue shift in the SPR during irradiation is likely due to the reversible conversion of initial larger-sized anisotropic shapes to smaller anisotropic shapes or partial conversion to spherical shapes caused by continuous irradiation. EDS spectra revealed the chemical composition of these NIRAuNMs (Figure 3). Au peak positions observed in the EDS spectrum are in good agreement with literature results [57,58]. As the NIRAuNM precursor contains sulfur, the absence of any sulfur signal in the EDS spectrum confirms that the precursor ligand has been driven out of the system and thus the particles are purely Au-based. Signals from C, O, Cu, and Si were due to the PNIPAm stabilizer and Cu grid used in the EDS analysis. Au peaks confirmed the elemental composition and purity of the nanoparticles. Figure 3 confirms the formation of stable NIR-absorbing anisotropic shapes within PNIPAm-co-allylamine microgels without the aid of any exogenous reducing or growth-assisting agents. To the best of our knowledge, this is the simple, straight-forward, and single-step synthetic technique for making a mixture of stable, NIRAuNMs within a/microgel medium.

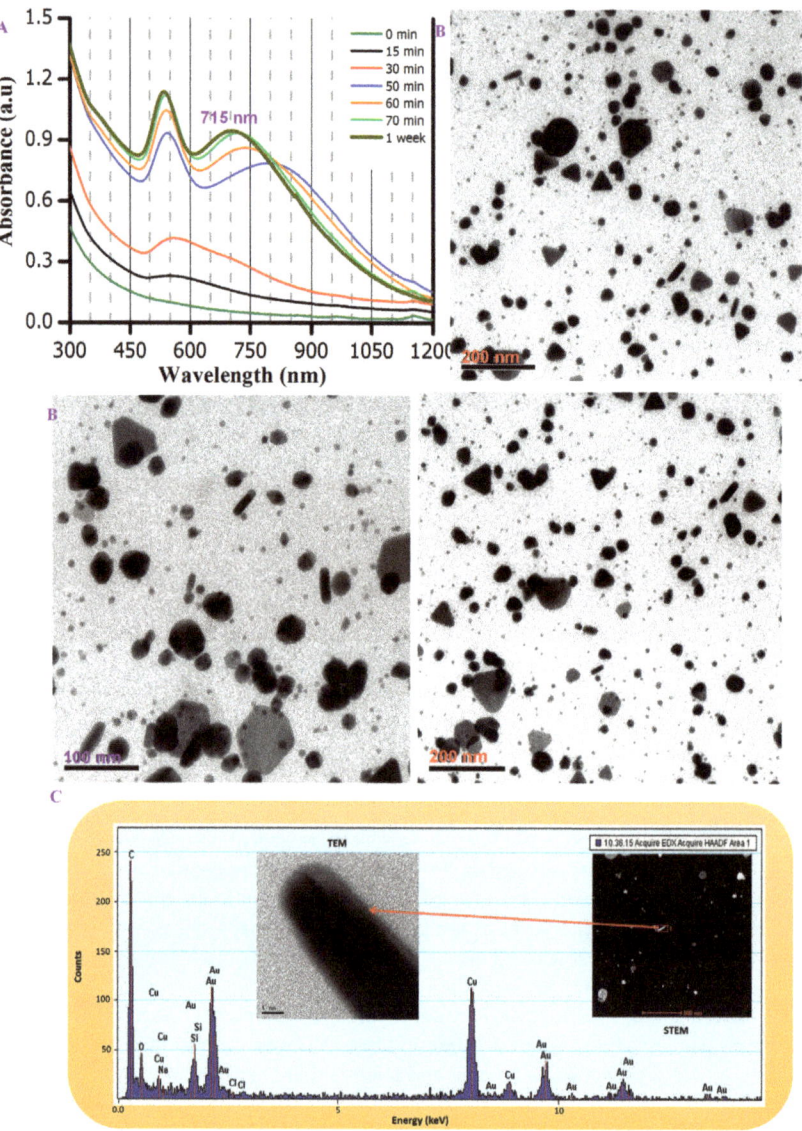

Figure 3. Characterization of NIR-absorbing anisotropic gold nanomosaic (NIRAuNM) formed within 0.5% wt/v of PNIPAm-*co*-allylamine microgels. In this specific reaction, photolysis was used to reduce 0.023 moles of Au(Me$_2$S)Cl in the aqueous microgels medium by a single-step method. (**A**) Time-dependent absorption spectra, (**B**) TEM images, and (**C**) EDS data with TEM and scanning transmission electron microscope (STEM) images. The STEM image in the inset is collected using a high-angle annular dark-filed (HAADF) detector.

To understand the effect of Au(I) concentration on the tunability of the NIR SPR, the reaction was repeated at two different Au(Me$_2$S)Cl concentrations other than the one described in Figure 3. Figure 4 shows the formation of NIRAuNM at a higher concentration compared to the sample in Figure 3. The time-dependent absorption spectra in Figure 4 are like those noticed in Figure 3. Specifically, both figures show an initial evolution of a visible absorption peak, followed by the evolution of a NIR peak, followed by a red-shift in the NIR peak maxima with continuous irradiation, culminating with an SPR peak in the NIR region ($\lambda_{max} > 650$ nm). At the higher concentration of Au(Me$_2$S)Cl, the sample exhibited a red-shifted NIR absorption peak maximum at around 825 nm compared to the 715 nm NIR peak noticed in the sample with a lower concentration of Au(Me$_2$S)Cl. The two samples established the correlation between Au(I) concentration and the size of the particles, consistent with their SPR spectra. At lower concentrations of Au(I), the NIRAuNMs exhibited a NIR peak maximum around 715 nm, whereas the higher Au(I) concentration resulted in a red-shifted NIRAuNM with a peak maximum at 825 nm. Additionally, comparing the TEM images in Figures 3 and 4 showed that the sample containing the higher concentration of Au(I) contained larger anisotropic shapes with longitudinal lengths over 100 nm for multiple particles compared to the prevalent 50 nm sizes at the lower Au(I) concentration. Evident from Figure 3, at the reaction's endpoint, the sample did not contain a dominant NIR peak. Additionally, absorption spectra from Figure 4 showed the successful enrichment of NIR absorbance by benchtop centrifugation. The sediment sample exhibited a dominant NIR peak compared to uncentrifuged samples.

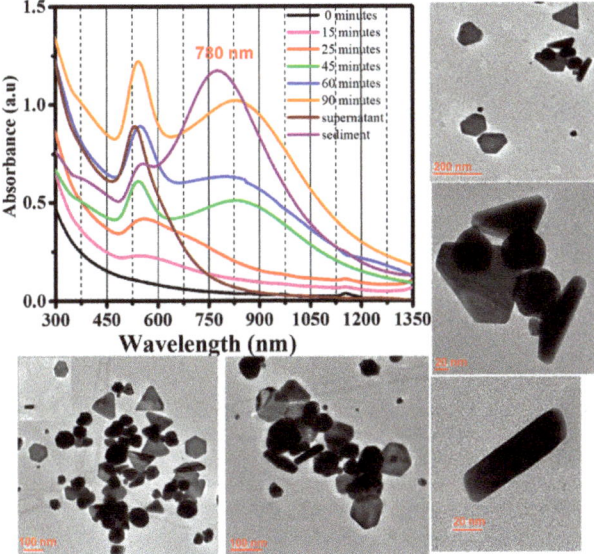

Figure 4. Characterization of NIRAuNM formed within 0.5% wt/v of PNIPAm-*co*-allylamine microgels by photolysis of 0.033 mmol of Au(Me$_2$S)Cl in the aqueous microgel medium by a single-step method. Time-dependent absorption spectra and TEM images are included.

As expected, a sample containing a lower content (0.016 mmol) of Au(I) compared to both previous samples exhibited a blue-shifted NIR absorption peak (Figure 5). Each TEM image, again even for this lower-Au-content composition, comprised a nanomosaic without a dominant geometry for the tesserae elements that comprised the mosaic with interesting polygonal shapes with an average size of 30 ± 7 nm for each tessera in this lower-Au-content sample–in contrast to the nanorods and nanotriangles that comprised the tesserae observed in the previous samples with greater Au content. This is again akin to the mosaic analogy that different mosaics have their elements of beauty although the collection of tesserae is different both within the same mosaic and between different mosaics. Still, it is often the case that the tesserae in the same mosaic exhibit greater similarity within one another (i.e., an assortment of polygonal shapes in Figure 5 vs. an assortment of nanorods and nanoprisms in Figures 3 and 4). Concluding from the absorption data and TEM images obtained from three different samples with varying concentrations of Au(I) precursor, it is clear that the size and SPR of anisotropic NIRAuNM are dependent on Au(I) concentration, higher Au(I) concentration resulted in larger and red-shifted NIRAuNM. UV/VIS/NIR and TEM data of different Au(I) concentration samples imply that photoirradiation initially results in the formation of spherical AuNPs that eventually grow into larger anisotropic structures that remain unaltered after their formation. Based on the existing literature overviewed above, we determined that it was a priority objective to investigate the feasibility of making NIR-absorbing anisotropic AuNPs by use of an Au(I) precursor and to capture the complete reaction in a single-step method that is absent of CTAB and other growth or reducing agents. Based upon the UV/VIS/NIR spectra, TEM images, and EDS spectra presented herein for the samples discussed, we believe we have demonstrated the achievement of this objective.

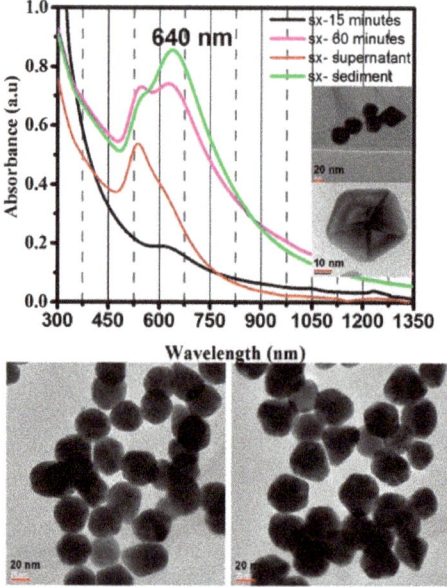

Figure 5. Characterization of NIRAuNM formed within 0.5% wt/v of PNIPAm-co-allylamine microgels by photolysis of 0.016 mmol of Au(Me$_2$S)Cl in aqueous microgels media by a single-step method. Time-dependent absorption spectra and TEM images are included.

Due to its low stability and sensitivity to water and temperature, we conjectured that Au(Me$_2$S)Cl could be reduced to Au(0) even under other experimental conditions besides photolysis. Using our single-step methodology, the synthesis of NIRAuNM containing mixed anisotropic shapes was also found to be driven by thermolysis and sonolysis conditions (Figures S4–S6). Based on the absorption spectra as noted in Figure S4, the thermolysis procedure emerged as a more facile and promising process compared to photoirradiation for making strong NIR-absorbing anisotropic AuNPs. Samples subjected to thermolysis exhibited the NIR peak as their major peak even without requiring centrifugation. However, for yet unidentified reasons, TEM images (Figures S4 and S5) revealed large, polyhedral nanostructures along with hitherto unreported tailed structures. EDS (Figure S5) showed no traces of contamination or sulfur, confirming the structures to be pure AuNPs. Particles prepared by the sonolysis process also exhibited a mixture of shapes, akin to the nanotesserae observed by photolysis (Figures S4 and S6). These results indicate that under the appropriate conditions, i.e., light, thermal, and kinetic energy, one can reduce the Au(Me$_2$S)Cl precursor to Au(0), and when this precursor is reduced in an appropriate stabilizing medium, spherical or anisotropic AuNPs are formed.

Evaluating the shelf-life stability of AuNPs is crucial in establishing our method's viability for producing AuNPs toward commercial and/or clinical applications. Samples with different $Au(Me_2S)Cl$ concentrations were synthesized within PNIPAm-*co*-allylamine microgels by photoirradiation and heating. Long-term stability was evaluated by directly comparing their absorption spectra at different time intervals. All tested samples were stored under ambient conditions. Figure 6 shows changes in absorption spectra for NIR-absorbing AuNP samples. Selected samples were planned to be tested for shelf-life stability after 3 months of storage under ambient conditions; however, after noticing their unexpected, unchanged absorption profile, samples were placed into ambient storage, and unintentionally left there for 7 years, at which time, they underwent additional testing. Overall, the absorption spectra in Figure 6 showed no changes between days 1 (solid line) vs. day 90 (dashed line), indicating that these samples did not undergo any chemical or physical changes in composition or AuNP morphology (i.e., these data suggested that the samples exhibited no decomposition or aggregation tendency after the first 90 days of storage). Incredibly, the negligible changes that were noticed after 7 years of ambient storage indicate their strong commercial utility. Only two minor changes were observed. The first was an increase in the visible absorption peak, and the second was a rise in the baseline absorbance at wavelength ≥1000 nm (dotted lines, Figure 6). We assume these minor changes could be due to the rather slow conversion of minute amounts of anisotropic particles to spherical particles. Future work will involve analysis following NIST stability testing protocols to estimate the shelf life of these highly stable NIRAuNM. We believe the extraordinary shelf-life stability of the NIRAuNM synthesized using the single-step method, containing no CTAB or any additional reducing agents, merits fine-tuning the reaction parameters. This fine-tuning will define the synthesis conditions necessary to control the shape- and size-selective NIR-absorbing anisotropic AuNPs, while utilizing the highly desired, mild chemical environment as opposed to the harsh surfactants and reducing agents.

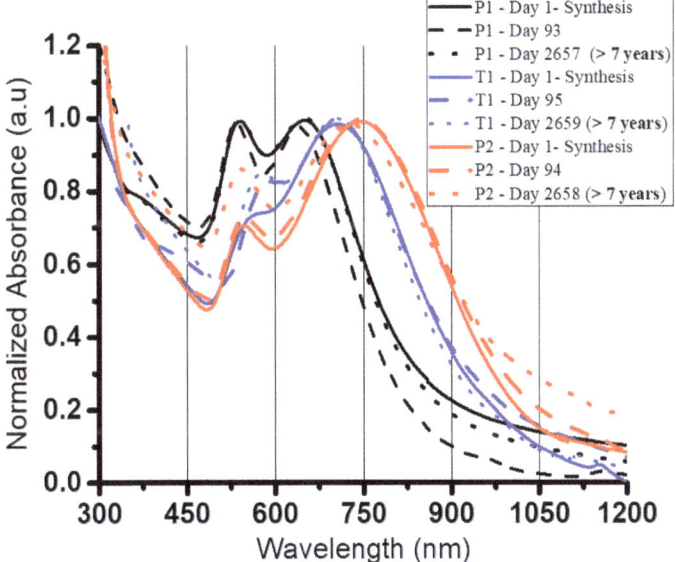

Figure 6. Demonstration of extreme time-dependent stability of NIRAuNM stabilized within PNIPAm-*co*-allylamine microgels. P1, T1, and P2 refer to NIRAuNM samples prepared by photochemistry, heating, and photochemistry, respectively, within PNIPAM-*co*-allylamine microgels media.

3.5. Demonstrating Broad Applications by Altering the Polymer Stabilizer

Encapsulating AuNPs within polymer matrices was found to be an effective way to enhance the stability and functions of metal nanoparticles. Conjugation of polymers to AuNPs and/or using them as templates allows one to build structural and functional units useful for many optoelectronic and biological applications [59]. We tested the feasibility, versatility, and suitability of our methodology for in situ formation of stable AuNPs within various polymers, surfactants, and biological media. Stabilizing matrices were selected based on chemistry and application significance, i.e., CS was selected for its biocompatibility, SDS for its surfactant chemistry, alginic acid for its acid (–COOH) chemistry, and HPC and PVA for their hydroxy (–OH) chemistry. The pH-sensitive PAA was selected for its broad usage in household/personal care products, moisturizers, and super porous microgels. The binding and coating capabilities of PVA are efficiently utilized in the food industry [60]. Agar, the gelatinous polysaccharide which solidifies at 32–40 °C is a crucial component in many biological assays [61]. HPC is a derivative of cellulose, which is soluble in water as well as many organic solvents, is typically used in tablet binding, tablet coating, and as an ophthalmic protectant and lubricant [62]. As one of the most important nutrients in cell culture studies, BSA [63] is a crucial protein in various biological studies. In the existing literature, a few reports exist for making AuNPs using the above stabilizing media [63–68]. Figure 7 illustrates the formation of spherical AuNPs within these stabilizers by photoirradiation or by heating. For yet unidentified reasons, some polymers have exhibited the formation of AuNPs by photoirradiation, while others have formed AuNPs through heating. Table 2 summarizes the optical and morphological properties of these different AuNPs. TEM images revealed some anisotropic structures, which contrasted with the single SPR peak. The formation of nonspherical particles in some of these media is hypothesized to be polymer- and Au(I)-concentration-dependent, which is currently under investigation. Visible colors, the evolution of SPR peaks, and TEM images confirmed the formation of AuNPs regardless of the stabilizer or energy source and using $Au(Me_2S)Cl$ as the precursor without additional reagents. TEM images showed AuNPs with sizes ranging from 5 to 50 nm formed within these stabilizers. From the UV–VIS and TEM data, the relation between the size of the particles and the chemistry of the stabilizers was not fully established; however, we observed that polymers with a negative surface charge tend to stabilize AuNPs with blue-shifted, narrow SPR peaks and exhibit narrowly dispersed particle sizes. The exception to this observation was the CSN polymer for reasons not yet understood. Alginic acid-stabilized samples showed a narrow SPR peak at 525 nm with TEM images for the same samples revealing particles with sizes ranging between 5 and 10 nm. Samples stabilized in SDS, a negatively charged surfactant, also exhibited narrow SPR with a peak maximum at 528 nm and particle size ranging from 5 to 10 nm. In contrast, HPC and BSA formed AuNPs that exhibited red-shifted, broader SPR peaks, with particle sizes ranging between 30 and 40 nm. Under similar experimental conditions, we have not noticed any formation of AuNPs within these media using $HAuCl_4$ as a precursor without the aid of additional chemical reagents. By demonstrating the formation of AuNPs within this wide variety of media, the extensive applicability of using $Au(Me_2S)Cl$ as a precursor for making spherical AuNPs without any reducing or assisting chemical reagents is validated. This demonstration will provide flexibility for nanoparticle researchers to select and grow AuNPs within desired stabilizing media based on their requirements and application.

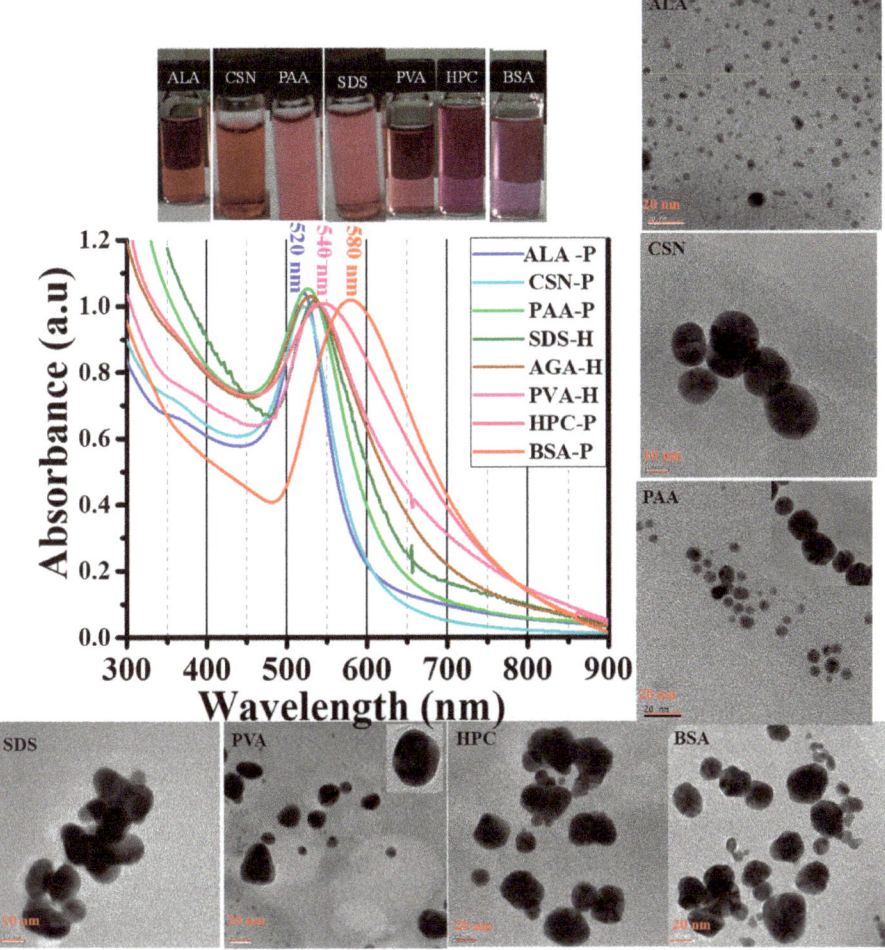

Figure 7. Characterization of spherical AuNPs stabilized in different polymers under photoirradiation (P) and heating (H) by daylight images, UV/VIS absorption spectra, and TEM images. ALA = alginic acid; CSN = chitosan; PAA = polyacrylic acid; SDS = sodium dodecyl sulfate; PVA = polyvinyl alcohol; HPC = hydroxypropyl cellulose; BSA = bovine serum albumin.

Table 2. Optical and morphological properties of AuNPs obtained under various experimental conditions within the wide range of stabilizing media (using Figure 7 data).

Stabilizing Media	Experimental Condition (Time, Minutes)	SPR λ_{max} * (nm)	FWHM * (nm)	FWHM * (cm^{-1})	TEM d_{avg} (nm)
Alginic acid (ALA)	Photoirradiation (15 min)	521	96	3680	4.1 ± 1.6
Chitosan (CSN)	Photoirradiation (45 min)	522	102	3883	19.8 ± 1.6
Polyacrylic acid (PAA)	Photoirradiation (15 min)	527	130	4864	6.5 ± 2.2
Sodium dodecyl sulfate (SDS)	Heating (10 min)	535	122	4222	Nonspherical, fused 20 ± 4
Polyvinyl alcohol (PVA)	Heating (20 min)	538	166	5772	Nonspherical, 25 ± 5
Hydroxypropyl cellulose (HPC)	Photoirradiation (30 min)	547	210	6764	Nonspherical, fused, 30 ± 5
Bovine serum albumin (BSA)	Photoirradiation (90 min)	580	178	5142	Nonspherical, 35 ± 5

* SPR = surface plasmon resonance, peak maxima; FWHM = full-width-half-max (nanometers (nm) and wavenumbers (cm^{-1})). The heating and photoirradiation time varied depending on the nature of the polymer stabilizer.

3.6. Photothermally Driven Release of a Model Dye from NIRAuNM Containing PNIPAm–Co-Allylamine (Hybrid) Microgels

The ability of metallic nanoparticles to transduce absorbed light into heat has been used for direct cell killing and drug delivery applications [10,19,56,57]. For drug delivery and PPTT, plasmonic nanoparticles or dyes which absorb in the NIR region are considered superior to visible-absorbing NPs for numerous reasons [12,14,57]. Thermoresponsive hydrogel microparticles, which exhibit volume-phase transitions, particularly photothermally modulated phase or size transitions induced by guest metallic nanoparticles are also known for their potential use in "smart," "switchable" devices [45,69–71]. To the best of our knowledge, until now only two groups have demonstrated a volume-phase transition in PNIPAm particles using NIR-sensitive AuNPs, the Halas and West group, who demonstrated photothermal phase transition and drug delivery using Au nanoshells, and the Kumacheva group, who demonstrated the photothermally driven swelling–shrinking ability of PNIPAm microgels by loading CTAB-stabilized AuNRs [70,72]. The major distinction and advantage of our NIRAuNMs are that they exhibit a large absorption cross-section (700–1200 nm) that facilitates the use of inexpensive white light/broad-band lamp sources instead of expensive, wavelength-specific monochromatic lasers for exciting the surface plasmon electrons.

Herein, in situ stabilized, CTAB-free NIRAuNMs were employed in a proof-of-concept experiment, which demonstrated their ability to release a molecular dye (PtPOP) based on photothermally driven "shrinking" of PNIPAm-co-allylamine microgel particles. A control microgel containing no AuNPs was tested under identical experimental conditions. The control and hybrid microgels showed similar phase transition temperatures (32 °C, Figure S1). Based on LCST data, the microgel samples were maintained at 32 °C using circulating water flow. A 100-W quartz tungsten halogen lamp was selected as the light source. The irradiance curve for the lamp is shown in Figure S7. Lamp output under experimental conditions was measured using a light-output meter and was determined to be 0.13 W/cm^2. A converging lens and a 500 nm cutoff filter were used to focus the radiation from the lamp onto the sample vial and to eliminate any photothermal effect of higher energy, i.e., UV/VIS absorption of the NIRAuNM sample on photothermal studies. The experiments were conducted by placing the sample test tube in the sample holder of a dynamic light scattering instrument (AVL-5000, Langen, Germany,) followed by irradiation with the NIR lamp. The constant water flow helped to maintain the sample temperature uniformly at 32 °C. Heating cycles were separated by 1-hour intervals to allow the samples to cool to ambient temperature for deswelling. The UV/VIS/NIR spectra of hybrid microgel samples used for both volume-size change and dye release studies are shown in Figure S8. Figure 8 shows the changes in the average hydrodynamic radius of hybrid and control microgel particles upon irradiation with a NIR lamp source. The greater decrease in size of PNIPAm microgels containing NIRAuNMs relative to the control gel particles containing no AuNPs indicated PPTT activity of NIRAuNMs. Microgel particles containing gold nanoparticles exhibited an average decrease of 14.6 ± 2.9 nm and 14.7 ± 1.5 nm in hydrodynamic radius (R_h) after the first 30 min and after the second 30 min of exposure, respectively, for three cycles. At the end of 60 min, the total decrease in the size of the hybrid microgels was found to be 26.72 ± 1.35 nm accounting for 3 cycles. In contrast, the unloaded control microgels exhibited a marginal decrease of 3.5 ± 1.2 nm and 5.3 ± 1.2 nm in R_h after 2 cycles of irradiation, under identical experimental conditions. This order of magnitude difference in R_h changes of hybrid microgels compared to control microgels demonstrates the photothermal activity of NIRAuNMs. Further validation of photothermal behavior was demonstrated by the release of a molecular dye, ($K_4[Pt_2(P_2O_5H_2)_4] \cdot 2H_2O$) (also known as Pt-POP) from hybrid microgels upon NIR irradiation (Figure 9). Retention of the NIRAuNMs and the dye (Pt-POP) within hybrid microgels after stirring and centrifugation was verified by UV/VIS/NIR spectra (Figure S8). UV/VIS/NIR spectra of hybrid and control microgels after loading Pt-POP exhibited a characteristic UV transition band at 380 nm (Figure S8) with similar absorbance, indicating the presence of a similar concentration of the dye in both hybrid and control microgel particles. For demonstrating photothermal release, both the microgel samples were enclosed in 3000 Da dialysis tubing and then subjected to irradiation by maintaining the temperature at 32 °C. Dye release from microgel particles was monitored by measuring the changes in UV–VIS absorption and photoluminescence of the water sample in which the dialysis tube was immersed (schematic in Figure 9A,B). Initially, both samples exhibited an identical baseline and no absorption at 367 nm. After 30 and 45 min of irradiation, the percentage variation in absorbance at 367 nm from hybrid microgel samples was 165% and 164%, respectively. This is a clear indication of Pt-POP dye release from hybrid microgel particles in contrast to an insignificant release of dye from the control microgel particles (Figure 9C). In the evaluation of individual absorbance changes at 367 nm for control and hybrid samples, the absorbance of the hybrid sample changed from 0.0225 to 0.4415 (arbitrary units), whereas the absorbance of the control microgels changed marginally from 0.0225 to 0.0431 in 45 min of irradiation, indicating an order of magnitude difference in absorbance changes for hybrid microgels compared to control microgels. It can be noticed from the absorbance changes (Figure 9) that potentially, most of the dye was released within the first 15 min. As Pt-POP exhibited strong green emission, a strong difference in photoluminescence emission intensity was also noticed from hybrid vs. control microgels (Figure 9D). There is an order of magnitude (or about 90%) variation in emission intensity between hybrid and control microgels, like absorbance changes. These dye release data not only demonstrate the release of the dye molecule (Pt-POP) due to photothermally driven size changes but also reconfirm photothermally driven shrinking effect in hybrid PNIPAm microgels due to the presence of NIRAuNMs. Light-activated therapies to kill diseased cells and tissues in a noninvasive manner using exogenous agents with large absorption cross-section are well known [56]; however, most demonstrations have been performed using CTAB-stabilized AuNRs. In contrast, based on our ongoing cytotoxicity studies with CTAB-free anisotropic AuNPs, that have already demonstrated more than 50% lower cytotoxicity vs. CTAB-stabilized AuNRs, we strongly believe that our CTAB-free NIRAuNMs with a large absorption cross-section, demonstrating photothermally driven size changes and dye release, are expected to exhibit potential beneficial effects as photothermal agents for cell killing studies, once the cytotoxicity of our AuNPs is fully established.

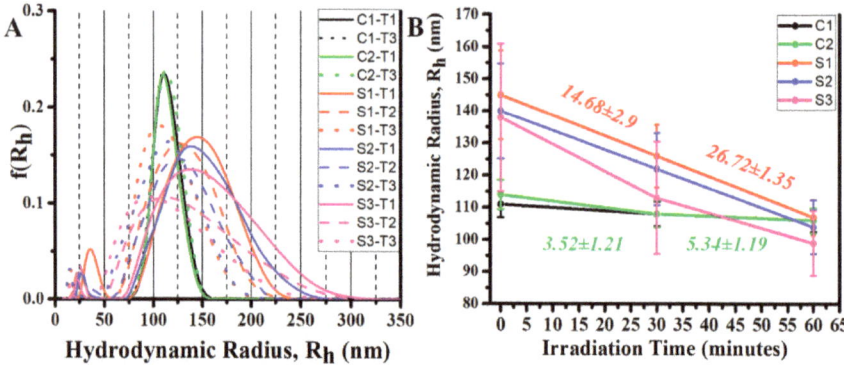

Figure 8. Demonstration of size shrinkage hybrid PNIPAm-*co*-allylamine microgels containing NIR-absorbing AuNM (hybrid microgels) on irradiation with NIR light source. (**A**) Light scattering data representing the changes in hydrodynamic radius of PNIPAm-*co*-allylamine microgels containing NIRAuNMs (S1–S3) vs. control microgels containing no AuNPs (C1–C2). S–irradiation cycle and T–irradiation time (0, 30, and 60 min). Control microgels data for two cycles of irradiation, whereas hybrid microgels are exposed to three cycles of irradiation. (**B**) Changes in hydrodynamic radius (R_h) of the hybrid microgels vs. irradiation time. C and S represent control and hybrid microgels, respectively, and 1, 2, and 3 represent cycles of irradiation.

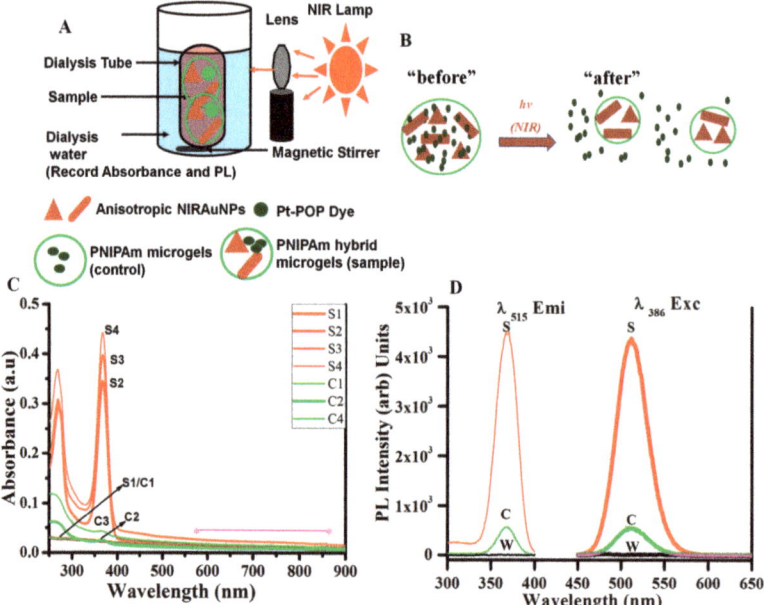

Figure 9. Demonstration of the release of a dye molecule from hybrid PNIPAm-*co*-allylamine microgels containing NIR-absorbing AuNM (hybrid microgels) on irradiation with NIR light source. (**A**) Schematic illustration of dye-release studies from the hybrid microgels containing NIRAuNMs and Pt-pop dye. (**B**) Schematics of dye release "before" and "after" irradiation with the NIR light source. (**C**) Changes in absorption spectra at 0, 15, 30, and 45 min (1,2, 3, and 4) of irradiation for control and hybrid microgels. (**D**) Photoluminescence spectra of dialysis water at 45 min of irradiation (solid lines: emission spectra and dashed lines: excitation spectra). W–blank water, C–control microgel, and S–hybrid microgel.

4. Conclusions

The present investigation demonstrates two important discoveries: (1) development and use of an unexplored methodology wherein an Au(I) complex serve as a gold precursor to generate AuNPs of different sizes and shapes (nanomosaics) in various stabilizing media and (2) the first-ever direct formation of NIR-absorbing AuNPs within thermoresponsive PNIPAm microgels. The facile wet photochemical method resulted in NIR-absorbing Au nanomosaic (NIRAuNM) of diverse anisotropic sizes and shapes and a corresponding wide absorption cross-section. No exogenous reducing agents are needed to reduce the gold precursor. The Au(Me$_2$S)Cl complex, a commercially available well-known starting material for Au(I) complexes, has proven to be an effective precursor for making both spherical and anisotropic AuNPs by tuning experimental conditions. The instantaneous reaction of gold(I) sulfide in aqueous media is shown to be responsible for the reduction process without exogenous reducing agents. The flexibility of the reduction of Au(Me$_2$S)Cl to form AuNPs within a wide variety of media is demonstrated. Even with a mixture of shapes to compose nanotesserae, a direct correlation is noticed between the size of anisotropic AuNPs on the one hand (longest dimension for representative tesserae of each sample) and the NIR SPR peak maximum on the other hand. Additionally, a strong direct correlation is observed between the precursor concentration and average longitudinal length and NIR SPR of the anisotropic structures. The higher concentration of Au(I) resulted in large size particles with red-shifted NIR absorption. The demonstration of photothermally driven shrinkage in size followed by the release of a dye from the hybrid microgels exhibits a proof-of-concept result toward potential drug release studies in the future, but for this, higher LCST slightly above body temperature is required. The proof-of-concept result, nonetheless, led to validation studies of the photothermal transduction property of NIRAuNM produced by our distinct one-step photochemical methodology. Based on our ongoing cytotoxicity tests and because these particles do not rely on CTAB or additional chemicals, they are expected to be far less toxic compared to CTAB-containing NIRAuNPs. Of consequence is our development of this method that uses conditions comparatively milder than the literature standard for the formation of different sizes and shapes of AuNPs. In this regard, we suggest our method will add to the existing "green" synthesis methods, and thus will have an impact on reducing the environmental footprint of these technologies. Finally, the preparation of specific drug delivery systems with a variety of model drugs is underway, taking advantage of the approach herein.

Supplementary Materials: The following are available online at http://www.mdpi.com/2079-4991/10/7/1251/s1, Figure S1: Light scattering data representing the changes in hydrodynamic radius of PNIPAm-*co*-allylamine microgels containing NIRAuNMs vs. control microgels containing no AuNPs. Figure S2: Additional TEM and FE-SEM images of isotropic, spherical AuNPs stabilized within PNIPAm-*co*-allylamine microgels, produced by photolysis. Figure S3: Absorption spectra of AuNPs formed using Au(Me$_2$S)Cl precursor using PNIPAm-*co*-acrylic acid microgels. The traces illustrate the changes in absorbance of AuNPs with respect to irradiation time. Figure S4: Characterization of NIRAuNM formed within 0.5% wt/v of PNIPAm-co-allylamine microgels by thermolysis (top) and sonolysis (bottom) of 0.033 mmol of Au(Me$_2$S)Cl in aqueous microgel media by a single-step method. Absorption spectra and TEM micrographs are shown. Figure S5: TEM micrographs and EDS spectrum of anisotropic, polyhedral, tailed gold nanostructures obtained by thermolysis. Figure S6: Absorption spectra and TEM micrographs of anisotropic AuNPs obtained by sonolysis. Figure S7: Irradiance curve for quartz tungsten halogen (QTH) lamp (100 W) used as a radiation source to demonstrate photothermal volume phase transition and dye-release studies (taken from Newport website, model 6333). Figure S8: Absorption spectra of PNIPAm-*co*-allylamine microgel samples containing NIRAuNMs vs. control microgels containing no AuNPs.

Author Contributions: Conceptualization, M.A.O. and S.B.M.; project administration, M.A.O., S.B.M., and Z.H.; supervision, M.A.O., S.B.M., and Z.H.; investigation, S.B.M., O.E., and M.A.O.; methodology, S.B.M.; experiments, data generation, and analysis, S.B.M.; resources, M.A.O. and S.B.M.; writing–original draft preparation, S.B.M.; writing–review and editing, S.B.M., M.A.O., B.L.K., N.M., and D.P.S.; and funding acquisition, M.A.O. and Z.H. All authors have read and agreed to the published version of the manuscript.

Funding: The authors also acknowledge financial support from the United States' National Science Foundation (Grants CHE-1413641 and CHE-1545934) and Robert A. Welch Foundation (Grant B-1542) awards.

Acknowledgments: The authors would also thank Moon Kim from the University of Texas at Dallas for FESEM measurements. We also thank Donald Benton and Brooke Otten for editorial comments. The authors gratefully acknowledge the Materials Research Facility at the University of North Texas for SEM, TEM, and EDS instrument access.

Conflicts of Interest: The authors declare no conflicts of interest.

References

1. Nayak, S.; Lyon, L.A. Soft Nanotechnology with Soft Nanoparticles. *Angew. Chem. Int.* **2005**, *44*, 7686–7708. [CrossRef]
2. Chai, Q.; Jiao, Y.; Yu, X. Hydrogels for Biomedical Applications: Their Characteristics and the Mechanism Behind Them. *Gels* **2017**, *3*, 6. [CrossRef]
3. Wang, J.; Gan, D.; Lyon, L.A.; El-Sayed, A.M. Temperature-Jump Investigations of the Kinetics of Hydrogel Nanoparticle Volume Phase Transitions. *J. Am. Chem. Soc.* **2001**, *123*, 11284–11289. [CrossRef]
4. Hu, Z.; Huang, G. A New Route to Crsytalline Hydrogels, Guided by a Phase Diagram. *Angew. Chem. Int.* **2003**, *42*, 4799–4802. [CrossRef] [PubMed]
5. Choi, M.; Choi, W.J.; Kim, S.; Nizamoglu, S.; Yun, H.S. Light-Guiding Hydrogels for Cell-based Sensing and Optgenetic Synthesis In Vivo. *Nat. Photonics* **2013**, *7*, 987–994. [CrossRef]
6. Jiang, X.; Xiong, D.; An, Y.; Zheng, P.; Zhang, W.; Shi, L. Thermoresponsive Hydrogel of Poly(Glycidyl Methacrylate-Co-N-Isopropylacrylamide) as a Nanoreactor of Gold Nanoparticles. *J. Polym. Sci. A Polym. Chem.* **2007**, *45*, 2812–2819. [CrossRef]
7. Li, Y.; Hong, X.M.; Collard, D.M.; El-Sayed, M.A. Suzuki Cross-Coupling Reactions Catalyzed by Palladium Nanoparticles in Aqueous Solution. *Org. Lett.* **2000**, *2*, 2385–2388. [CrossRef]
8. Caló, E.; Khutoryanskiy, V.V. Biomedical Applications of Hydrogels: A Review of Patents and Commercial Products. *Eur. Polym. J.* **2015**, *65*, 252–267. [CrossRef]
9. Marquez, G.; Wang, L.V.; Wang, C.; Hu, Z. Development of Tissue-Simulating Optical Phantoms: Poly-N-Isopropylacrylamide Solution Entrapped inside a Hydrogel. *Phys. Med. Biol.* **1999**, *44*, 309–318. [CrossRef] [PubMed]
10. Link, S.; El-Sayed, M.A. Shape and Size Dependence of Radiative, Non-Radiative and Photothermal Properties of Gold Nanocrystals. *Int. Rev. Phys. Chem.* **2000**, *19*, 409–453. [CrossRef]
11. Perezjuste, J.; Pastorizasantos, I.; Lizmarzan, L.; Mulvaney, P. Gold Nanorods: Synthesis, Characterization and Applications. *Coord. Chem. Rev.* **2005**, *249*, 1870–1901. [CrossRef]
12. Pissuwan, D.; Valenzuela, S.M.; Cortie, M.B. Prospects for Gold Nanorod Particles in Diagnostic and Therapeutic Applications. *Biotechnol. Genet. Eng. Rev.* **2008**, *25*, 93–112. [CrossRef] [PubMed]
13. Weissleder, R. A Clearer Vision for in Vivo Imaging. *Nat. Biotechnol* **2001**, *19*, 316–317. [CrossRef] [PubMed]
14. Pissuwan, D.; Valenzuela, S.M.; Killingsworth, M.C.; Xu, X.; Cortie, M.B. Targeted Destruction of Murine Macrophage Cells with Bioconjugated Gold Nanorods. *J. Nanopart Res.* **2007**, *9*, 1109–1124. [CrossRef]
15. Huang, X.; Jain, P.K.; El-Sayed, I.H.; El-Sayed, M.A. Determination of the Minimum Temperature Required for Selective Photothermal Destruction of Cancer Cells with the Use of Immunotargeted Gold Nanoparticles. *Photochem Photobiol* **2006**, *82*, 412. [CrossRef] [PubMed]
16. Dreaden, E.C.; Mackey, M.A.; Huang, X.; Kang, B.; El-Sayed, M.A. Beating Cancer in Multiple Ways Using Nanogold. *Chem. Soc. Rev.* **2011**, *40*, 3391. [CrossRef] [PubMed]
17. Wu, H.-Y.; Chu, H.-C.; Kuo, T.-J.; Kuo, C.-L.; Huang, M.H. Seed-Mediated Synthesis of High Aspect Ratio Gold Nanorods with Nitric Acid. *Chem. Mater.* **2005**, *17*, 6447–6451. [CrossRef]
18. Wang, Y.; Wang, F.; Guo, Y.; Chen, R.; Shen, Y.; Guo, A.; Liu, J.; Zhang, X.; Guo, S. Controlled Synthesis of Monodispersed Gold Nanorods with Different Aspect Ratios in the Presence of Aromatic Derivatives. *J. Nanoparticle Res.* **2014**, *16*, 2806. [CrossRef]
19. Dreaden, E.C.; Alkilany, A.M.; Huang, X.; Murphy, C.J.; El-Sayed, M.A. The Golden Age: Gold Nanoparticles for Biomedicine. *Chem. Soc. Rev.* **2012**, *41*, 2740–2779. [CrossRef] [PubMed]
20. Chang, S.-S.; Shih, C.-W.; Chen, C.-D.; Lai, W.-C.; Wang, C.R.C. The Shape Transition of Gold. *Nanorods Langmuir* **1999**, *15*, 701–709. [CrossRef]
21. Alkilany, A.M.; Murphy, C.J. Toxicity and Cellular Uptake of Gold Nanoparticles: What We Have Learned so Far? *J. Nanopart Res.* **2010**, *12*, 2313–2333. [CrossRef] [PubMed]
22. Isomaa, B.; Reuter, J.; Djupsund, B.M. The Subacute and Chronic Toxicity of Cetyltrimethylammonium Bromide (CTAB), a Cationic Surfactant, in the Rat. *Arch. Toxicol.* **1976**, *35*, 91–96. [CrossRef] [PubMed]
23. Li, N.; Zhao, P.; Astruc, D. Anisotropic Gold Nanoparticles: Synthesis, Properties, Applications, and Toxicity. *Angew. Chem. Int. Ed.* **2014**, *53*, 1756–1789. [CrossRef]

24. Bandyopadhyay, S.; Sharma, A.; Glomm, W. The Influence of Differently Shaped Gold Nanoparticles Functionalized with NIPAM-Based Hydrogels on the Release of Cytochrome C. *Gels* **2017**, *3*, 42. [CrossRef]
25. Rostro-Kohanloo, B.C.; Bickford, L.R.; Payne, C.M.; Day, E.S.; Anderson, L.J.E.; Zhong, M.; Lee, S.; Mayer, K.M.; Zal, T.; Adam, L.; et al. The Stabilization and Targeting of Surfactant-Synthesized Gold Nanorods. *Nanotechnology* **2009**, *20*, 434005. [CrossRef]
26. Choi, B.-S.; Iqbal, M.; Lee, T.; Kim, Y.H.; Tae, G. Removal of Cetyltrimethylammonium Bromide to Enhance the Biocompatibility of Au Nanorods Synthesized by a Modified Seed Mediated Growth Process. *J. Nanosci. Nanotechnol.* **2008**, *8*, 4670–4674. [CrossRef]
27. Todor, I.; Szabo, L.; Marisca, O.T.; Chis, V.; Leopold, N. Gold nanoparticle assemblies of controllable size obtained by hydroxylamine reduction at room temperature. *J. Nanopart. Res.* **2014**, *16*, 2740. [CrossRef]
28. Shankar, S.S.; Rai, A.; Ankamwar, B.; Singh, A.; Ahmad, A.; Sastry, M. Biological Synthesis of Triangular Gold Nanoprisms. *Nat. Mater.* **2004**, *3*, 482–488. [CrossRef] [PubMed]
29. Narayanan, K.B.; Sakthivel, N. Phytosynthesis of Gold Nanoparticles Using Leaf Extract of Coleus Amboinicus Lour. *Mater. Charact.* **2010**, *61*, 1232–1238. [CrossRef]
30. Kitching, M.; Ramani, M.; Marsili, E. Fungal Biosynthesis of Gold Nanoparticles: Mechanism and Scale up: Fungal Biosynthesis of AuNPs. *Microb. Biotechnol.* **2015**, *8*, 904–917. [CrossRef]
31. Fazal, S.; Jayasree, A.; Sasidharan, S.; Koyakutty, M.; Nair, S.V.; Menon, D. Green Synthesis of Anisotropic Gold Nanoparticles for Photothermal Therapy of Cancer. *Acs Appl. Mater. Interfaces* **2014**, *6*, 8080–8089. [CrossRef]
32. Dong, S.; Tang, C.; Zhou, H.; Zhao, H. Photochemical Synthesis of Gold Nanoparticles by the Sunlight Radiation Using a Seeding Approach. *Gold Bull.* **2004**, *37*, 187–195. [CrossRef]
33. Eustis, S.; Hsu, H.-Y.; El-Sayed, M.A. Gold Nanoparticle Formation from Photochemical Reduction of Au 3+ by Continuous Excitation in Colloidal Solutions. A Proposed Molecular Mechanism. *J. Phys. Chem. B* **2005**, *109*, 4811–4815. [CrossRef] [PubMed]
34. Pal, A. Photochemical Synthesis of Gold Nanoparticles via Controlled Nucleation Using a Bioactive Molecule. *Mater. Lett.* **2004**, *58*, 529–534. [CrossRef]
35. Kim, F.; Song, J.H.; Yang, P. Photochemical Synthesis of Gold Nanorods. *J. Am. Chem. Soc.* **2002**, *124*, 14316–14317. [CrossRef] [PubMed]
36. Zhu, J.; Shen, Y.; Xie, A.; Qiu, L.; Zhang, Q.; Zhang, S. Photoinduced Synthesis of Anisotropic Gold Nanoparticles in Room-Temperature Ionic Liquid. *J. Phys. Chem. C* **2007**, *111*, 7629–7633. [CrossRef]
37. Zhai, Y.; DuChene, J.S.; Wang, Y.-C.; Qiu, J.; Johnston-Peck, A.C.; You, B.; Guo, W.; DiCiaccio, B.; Qian, K.; Zhao, E.W.; et al. Polyvinylpyrrolidone-Induced Anisotropic Growth of Gold Nanoprisms in Plasmon-Driven Synthesis. *Nat. Mater.* **2016**, *15*, 889–895. [CrossRef] [PubMed]
38. Ahmed, M.; Narain, R. Rapid Synthesis of Gold Nanorods Using a One-Step Photochemical Strategy. *Langmuir* **2010**, *26*, 18392–18399. [CrossRef]
39. Abdelrasoul, G.N.; Cingolani, R.; Diaspro, A.; Athanassiou, A.; Pignatelli, F. Photochemical Synthesis: Effect of UV Irradiation on Gold Nanorods Morphology. *J. Photochem. Photobiol. A Chem.* **2014**, *275*, 7–11. [CrossRef]
40. Zhang, Y.; Liu, K.; Guan, Y.; Zhang, Y. Assembling of Gold Nanorods on P(NIPAM-AAPBA) Microgels: A Large Shift in the Plasmon Band and Colorimetric Glucose Sensing. *RSC Adv.* **2012**, *2*, 4768–4776. [CrossRef]
41. Zhang, H.; Guo, S.; Fu, S.; Zhao, Y. A Near-Infrared Light-Responsive Hybrid Hydrogel Based on UCST Triblock Copolymer and Gold Nanorods. *Polymer* **2017**, *9*, 238. [CrossRef] [PubMed]
42. Contreras-Caceres, R.; Pastoriza-Santos, I.; Perez-Juste, J.; Fernandez-Barbero, A.; Liz-Marzan, L. Au@pNIPAM Thermosensitive Nanostructures: Control Over Shell Cross-linking, Overall Dimensions, and Core Growth. *Adv. Funct. Mat.* **2009**, *19*, 3070–3076. [CrossRef]
43. Kawano, T.; Niidome, Y.; Mori, T.; Katayama, Y.; Niidome, T. PNIPAM Gel-Coated Gold Nanorods for Targeted Delivery Responding to a Near-Infrared Laser. *Bioconjugate Chem.* **2009**, *20*, 209–212. [CrossRef] [PubMed]
44. Jiang, C.; Qian, Y.; Gao, Q.; Dong, J.; Qian, W. In Situ Controllable Preparation of Gold Nanorods in Thermo-Responsive Hydrogels and Their Application in Surface Enhanced Raman Scattering. *J. Mater. Chem.* **2010**, *20*, 8711. [CrossRef]

45. Fernández-López, C.; Polavarapu, L.; Solís, D.M.; Taboada, J.M.; Obelleiro, F.; Contreras-Cáceres, R.; Pastoriza-Santos, I.; Pérez-Juste, J. Gold Nanorod–PNIPAM Hybrids with Reversible Plasmon Coupling: Synthesis, Modeling, and SERS Properties. *Acs Appl. Mater. Interfaces* **2015**, *7*, 12530–12538. [CrossRef] [PubMed]
46. Vogler, A.; Quett, C.; Kunkely, H. Photochemistry of Azide Complexes of Gold, Silver, Platinum, and Palladium. Generation of the Metallic State. *Ber. Bunsengesphys. Chem.* **1988**, *92*, 1486–1492. [CrossRef]
47. Kim, J.-U.; Cha, S.-H.; Shin, K.; Jho, J.Y.; Lee, J.-C. Synthesis of Gold Nanoparticles from Gold(I)-Alkanethiolate Complexes with Supramolecular Structures through Electron Beam Irradiation in TEM. *J. Am. Chem. Soc.* **2005**, *127*, 9962–9963. [CrossRef]
48. Lu, X.; Tuan, H.-Y.; Korgel, B.A.; Xia, Y. Facile Synthesis of Gold Nanoparticles with Narrow Size Distribution by Using AuCl or AuBr as the Precursor. *Chem. Eur. J.* **2008**, *14*, 1584–1591. [CrossRef]
49. Elbjeirami, O.; Omary, M.A. Photochemistry of Neutral Isonitrile Gold(I) Complexes: Modulation of Photoreactivity by Aurophilicity and π-Acceptance Ability. *J. Am. Chem. Soc.* **2007**, *129*, 11384–11393. [CrossRef]
50. Marpu, S.B. Biocompatible Hybrid Nanomaterials Involving Polymers and Hydrogels Interfaced with Phosphorescent Complexes and Toxin-Free Metallic Nanoparticles for Biomedical Applications. Ph.D. Thesis, Denton, TX, USA, August 2011.
51. Gao, J.; Frisken, B.J. Influence of Reaction Conditions on the Synthesis of Self-Cross-Linked N-Isopropylacrylamide Microgels. *Langmuir* **2003**, *19*, 5217–5222. [CrossRef]
52. Xia, X.; Hu, Z.; Marquez, M. Physically Bonded Nanoparticle Networks: A Novel Drug Delivery System. *J. Control. Release* **2005**, *103*, 21–30. [CrossRef] [PubMed]
53. Tang, S.; Hu, Z.; Zhou, B.; Cheng, Z.; Wu, J.; Marquez, M. Melting Kinetics of Thermally Responsive Microgel Crystals. *Macromolecules* **2007**, *40*, 9544–9548. [CrossRef]
54. Zhou, J.; Wang, G.; Marquez, M.; Hu, Z. The Formation of Crystalline Hydrogel Films by Self-Crosslinking Microgels. *Soft Matter* **2009**, *5*, 820. [CrossRef]
55. WHO | JECFA. Available online: https://apps.who.int/food-additives-contaminants-jecfa-database/chemical.aspx?chemID=1966 (accessed on 19 June 2020).
56. Tong, L.; Zhao, Y.; Huff, T.B.; Hansen, M.N.; Wei, A.; Cheng, J.-X. Gold Nanorods Mediate Tumor Cell Death by Compromising Membrane Integrity. *Adv. Mater.* **2007**, *19*, 3136–3141. [CrossRef]
57. Huang, X.; Neretina, S.; El-Sayed, M.A. Gold Nanorods: From Synthesis and Properties to Biological and Biomedical Applications. *Adv. Mater.* **2009**, *21*, 4880–4910. [CrossRef]
58. Energy Dispersive X-Ray Periodic Table, Hitachi. Available online: https://www.bruker.com/fileadmin/user_upload/8-PDF-Docs/X-rayDiffraction_ElementalAnalysis/HH-XRF/Misc/Periodic_Table_and_X-ray_Energies.pdf (accessed on 18 January 2020).
59. Shan, J.; Tenhu, H. Recent Advances in Polymer Protected Gold Nanoparticles: Synthesis, Properties and Applications. *Chem. Commun.* **2007**, 4580–4598. [CrossRef]
60. Saxena, S.K. Polyvinyl Alcohol, Chemical and Technical Assessment. FAO. 2004. Available online: http://www.fao.org/fileadmin/templates/agns/pdf/jecfa/cta/61/PVA.pdf (accessed on 19 June 2010).
61. Brody, J.R.; Kern, S.E. History and Principles of Conductive Media for Standard DNA Electrophoresis. *Anal. Biochem.* **2004**, *333*, 1–13. [CrossRef]
62. Pharm, K. *Hydroxypropyl Cellulose*; Hercules Incorporated: Wilmington, DE, USA, 2004; p. 494. Available online: https://www.stobec.com/DATA/PRODUIT/1557~{}v~{}data_8524.pdf (accessed on 21 June 2010).
63. Housni, A.; Ahmed, M.; Liu, S.; Narain, R. Monodisperse Protein Stabilized Gold Nanoparticles vis a Simple Photochemical Process. *J. Phys. Chem. C* **2008**, *112*, 12282–12290. [CrossRef]
64. Jans, H.; Jans, K.; Lagae, L.; Borghs, G.; Maes, G.; Huo, Q. Poly(acryliac acid)-stabilized Colloidal Gold Nanoparticles: Synthesis and Properties. *Nanotechnology* **2010**, *21*, 455702. [CrossRef]
65. Khanna, P.; Gokhale, R.; Subbarao, V.; Vishwanath, A.K.; Das, B.; Satyanarayana, C. PVA Stabilized Gold Nanoparticles by use of Unexplored Albeit Conventional Reducing Agent. *Mater. Chem. Phys.* **2005**, *92*, 229–233. [CrossRef]
66. Kuo, C.-H.; Chiang, T.-F.; Chen, L.-J.; Huang, M.H. Synthesis of Highly Faceted Pentagonal and Hexagonal-Shaped Gold Nanoparticles with Controlled Sized by Sodium Dodecyl Sulfate. *Langmuir* **2004**, *20*, 7820–7824. [CrossRef] [PubMed]

67. Pucci, A.; Bernabò, M.; Elvati, P.; Meza, L.I.; Galembeck, F.; Leite, C.A.D.P.; Tirelli, N.; Ruggeri, G. Photoinduced Formation of Gold Nanoparticles into Vinyl Alcohol Based Polymers. *J. Mater. Chem.* **2006**, *16*, 1058–1066. [CrossRef]
68. Pal, A.; Esumi, K.; Pal, T. Preparation of Nanosized Gold Particles in a Biopolymer Using UV Photoactivation. *J. Colloid Interface Sci.* **2005**, *288*, 396–401. [CrossRef] [PubMed]
69. Das, M.; Mordoukhovski, L.; Kumacheva, E. Sequestering Gold Nanorods by Polymer Microgels. *Adv. Mater.* **2008**, *20*, 2371–2375. [CrossRef]
70. Gorelikov, I.; Field, L.M.; Kumacheva, E. Hybrid Microgels Photoresponsive in the Near-Infrared Spectral Range. *J. Am. Chem. Soc.* **2004**, *126*, 15938–15939. [CrossRef] [PubMed]
71. Shiotani, A.; Mori, T.; Niidome, T.; Niidome, Y.; Katayama, Y. Stable Incorporation of Gold Nanorods into N-Isopropylacrylamide Hydrogels and Their Rapid Shrinkage Induced by a Near-Infrared Laser Irradiation. *Langmuir* **2007**, *23*, 4012–4018. [CrossRef]
72. Hirsch, R.L.; Gobin, M.A.; Lowery, R.A.; Tam, F.; Drezek, A.R.; Halas, J.N.; West, L.J. Metal Nanoshells. *Ann. Biomed. Eng.* **2006**, *34*, 15–22. [CrossRef]

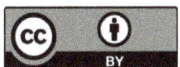

© 2020 by the authors. Licensee MDPI, Basel, Switzerland. This article is an open access article distributed under the terms and conditions of the Creative Commons Attribution (CC BY) license (http://creativecommons.org/licenses/by/4.0/).

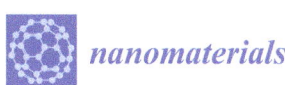

Article

Photostable and Small YVO$_4$:Yb,Er Upconversion Nanoparticles in Water

Masfer Alkahtani [1,2,*], Anfal Alfahd [1], Najla Alsofyani [1], Anas A. Almuqhim [1], Hussam Qassem [1], Abdullah A. Alshehri [3], Fahad A. Almughem [3] and Philip Hemmer [2,4,5]

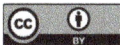

Citation: Alkahtani, M.; Alfahd, A.; Alsofyani, N.; Almuqhim, A.A.; Qassem, H.; Alshehri, A.A.; Almughem, F.A.; Hemmer, P. Photostable and Small YVO$_4$:Yb,Er Upconversion Nanoparticles in Water. *Nanomaterials* 2021, 11, 1535. https://doi.org/10.3390/nano11061535

Academic Editor: James C L Chow

Received: 18 May 2021
Accepted: 8 June 2021
Published: 10 June 2021

Publisher's Note: MDPI stays neutral with regard to jurisdictional claims in published maps and institutional affiliations.

Copyright: © 2021 by the authors. Licensee MDPI, Basel, Switzerland. This article is an open access article distributed under the terms and conditions of the Creative Commons Attribution (CC BY) license (https:// creativecommons.org/licenses/by/ 4.0/).

[1] National Center for Renewable Energy, King Abdulaziz City for Science and Technology (KACST), Riyadh 11442, Saudi Arabia; aalfahd@kacst.edu.sa (A.A.); nalsofyani@kacst.edu.sa (N.A.); amukhem@kacst.edu.sa (A.A.A.); hqasem@kacst.edu.sa (H.Q.)
[2] Institute for Quantum Science and Engineering, Texas A&M University, College Station, TX 77843, USA; prhemmer@exchange.tamu.edu
[3] National Center for Pharmaceutical Technology, King Abdulaziz City for Science and Technology (KACST), Riyadh 11442, Saudi Arabia; abdualshehri@kacst.edu.sa (A.A.A.); falmughem@kacst.edu.sa (F.A.A.)
[4] Department of Electrical and Computer Engineering, Texas A&M University, College Station, TX 77843, USA
[5] Zavoisky Physical-Technical Institute, Federal Research Center "Kazan Scientific Center of RAS", 420029 Kazan, Russia
* Correspondence: mqhtani@kacst.edu.sa; Tel.: +966-553322891

Abstract: In this work, we report a simple method of silica coating of upconversion nanoparticles (UCNPs) to obtain well-crystalline particles that remain small and not agglomerated after high-temperature post-annealing, and produce bright visible emission when pumped with near-infrared light. This enables many interesting biological applications, including high-contrast and deep tissue imaging, quantum sensing and super-resolution microscopy. These VO$_4$-based UNCPs are an attractive alternative to fluoride-based crystals for water-based biosensing applications.

Keywords: upconversion nanoparticles; silica-coated UCNPs; bio-imaging; bio-application

1. Introduction

Lanthanide-doped upconversion nanoparticles (UCNPs) absorb one or more low-energy NIR photons to emit one high-energy visible photon [1–4]. This property greatly suppresses the biofluorescence background that limits other fluorescent probes. As a result, interest in UCNPs is rapidly growing for numerous biological applications, such as in background-free imaging, quantum sensing, drug delivery, and super-resolution microscopy [5–7]. Compared to upconversion dyes and quantum dots (QDS), UCNPs achieve efficient upconversion at low pump laser intensities, comparable to single-photon down-converting systems. This is because they have real long-lived metastable states with lifetimes on the microsecond scale. As a result, UCNPs provide photostable and tunable photoluminescence when excited within the tissue optical transparency window by inexpensive continuous-wave NIR lasers [8–13]. Furthermore, UCNPs have shown minimal toxicity to biological tissues, which makes them one of the safest fluorescent probes [11,14–17].

Lanthanide ions doped in fluoride crystals are known as the best and most efficient UCNPs in many interesting applications, with strong up-conversion luminescence (UCL) [8,9]. This is because fluoride crystals have a relatively low phonon energy so that the intermediate state can only decay by highly multi-phonon relaxations [18–20]. They work efficiently in organic solvents such as cyclohexane, but their UCL was reported to drop significantly when dispersed in water [21]. This is due to quenching of the intermediate state by water in contact with the surface of the UCNP, also to defects inherent to their low synthesis temperature [8]. To overcome these limitations, the use of core/shell or core/multi-shell strategies [8,9,11], and hydrophilic surface modification protocols [22], have been used. While successful, these significantly complicate their chemical synthesis.

So far, the best alternative to fluoride-based UCNPs is lanthanide ions doped in oxide crystals such as YVO_4 nanoparticles, which have shown a good upconversion efficiency in water, even for small particles without any surface modifications [18,23,24]. In general, oxide nanoparticles are obtained by colloidal synthesis at lower temperatures than fluoride-based UCNPs, and this gives them poor overall crystallinity and defect-enhanced surface quenching effects, which greatly reduces their UCL efficiency [23–25]. Post-annealing at high temperature is an effective solution to this problem [18,24,25]. However, the post-annealing process leads to unequal particle sizes and agglomerations. Many studies have reported that this challenge can be overcome by silica encapsulation during high temperature annealing, which allows the recovery of good crystalline properties without an excessive size increase [18,25]. However, most of these studies start with relatively large particles (50 nm average size) instead of the ultra-small and well-dispersed UCNPs that are desirable for many biosensing applications [18,23,25–27].

In this work, we report an easy and efficient method to synthesize a small (10 nm) VO_4-based UCNP, based on citrate size capping followed by a silica encapsulation for a protected calcination process. The recovered UCNPs retained their original small size with good up-conversion efficiency. The resulting UCNP particles are highly water dispersible, as desired for in vivo imaging.

2. Materials and Methods

2.1. Synthesis of YVO_4: Er^{+3}, Yb^{+3} Nanoparticles

Raw materials for this experiment, $Y(NO_3)_3$ $4H_2O$, $Yb(NO_3)_3$ $5H_2O$, $Er(NO_3)_3$ $5H_2O$, sodium citrate, sodium orthovanadate (Na_3VO_4), and tetraethylorthosilicate (TEOS 98%) were purchased from Sigma Aldrich (St. Louis, MO, USA). In a water bath at 60 °C, a solid mixture of $Y(NO_3)_3$ $4H_2O$ (0.270 g, 7.78×10^{-4} mol), $Yb(NO_3)_3$ $5H_2O$ (0.089 g, 1.99×10^{-4} mol) and $Er(NO_3)_3$ $5H_2O$ (0.0089 g, 2.0×10^{-5} mol) was dissolved in 10 mL of deionized water. The resulting solution of $Ln(NO_3)_3$ was added to an aqueous solution of (0.1 M) sodium citrate (0.22 g in 7.5 mL of deionized water) under vigorous stirring. During the addition, a white precipitate of lanthanide citrate was immediately formed. An aqueous solution of sodium orthovanadate (Na_3VO_4) (0.1 M, pH = 12) was prepared by dissolving 0.1839 g of Na_3VO_4 in 10 mL of deionized water and then added dropwise to the above mixture until the precipitate was completely dissolved. After constant stirring for 1 h at 60 °C, the final YVO_4:YbEr nanoparticles were obtained in a clear solution, with a pH of 8.0.

2.2. Synthesis of YVO_4: Er^{+3}, Yb^{+3}@SiO_2 Core-Shell Structured Nanoparticles

YVO_4: Er^{+3}, Yb^{+3} (10 mL) was added to 40 mL of ethanol and ultrasonicated for 30 min. Afterwards, 1 mL of ammonia (full concentration) plus 0.15 mL of tetraethylorthosilicate (TEOS 98%) were added to above solution and stirred at room temperature for 4 h. The resulting nanoparticles coated with silica were collected by centrifugation at 6000 rpm for 10 min, washed three times with ethanol/water (1:1 v/v), and then dried at 60 °C overnight. The white powder was then calcinated at 700–750 °C for 2 h.

2.3. Silica Shell Removal by NaOH Solution

The calcinated particles were dispersed in aqueous NaOH solution (10 mL, 0.5 M) under stirring for 4 h to remove the silica matrix from particles. The nanoparticles were collected by centrifugation and washed three times with deionized water. The final product was dispersed in deionized water.

2.4. In Vitro Cytotoxicity Assays for Synthesized UCNPs

The investigation of nanoparticles interactions with living tissues is an essential way to evaluate the toxicity, in vitro. The biotoxicity of the UCNPs was performed against two living cellular models supplied from the American Type Culture Collection (ATCC, Manassas, VA, USA), which are mouse skin cancer cell line (B16-F10, ATCC number: CRL-6475) and human lung carcinoma cell line (A549, ATCC number: CCL-185). Both cells were used between passages 7 and 20, and regularly maintained in complete cell culture growth medium composed of Dulbecco's modified Eagle's medium (DMEM), 1% (v/v) antibiotic solution (penicillin–streptomycin combination) and 10% (v/v) fetal bovine serum (FBS).

In vitro cytotoxicity of the UCNPs was evaluated using two colorimetric assays to quantify UCNPs effect on the cellular membrane integrity and the cellular metabolic activity of B16-F10 and A549 cells. Lactate dehydrogenase (LDH) enzyme is a cytoplasmic enzyme that can be released and quantified in cell culture media when the treated cellular membrane is being disrupted using LDH assay kit (Sigma-Aldrich, Poole, UK). The cell viability can be detected also using 3-(4,5-dimethylthiazol2-yl)-5-(3-carboxymethoxyphenyl)-2-(4-sulfophenyl)-2H-tetrazolium (MTS)assay. The MTS assay was used to evaluate the cellular metabolic activity of the cell lines using MTS cell proliferation reagent (Promega, Southampton, UK). In a 96-well plate, B16-F10 and A549 cells were initially counted and seeded (100 µL/well, seeding density of 1×10^4 cells/well), and then incubated overnight at 37 °C. Increasing doses of the UCNPs (from 0.39 to 800 µg/mL) were then applied to B16-F10 and A549 cells and incubated at 37 °C for 4 h in the presence of complete cell culture growth medium. In nanoparticle-free wells, 0.2% (v/v) Triton X-100 lysis solution and DMEM were applied to cells as a positive and a negative cytotoxicity control, respectively.

Following the incubation of the UCNPs with both cells, the LDH assay was conducted in a new 96-well plate to transfer 50 µL of the treated samples containing DMEM and the cytoplasmic LDH enzyme, which are being released from the disrupted cellular membrane. Next, 100 µL of the LDH reaction mixture was then pipetted into each well and incubated at room temperature for 30 min. Next, the absorbance at 490 nm was measured using the microplate reader (Cytation™ 3, BioTek Instruments Inc., Winooski, VT, USA). The percentage of LDH release and cell viability were calculated using the following Equations:

$$LDH\ release\ (\%) = (S - H) / (T - H) \times 100 \qquad (1)$$

$$Cell\ viability\ (\%) = 100 - LDH\ release\ (\%) \qquad (2)$$

where S is the absorbance of the cells treated with the UCNPs, H is the absorbance of the negative cytotoxicity control, and T is the absorbance of the positive cytotoxicity control.

For the MTS assay, the samples were removed from the wells and 100 µL of fresh complete cell culture medium mixed with 20 µL of the MTS solution was then pipetted into each well. The plates were then incubated at 37 °C for a further 3 h. Cytation™ 3 microplate reader was then used to measure the MTS absorbance at 490 nm. The percentage of cell viability was calculated using the following equation:

$$Cell\ viability\ (\%) = (S - T) / (H - T) \times 100 \qquad (3)$$

3. Results and Discussion

Experimentally, YVO$_4$:Yb,Er UCNPs were synthesized following a modified sodium citrate synthesis protocol reported in [28]. The sodium citrate protocol was chosen as the citrate complexing agent, which are known to limit the size of particles during growth to less than 10 nm, and also to increase their stability. Briefly, an appropriate amount of lanthanide ions salt was dissolved into deionized water (DI) and mixed with sodium citrate to form a lanthanide citrate mixture (see Material and Methods section for details). Then, an aqueous solution of sodium orthovanadate salt was added dropwise to the lanthanide citrate mixture to form ultrasmall YVO$_4$:Yb,Er UCNPs, after constant stirring for one hour at 60 °C. The synthesized UCNPs showed an average size less than 10 nm, but with poor optical and crystal structure properties. Therefore, protected high-temperature annealing is required.

For this purpose, we designed two experiments with and without silica coating, as illustrated in Figure 1a,b. In sample 1, illustrated in Figure 1a, the prepared particles were coated with silica in a core/shell structure following a silica-coating procedure reported in [25] and detailed in the Material and Methods section. The silica-coated UCNPs were then annealed to 750 °C for 2 h in air, using a high-temperature tube furnace. The silica coating was then partially removed by an NaOH solution incubation treatment to obtain dispersed and highly crystalline YVO_4:Yb,Er nanoparticles, as illustrated in a the transmission electron microscope (TEM) image shown in Figures 1a and 2. The final silica-coating thickness can be controlled by either the concentration of the NaOH solution or the incubation time as suggested in [25]. To appreciate the important role of silica encapsulation during high-temperature annealing, the prepared UCNPs in sample 2 were directly annealed to 750 °C for 2 h without silica coating. As a result, a large size distribution and significant agglomeration was seen in the TEM image in Figure 1b. Because sample 2 was introduced for comparison only, it will not be investigated any further.

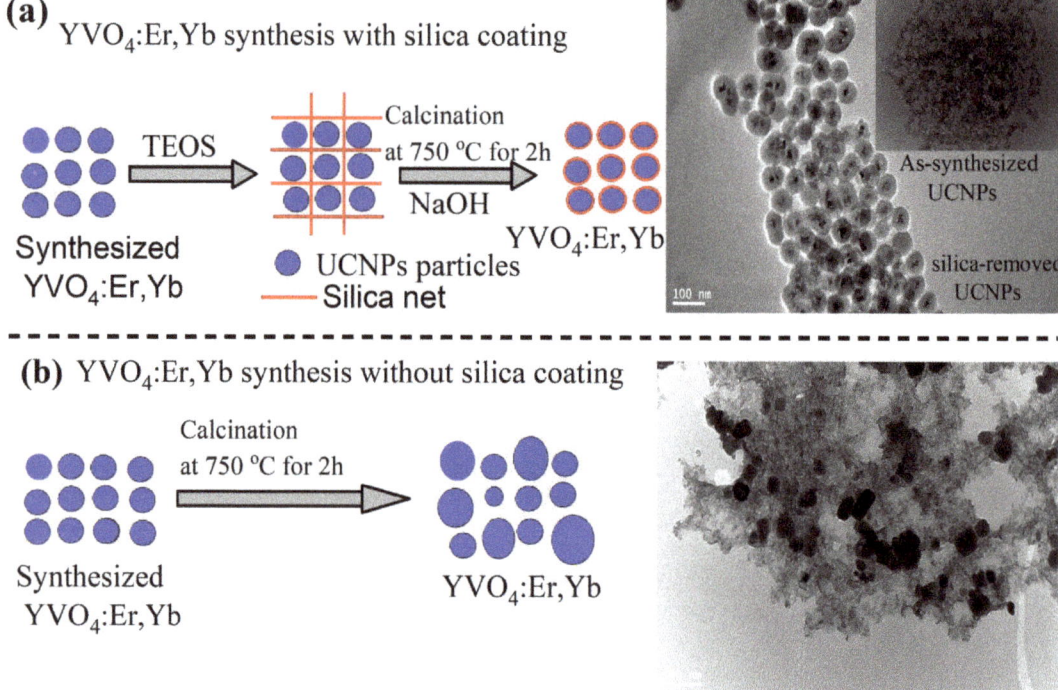

Figure 1. An illustration of high-temperature calcination of YVO_4:Yb,Er UCNPs. (**a**) Protected calcination of UCNPs by silica coating resulting in well size-controlled and dispersed UCNPs particles. (**b**) Direct calcination process of the UCNPs to 750 °C for 2 h without silica coating, which results in a large size distribution and agglomerated UCNPs.

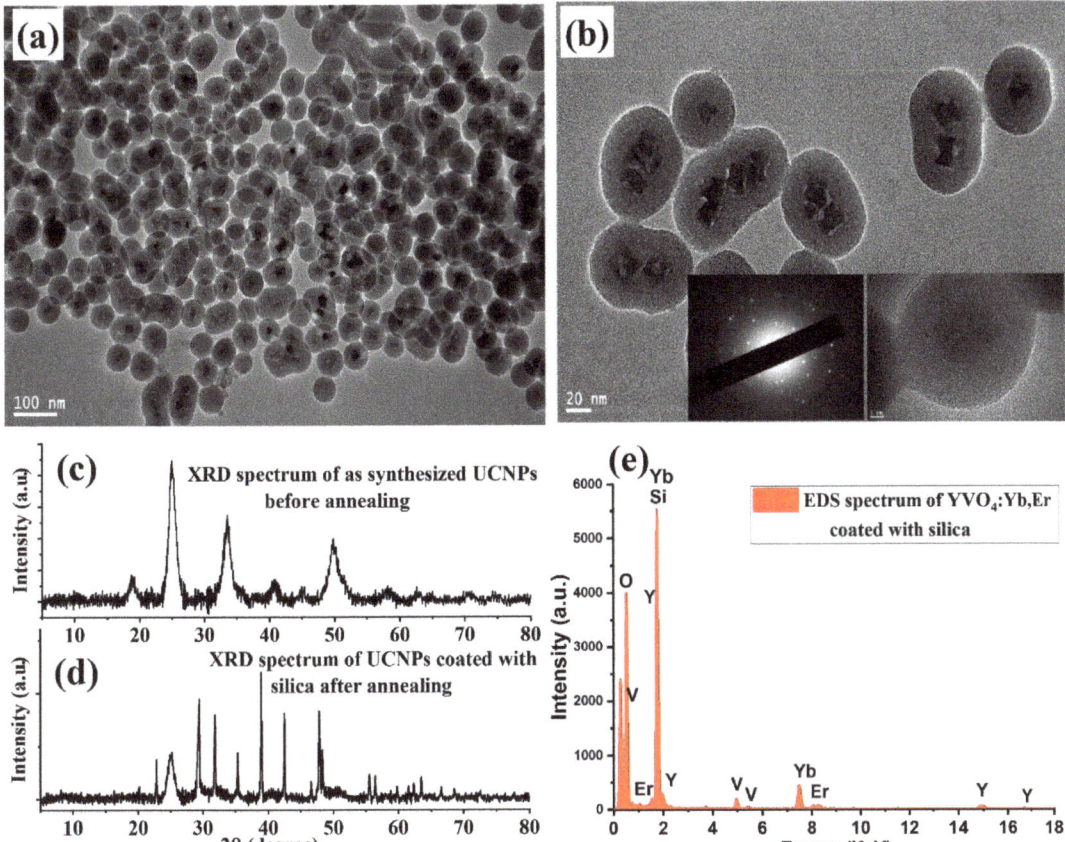

Figure 2. Structural analysis and characterization of YVO$_4$:Yb, Er UCNPs. (**a**) Low magnification TEM image of well-crystalline and small size UCNPs obtained by the protected calcination process. (**b**) High magnification of the synthesized UCNPs. (**c**,**d**) XRD data of UCNPs before and after high-temperature treatment. (**e**) Energy-dispersive X-ray (EDX) spectrum recorded and analyzed from the synthesized UCNPs.

The shape, size, and elemental composition of the synthesized silica-coated UCNP particles were characterized using a JEM-2100F TEM microscope (JEOL, Peabody, MA, USA) operating at an acceleration voltage of 200 kV TEM microscope. For this, a 1 µL sample was dropped onto carbon TEM grids for imaging. Low- and high-magnification TEM images showed dispersed and well-crystalline UCNP particles, with average sizes of 10–15 nm, as demonstrated in Figure 2a,b. The crystallinity of the synthesized YVO$_4$:Yb,Er nanoparticles before and after the protected calcination treatment was investigated using X-ray diffraction (XRD, Malvern, Westborough, MA, USA). Figure 2c shows weak and broad XRD intensity peaks of the synthesized UCNPs before high-temperature annealing treatment, due to the poor overall crystallinity. After protected high-temperature annealing at 750 °C, the XRD patterns revealed strong and sharp peak intensity after calcination, as illustrated in Figure 2d. The narrow XRD peaks indicate well-crystalline particles, which can result in good optical properties. The energy-dispersive X-ray (EDX) spectrum revealed the expected composition elements of the synthesized UCNPs, as illustrated in Figure 2e.

Next, to study the optical properties of the synthesized UCNPs, 1 µL of the sample was spin-coated on a quartz slide to make a thin layer of the sample for optical characterizations. The spin-coating technique was used to avoid agglomeration during drying. The UCNPs sample was then placed on a custom-made confocal laser-scanning microscope equipped with a continuous wave (CW) 980 nm NIR laser excitation, optical spectrometer, and a single-photon counter, as illustrated in Figure 3a. Figure 3b shows the optical scan of the spin-coated UCNPs under a 980 nm laser at an illumination intensity of 8 kW/cm^2. The optical spectrum from each spot in the image revealed a clear UCL spectrum, with two strong green emissions peaked at 520 nm and 550 nm, and a weak red emission peaked at 650 nm, as shown in Figure 3c. The photostability of the UCL green emission, which peaked at 525 and 550 nm from individual UCNP particles (after high-temperature treatment) in the optical scan, was evaluated over 15 min. Figure 3c (inset) showed neither photobleaching nor blinking from the synthesized UCNPs under continuous NIR excitation. In contrast, synthesized UCNPs (before high-temperature treatment) showed a very weak UCL spectrum, as shown in Figure 3c.

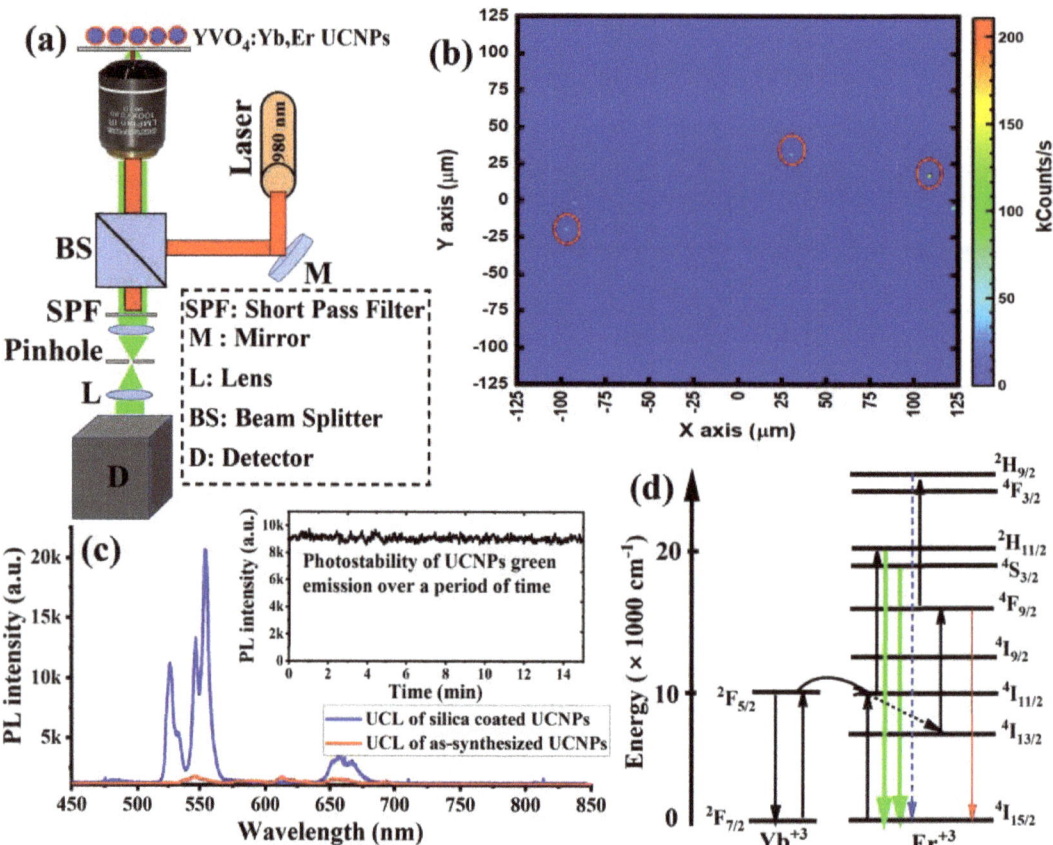

Figure 3. (a) An illustration of optical setup used for optical characterizations in this study. The optical setup consists of 980 nm excitation laser, custom-built confocal microscope, and spectrometer. (b) Optical scan of the spin-coated UCNPs under 980 nm laser illumination. (c) Upconversion luminescence (UCL) spectrum of the synthesized UCNPs before and after high-temperature treatment. UCL of synthesized UCNPs showed a very weak spectrum due to overall poor crystallinity. The fluorescence of the UCNPs after high-temperature treatment showed two strong green emissions at 525 nm and 550 nm, and a weak emission at 650 nm. (d) Electronic structure and upconversion energy transfer processes between energy synthesizer (Yb^{+3}) and activator ion (Er^{+3}) under 980 nm laser excitation (photon upconversion).

Figure 3d explains the UCL optical process in UCNPs. In this optical process, initially, Yb^{+3} ions absorb the first NIR photon of the 980 nm laser to populate the $(^2F_{5/2})$ Yb^{+3} excited state. After that, energy transfer from this state promotes Er^{+3} ions to its quasi-resonant metastable state $^4I_{11/2}$. Due to a two-photon optical process, a second NIR photon absorption re-excites the Yb^{+3} back to the $(2F_{5/2})$ Yb^{+3} excited state, and energy transfer further excites the Er^{+3} ($^4I_{11/2}$) metastable state to a higher excited ($^4F_{7/2}$) Er^{+3} state. After the two-photon excitation is complete, the highly excited state ($^4F_{7/2}$) of Er^{+3} then relaxes to ($^2H_{11/2}$, $^4S_{3/2}$, and $^4F_{9/2}$) Er^{+3} states through multi-phonon relaxations. Consequently, radiative transitions then occur to the ground state $^4I_{15/2}$ of the Er^{+3}, according to the following transitions: $^2H_{11/2} \rightarrow {}^4I_{15/2}$, $^4S_{3/2} \rightarrow {}^4I_{15/2}$, and $^4F_{9/2} \rightarrow {}^4I_{15/2}$, which give green emission peaks at 525 nm and 550 nm, and red emission peaks at 650 nm.

As biocompatibility is the most important criteria for successful fluorescent markers, we performed an in vitro toxicity evaluation of the synthesized UCNPs to confirm the safety and the biocompatibility of the applied nanoparticles to biomedical applications. In this study, increased doses of the UCNPs were incubated with B16-F10 and A549 cell lines to identify the optimum doses that are able to fluoresce efficiently, while not showing cellular toxic effects, in vitro.

Figure 4a shows the cellular viability of B16-F10 and A549 cells following the treatment with the UCNPs for 4 h, and evaluated using LDH assay. The results exhibited high cell viability (above 80%) for applied doses (from 0.39 to 800 µg/mL).

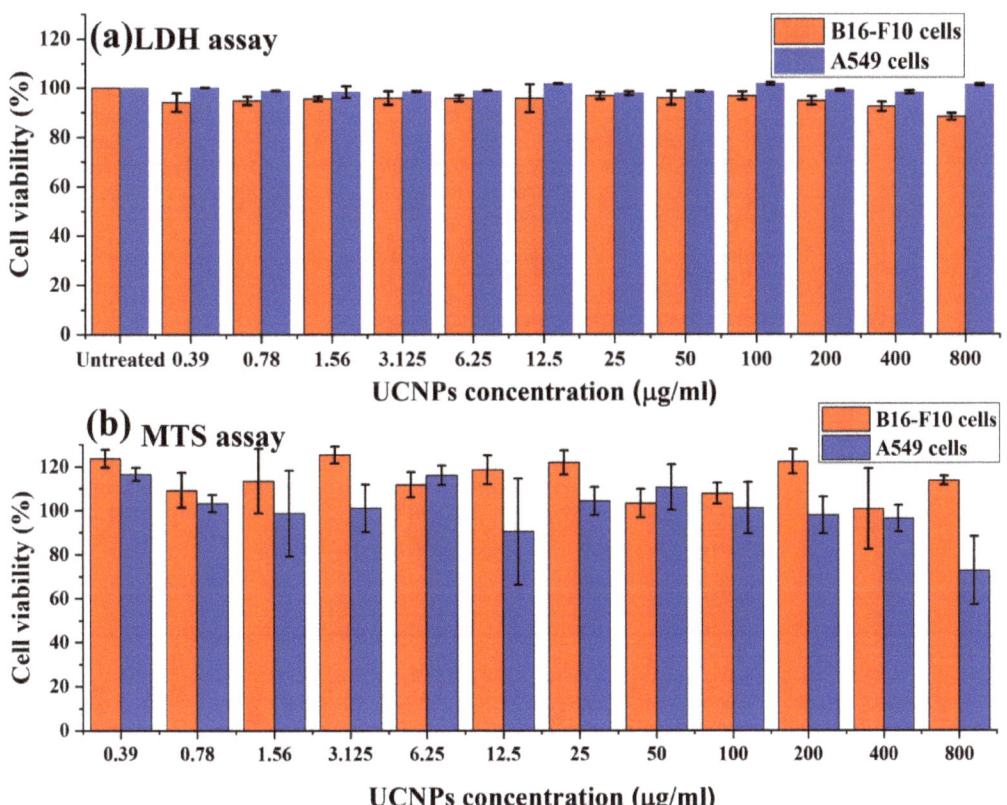

Figure 4. Cell viability of UCNPs after incubation with B16-F10 and A549 cells for 4 h. The data are the result of (a) LDH and (b) MTS assays, which are expressed as cell viability (%) and presented as the mean ± SD (n = 3).

Figure 4b shows the metabolic activity of B16-F10 and A549 cells in terms of the percentage of cell viability, assessed using MTS assay. The results demonstrated high metabolic activity of both cells and no negative effect of the UCNPs on the cell viability. However, increasing the dose from 400 µg/mL in A549 cells to 800 µg/mL showed a significant decrease in the cell viability from 96% to around 72%.

Following the cells exposure to the UCNPs, the overall results of the cellular viability assays demonstrated no observed change in the viability profile when increasing the concentration of applied nanoparticles, apart from the effect of the highest concentration used in A549 cells (800 µg/mL). The in vitro assessments of the UCNPs exhibited low cytotoxicity effects on B16-F10 and A549 cells, suggesting these fluorescent probe nanoparticles can be applied safely in the biomedical applications.

4. Conclusions

We have synthesized small, bright UCNPs that are well dispersed in water, following a simple and robust protected calcination process. The final particles were less than 10 nm in size and well-crystalline with bright up-conversion emission, without optical intermittency (blinking). These properties make them a good alternative to commonly used fluoride-based UCNPs in many biosensing applications. This protected calcination method is a robust and effective strategy to enhance the optical properties of small water-dispersible fluorescent markers.

Author Contributions: Conceptualization, M.A. and P.H.; data curation, M.A., A.A., N.A., A.A.A. (Anas A. Almuqhim), A.A.A. (Abdullah A. Alshehri) and F.A.A.; formal analysis, M.A., A.A.A. (Anas A. Almuqhim), H.Q., A.A., F.A.A. and P.H.; funding acquisition, M.A., H.Q. and P.H.; methodology, M.A., A.A., N.A., H.Q., A.A.A. (Abdullah A. Alshehri) and F.A.A.; project administration, P.H.; supervision, M.A. and P.H.; validation, M.A. and P.H.; visualization, A.A.A. (Abdullah A. Alshehri) and F.A.A.; writing—original draft, M.A., A.A., N.A., A.A.A. (Anas A. Almuqhim), H.Q., A.A.A. (Abdullah A. Alshehri), F.A.A. and P.H.; writing—review and editing, M.A., A.A.A. (Anas A. Almuqhim), H.Q., A.A.A. (Abdullah A. Alshehri), F.A.A. and P.H. All authors have read and agreed to the published version of the manuscript.

Funding: This work was funded by King Adulaziz City for Science and Technology (KACST), Saudi Arabia.

Institutional Review Board Statement: Not applicable.

Informed Consent Statement: Not applicable.

Data Availability Statement: The data presented in this study are available on request from the corresponding author.

Acknowledgments: We acknowledge the support of King Adulaziz City for Science and Technology (KACST), Saudi Arabia. P.H. acknowledges financial support from the Government of the Russian Federation (Mega-grant No. 14.W03.31.0028). Texas A&M University (T3 program) grant # 101.

Conflicts of Interest: The authors declare no conflict of interest.

References

1. Wen, S.; Zhou, J.; Zheng, K.; Bednarkiewicz, A.; Liu, X.; Jin, D. Advances in highly doped upconversion nanoparticles. *Nat. Commun.* **2018**, *9*, 2415. [CrossRef] [PubMed]
2. Liu, Y.; Lu, Y.; Yang, X.; Zheng, X.; Wen, S.; Wang, F.; Vidal, X.; Zhao, J.; Liu, D.; Zhou, Z.; et al. Amplified stimulated emission in upconversion nanoparticles for super-resolution nanoscopy. *Nature* **2017**, *543*, 229–233. [CrossRef] [PubMed]
3. Zhou, B.; Shi, B.; Jin, D.; Liu, X. Controlling upconversion nanocrystals for emerging applications. *Nat. Nanotechnol.* **2015**, *10*, 924–936. [CrossRef]
4. Wang, F.; Han, Y.; Lim, C.S.; Lu, Y.; Wang, J.; Xu, J.; Chen, H.; Zhang, C.; Hong, M.; Liu, X. Simultaneous phase and size control of upconversion nanocrystals through lanthanide doping. *Nature* **2010**, *463*, 1061–1065. [CrossRef]
5. Wilhelm, S. Perspectives for upconverting nanoparticles. *ACS Nano* **2017**, *11*, 10644–10653. [CrossRef]
6. Chan, E.M. Combinatorial approaches for developing upconverting nanomaterials: High-throughput screening, modeling, and applications. *Chem. Soc. Rev.* **2015**, *44*, 1653–1679. [CrossRef]
7. Liu, X.; Yan, C.-H.; Capobianco, J.A. Photon upconversion nanomaterials. *Chem. Soc. Rev.* **2015**, *44*, 1299–1301. [CrossRef]

8. Siefe, C.; Mehlenbacher, R.D.; Peng, C.S.; Zhang, Y.; Fischer, S.; Lay, A.; McLellan, C.A.; Alivisatos, P.; Chu, S.; Dionne, J.A. Sub-20 nm core–shell–shell nanoparticles for bright upconversion and enhanced förster resonant energy transfer. *J. Am. Chem. Soc.* **2019**, *141*, 16997–17005. [CrossRef] [PubMed]
9. Liu, Q.; Zhang, Y.; Peng, C.S.; Yang, T.; Joubert, L.-M.; Chu, S. Single upconversion nanoparticle imaging at sub-10 W cm−2 irradiance. *Nat. Photonics* **2018**, *12*, 548–553. [CrossRef] [PubMed]
10. Sreenivasan, V.K.A.; Zvyagin, A.; Goldys, E. Luminescent nanoparticles and their applications in the life sciences. *J. Phys. Condens. Matter* **2013**, *25*, 194101. [CrossRef]
11. Alkahtani, M.; Alsofyani, N.; Alfahd, A.; Almuqhim, A.A.; Almughem, F.A.; Alshehri, A.A.; Qasem, H.; Hemmer, P.R. Engineering red-enhanced and biocompatible upconversion nanoparticles. *Nanomaterials* **2021**, *11*, 284. [CrossRef] [PubMed]
12. Zhu, X.; Zhang, J.; Liu, J.; Zhang, Y. Recent progress of rare-earth doped upconversion nanoparticles: Synthesis, optimization, and applications. *Adv. Sci.* **2019**, *6*, 1901358. [CrossRef] [PubMed]
13. Li, Z.; Zhang, Y.; Jiang, S. Multicolor core/shell-structured upconversion fluorescent nanoparticles. *Adv. Mater.* **2008**, *20*, 4765–4769. [CrossRef]
14. Sun, Y.; Feng, W.; Yang, P.; Huang, C.; Li, F. The biosafety of lanthanide upconversion nanomaterials. *Chem. Soc. Rev.* **2014**, *44*, 1509–1525. [CrossRef] [PubMed]
15. Qian, H.; Guo, H.C.; Ho, P.C.-L.; Mahendran, R.; Zhang, Y. Mesoporous-silica-coated up-conversion fluorescent nanoparticles for photodynamic therapy. *Small* **2009**, *5*, 2285–2290. [CrossRef]
16. Dou, Q.Q.; Guo, H.C.; Ye, E. Near-infrared upconversion nanoparticles for bio-applications. *Mater. Sci. Eng. C* **2014**, *45*, 635–643. [CrossRef]
17. Loh, X.J.; Dou, Q.Q.; Ye, E.; Teng, C.P. Effective near-infrared photodynamic therapy assisted by upconversion nanoparticles conjugated with photosensitizers. *Int. J. Nanomed.* **2015**, *10*, 419–432. [CrossRef]
18. Mialon, G.; Tuerkcan, S.; Dantelle, G.; Collins, D.P.; Hadjipanayi, M.; Taylor, R.A.; Gacoin, T.; Alexandrou, A.; Boilot, J.-P. High up-conversion efficiency of YVO$_4$:Yb,Er nanoparticles in water down to the single-particle level. *J. Phys. Chem. C* **2010**, *114*, 22449–22454. [CrossRef]
19. Joubert, M.-F. Photon avalanche upconversion in rare earth laser materials. *Opt. Mater.* **1999**, *11*, 181–203. [CrossRef]
20. Goldner, P.; Pelle, F. Site selection and up-conversion studies in erbium and ytterbium doped CsCdBr. *J. Lumin.* **1993**, *55*, 197–207. [CrossRef]
21. Wilhelm, S.; Kaiser, M.; Würth, C.; Heiland, J.; Carrillo-Carrion, C.; Muhr, V.; Wolfbeis, O.S.; Parak, W.J.; Resch-Genger, U.; Hirsch, T. Water dispersible upconverting nanoparticles: Effects of surface modification on their luminescence and colloidal stability. *Nanoscale* **2015**, *7*, 1403–1410. [CrossRef]
22. Wiesholler, L.M.; Frenzel, F.; Grauel, B.; Würth, C.; Resch-Genger, U.; Hirsch, T. Yb,Nd,Er-doped upconversion nanoparticles: 980 nm versus 808 nm excitation. *Nanoscale* **2019**, *11*, 13440–13449. [CrossRef] [PubMed]
23. Alkahtani, M.H.; Gomes, C.L.; Hemmer, P.R. Engineering water-tolerant core/shell upconversion nanoparticles for optical temperature sensing. *Opt. Lett.* **2017**, *42*, 2451–2454. [CrossRef]
24. Alkahtani, M.H.; Alghannam, F.S.; Sanchez, C.; Gomes, C.L.; Liang, H.; Hemmer, P.R. High efficiency upconversion nanophosphors for high-contrast bioimaging. *Nanotechnology* **2016**, *27*, 485501. [CrossRef] [PubMed]
25. Mialon, G.; Gohin, M.; Gacoin, T.; Boilot, J.-P. High temperature strategy for oxide nanoparticle synthesis. *ACS Nano* **2008**, *2*, 2505–2512. [CrossRef] [PubMed]
26. Maurin, I.; Dantelle, G.; Boilot, J.-P.; Gacoin, T. A protected annealing process for the production of high quality colloidal oxide nanoparticles with optimized physical properties. *J. Mater. Chem. C* **2013**, *1*, 13–22. [CrossRef]
27. Liang, Y.; Noh, H.M.; Xue, J.; Choi, H.; Park, S.H.; Choi, B.C.; Kim, J.H.; Jeong, J.H. High quality colloidal GdVO$_4$:Yb,Er upconversion nanoparticles synthesized via a protected calcination process for versatile applications. *Mater. Des.* **2017**, *130*, 190–196. [CrossRef]
28. Huignard, A.; Buissette, V.; Laurent, G.; Gacoin, T.; Boilot, J.-P. Synthesis and characterizations of YVO$_4$:Eu colloids. *Chem. Mater.* **2002**, *14*, 2264–2269. [CrossRef]

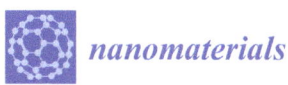

Article

Cell Volume (3D) Correlative Microscopy Facilitated by Intracellular Fluorescent Nanodiamonds as Multi-Modal Probes

Neeraj Prabhakar [1,2,*], Ilya Belevich [3], Markus Peurla [4,5,6], Xavier Heiligenstein [7], Huan-Cheng Chang [8], Cecilia Sahlgren [2], Eija Jokitalo [3] and Jessica M. Rosenholm [1]

1. Pharmaceutical Sciences Laboratory, Faculty of Science and Engineering, Åbo Akademi University, 20520 Turku, Finland; jerosenh@abo.fi
2. Cell Biology, Faculty of Science and Engineering, Åbo Akademi University, 20520 Turku, Finland; csahlgre@abo.fi
3. Electron Microscopy Unit, Helsinki Institute of Life Science—Institute of Biotechnology, University of Helsinki, FI-00014 Helsinki, Finland; ilya.belevich@helsinki.fi (I.B.); eija.jokitalo@helsinki.fi (E.J.)
4. Institute of Biomedicine, Faculty of Medicine, University of Turku, 20520 Turku, Finland; markus.peurla@utu.fi
5. Cancer Research Laboratory FICAN West, Institute of Biomedicine, University of Turku, 20520 Turku, Finland
6. Turku Bioscience Centre, University of Turku and Åbo Akademi University, 20520 Turku, Finland
7. CryoCapCell, 155 Boulevard de l'Hopital, 75013 Paris, France; xavier.heiligenstein@curie.fr
8. Institute of Atomic and Molecular Sciences, Academia Sinica, Taipei 10617, Taiwan; hchang@sinica.edu.tw
* Correspondence: nprabhak@abo.fi

Citation: Prabhakar, N.; Belevich, I.; Peurla, M.; Heiligenstein, X.; Chang, H.-C.; Sahlgren, C.; Jokitalo, E.; Rosenholm, J.M. Cell Volume (3D) Correlative Microscopy Facilitated by Intracellular Fluorescent Nanodiamonds as Multi-Modal Probes. *Nanomaterials* 2021, 11, 14. https://dx.doi.org/10.3390/nano11010014

Received: 18 November 2020
Accepted: 21 December 2020
Published: 23 December 2020

Publisher's Note: MDPI stays neutral with regard to jurisdictional claims in published maps and institutional affiliations.

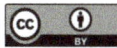

Copyright: © 2020 by the authors. Licensee MDPI, Basel, Switzerland. This article is an open access article distributed under the terms and conditions of the Creative Commons Attribution (CC BY) license (https://creativecommons.org/licenses/by/4.0/).

Abstract: Three-dimensional correlative light and electron microscopy (3D CLEM) is attaining popularity as a potential technique to explore the functional aspects of a cell together with high-resolution ultrastructural details across the cell volume. To perform such a 3D CLEM experiment, there is an imperative requirement for multi-modal probes that are both fluorescent and electron-dense. These multi-modal probes will serve as landmarks in matching up the large full cell volume datasets acquired by different imaging modalities. Fluorescent nanodiamonds (FNDs) are a unique nanosized, fluorescent, and electron-dense material from the nanocarbon family. We hereby propose a novel and straightforward method for executing 3D CLEM using FNDs as multi-modal landmarks. We demonstrate that FND is biocompatible and is easily identified both in living cell fluorescence imaging and in serial block-face scanning electron microscopy (SB-EM). We illustrate the method by registering multi-modal datasets.

Keywords: correlative microscopy; 3D CLEM; volume imaging

1. Introduction

Correlative light and electron microscopy (CLEM) combine the strengths of fluorescence and electron microscopy and this allows overcoming their respective limitations for cell imaging [1–3]. CLEM can be employed to study dynamics and localization of macromolecules and proteins with live cell light microscopy (LM) followed by electron microscopic (EM) examination of the ultrastructural morphology of the specific cell of interest [4–9]. Thus, functional and ultrastructural details of one cell are obtained by the integration of the two imaging modalities [10,11]. To date, numerous experimental CLEM approaches have been reported [5,12–14]. Apart from providing functional and ultrastructural information, recent CLEM methods have employed super-resolution fluorescence techniques to bridge the resolution gap between diffraction-limited fluorescence microscopy and EM [6,13,15–18]. However, the majority of developed CLEM methods are based on the correlation of LM with 2D images of thin cell sections imaged with transmission electron microscopy (TEM) [13,16,17,19–21]. Consequently, these CLEM methods provide very limited information on the z-axis direction, as TEM sections are generally restricted to slices of about 60–100 nm thickness and they may also be tilted relative to the image planes in the confocal image stack, resulting in uncertainty in the final correlation.

Considering the complex 3D organization of a cell, most of the critical 3D cellular information, especially in the z-direction, is generally under-explored. Therefore, 2D CLEM methods could be improved by employing instruments capable of performing 3D imaging [14,22–29], enabling CLEM methods to correlate 3D information from both LM and EM. Combining 3D fluorescence microscopy with 3D EM would significantly improve the technical possibilities for investigating complex cellular processes across the full volume of a cell [30].

Recently, several volume-CLEM methods that demonstrate 3D correlation have been presented [31–36]. Typically, there are common landmarks that are used as fiducials to facilitate correlation. These landmarks must be detectable with both imaging modalities. One such fluorescent and electron-dense CLEM marker is the fluorescent nanodiamond (FND) [19,37–44]. FNDs are non-toxic to cells, and being nanosized particles, they can be easily internalized in living cells via endocytosis [45–48]. FNDs have excellent photostability, and they have non-blinking far-red emission, which makes them well-suited for the imaging of living and fixed cells. We recently reported that FNDs are robust intracellular landmarks in 2D CLEM experiments [39].

In this article, a 3D CLEM method using on average 35 nm-sized FNDs as intracellular correlation landmarks for combining cell volume datasets from live-cell confocal microscopy and serial block-face scanning electron microscopy (SB-EM) is demonstrated.

2. Materials and Methods

2.1. FND Production

The synthesis and characterization of 35 nm FNDs have been previously reported [49]. A brief synthesis protocol is presented as follows. Synthetic type Ib diamond powders with a nominal size of 100 nm (MDA, Element Six) were purified in acids and suspended in water. A thin diamond film of ~50 μm thickness were made by depositing the diamond suspension on a silicon wafer. The diamond film was then treated by a 3-MeV proton beam and nitrogen-vacancy defect centers were created by annealing the proton beam-treated nanodiamonds. To produce 35 nm FNDs, the 100 nm FNDs were first mixed with NaF powders and crushed together with a hydraulic oil press under a pressure of 10 tons. Smaller FNDs were isolated by centrifugation after dissolving the mixture in hot water to remove NaF.

2.2. Cell Culture

MDA-MB-231 (Human breast adenocarcinoma) cells were obtained from Turku Bioscience Center, University of Turku and Åbo Akademi University, Finland. Cells were cultured in Dulbecco's modified Eagle's medium (DMEM (Lonza, Basel, Switzerland)) supplemented with 10% fetal bovine serum, 2 mM L-glutamine, and 1% penicillin-streptomycin (v/v), over μ-Dish 35 mm ibidi gridded dishes (ibidi GmbH, Gräfelfing, Germany). 10 μg/mL of 35 nm FNDs particles were prepared in 1 mL of cell growth media. Then, the cell media with particles was added to the cells growing. The cells were allowed to incubate with FNDs for 24 h. Staining with living cell dyes was performed as follows. The cells were washed three times with serum-free DMEM, after which 0.2 μL of Mitotracker (MitoTracker® Green, ThermoFisher Scientific Inc., Waltham, MA, USA) was first added to 1.5 mL of medium (without serum and antibiotics) and then drop by drop to the dish. MDA-MB-231 cells were incubated for 30 min at 37 °C.

2.3. 2D SEM

MDA-MB-231 (Human breast adenocarcinoma) cells were cultured in Dulbecco's modified Eagle's medium (DMEM, Lonza, Basel, Switzerland) supplemented with 10% fetal bovine serum, 2 mM L-glutamine, and 1% penicillin-streptomycin (v/v). Of 35 nm FNDs particles, 10 μg/mL were prepared in 1 mL of cell growth media. Then, the cell media with particles was added to the cells growing. The cells were allowed to incubate with FNDs for 24 h. Cells were fixed with 5% glutaraldehyde s-collidine buffer, postfixed with 2% OsO$_4$ containing 3% potassium ferrocyanide, dehydrated with ethanol, and flat embedded in a 45,359 Fluka Epoxy Embedding Medium kit. Thin sections were cut using an ultramicrotome to a thickness of 100 nm. The sections were stained using uranyl acetate and lead citrate to enable detection with SEM. The Zeiss LEO 1530 (Zeiss, Oberkochen, Germany) SEM instrument used was for imaging. The applied voltage was 15 kV, the detector was the in-lens detector. The secondary electron detector was placed in the electron optics column.

2.4. Confocal Microscopy

The living cell 3D imaging was performed with a Leica TCS SP5 confocal microscope (Leica Microsystems, Wetzlar, Germany), using a 63X oil objective. The cells were maintained at 37 °C, 5% CO$_2$ during the imaging. The MitoTracker® Green and the FNDs were excited by 488 nm argon laser. Fluorescence was collected at 510–550 nm and 650–730 nm with PMTs (Photomultiplier tubes) for MitoTracker® Green and FNDs, respectively. The MitoTracker® Green was recorded in 3D stacks together with FND landmarks in living cells. Live cell microscopy was performed for 2.5 min to obtain 35 stacks of step size 0.13 µm. The live cells were instantly fixed in a fixative mixture consisting of 2% glutaraldehyde, 2% PFA, 2 mM CaCl$_2$ in 0.1 M NaCac buffer, pH 7.4.

2.5. 3D SB-EM Sample Preparation

The specimens were prepared using a protocol modified from Deerinck et al. (2010) [50]. The cells were fixed for 30 min at RT with a fixative mixture consisting of 2% glutaraldehyde, 2% PFA, 2 mM CaCl$_2$ in 0.1 M NaCac buffer (pH 7.4) and washed five times with NaCac buffer containing 2 mM CaCl$_2$. The cells were postfixed for 1 h on an ice bath in a fume hood with 2% OsO, 1.5% K$_4$[Fe(CN)$_6$], 2 mM CaCl$_2$ in 0.1 M NaCac buffer, pH 7.4. The cells were washed 5 times with distilled water (DW). The cells were then incubated in 1% aqueous thiocarbohydrazide (TCH) for 10 min at RT. The cells were washed 5 times with DW. The cells were incubated in 1% OsO$_4$ in DW for 30 min at RT. The cells were washed 5 times with DW. The cells were incubated with 1% uranyl acetate at +4 °C overnight, washed 5 times with DW at RT, incubated in the pre-warmed lead aspartate solution at 60 °C oven for 30 min., and washed 5 times with DW followed by serial dehydration. The cells were dipped into an aluminium plate with a resin-acetone solution containing acetone with 50% (*v/v*) Epon resin to incubate for 1 h. Further, cells were incubated in 100% Epon resin and incubated for 1 h RT. The cells were allowed to polymerize in an oven at 60 °C for 28 h.

2.6. 3D SB-EM Imaging

The area of interest with the selected cells was trimmed from the plastic block and mounted onto a pin using conductive epoxy glue (model 2400; CircuitWorks, Kennesaw, GA, USA). The trimmed block was further trimmed as a pyramid and its sides were covered with silver paint (Agar Scientific Ltd., Stansted, UK). To improve conductivity, the whole assembly was platinum-coated using Quorum Q150TS (Quorum Technologies, Laughton, UK). SB-EM data sets were acquired with a FEG-SEM Quanta 250 (Thermo Fisher Scientific, FEI, Hillsboro, OR, USA), using a backscattered electron detector (Gatan Inc., Pleasanton, CA, USA) with 2.5-kV beam voltage, a spot size of 2.9, and a pressure of 0.15 Torr. The block faces were cut with 50-nm increments and imaged with XY resolution of 25 nm per pixel. The collected 16-bit images were processed for segmentation using an open-source software Microscopy Image Browser [51] as follows: (a) individual images were combined into 3D stacks; (b) the combined 3D-stack was aligned; (c) the contrast for the whole stack was adjusted, and (d) the images were converted to the 8-bit format.

2.7. Image Correlation

The multi-modal datasets were registered using the eC-CLEM plugin on the Icy bioimage analysis platform [52]. To match the large datasets on a laptop (i7, 16Gb RAM), the EM stack was binned 4 times. The FM stack was matched to the binned dataset using the FNDs as landmarks, targeting the center of the FNDs aggregates both in LM and EM using orthogonal views from Icy. Nine FNDs were sufficient to achieve the good overlay accuracy depicted in this manuscript. Rigid registration was performed despite a recommendation by the software to apply for non-rigid registration [53]. This decision was made after careful observation of the LM dataset. Since living cell imaging was performed on the 3D stack, the cell dynamics caused some of the FNDs to move during image acquisition. This natural movement was uneven in all FNDs. Local inaccuracies in this registration were coherent with the cell movement observed. The weighing of each landmark operated by eC-CLEM compensated for the shifts observed between the LM and the EM dataset and rigid registration lead to accurate full registration. To generate the final overlay, the transformation was applied to the LM dataset to match the original EM dataset using the "apply a reduced scaled transform to a full-size image" function from eC-CLEM (Advanced usage). This final overlay was used to generate movies in supplementary data.

3. Results
FND Facilitated 3D Cell Volume-CLEM

Our 3D CLEM workflow begins by seeding FND incubated MDA-MB-231 cells over gridded glass-bottom dishes designed for CLEM experiments. Two FND incubated living MDA-MB-231 cells shown in Figure 1a were selected for the 3D CLEM experiment. To demonstrate the usefulness of FNDs in the 3D CLEM experiment, MDA-MB-231 cells were stained with a mitochondrial marker dye MitoTracker (Figure 1b,c).

Confocal image stacks of the whole cell volumes were acquired from both the MitoTracker (green) and the FND (red) signals (Figure 1d–f and Video S1). MitoTracker signal was seen widespread in cytoplasmic space (Figure 1d). The fluorescence signal from FNDs (Figure 1e) was mostly localized to a few spots suggesting their confinement in vesicles. Following earlier results FNDs are internalized by clathrin-mediated endocytosis [45,46] and they tend to aggregate inside endosomal vesicles (Figure S1) and subsequently slowly exocytose from cells [45,47]. The aggregation of FNDs in cellular vesicles brings added benefit from a CLEM perspective [39] because, in comparison to single FNDs, the high concentration of FNDs aggregated inside vesicles provides better contrast both in fluorescence microscopy and in EM. Besides, the confinement of FNDs in vesicles prevents their movement in the sample processing steps after the confocal imaging enabling more reliable correlation of EM images.

3D localization of FNDs for the MitoTracker fluorescence signal can be seen in Video S2. These 3D confocal datasets were used for software-based correlation with SB-EM datasets. After confocal imaging, the selected cells were fixed, stained, and embedded for SB-EM (Figure 1g). The use of gridded glass-bottom dishes allowed easy identification of the cells of interest within the plastic block and trimming the blocks accordingly. The trimmed area was mounted on a pin and imaged in SEM. The mounted block-face overview image before SB-EM is displayed in Figure 1h.

The two selected cells were identified (Figure 1h) using a 15 kV electron beam. The collection of 3D EM data was performed with an SEM instrument equipped with a system for serial block-face SEM (SB-EM). In SB-EM, an ultramicrotome performed automated sectioning of whole-cell volume by cutting thin sections ($\geq$50 nm) from the sample's block-face (Video S3). Consequently, after each cut, a high-resolution image of the freshly made block-face was acquired using a backscattered electron detector to form a 3D image stack. SB-EM imaging provided a three-dimensional dataset of the selected cells with a resolution to recognize the structure of interest (mitochondria) and FNDs aggregated in vesicular structures for CLEM (Figure 2).

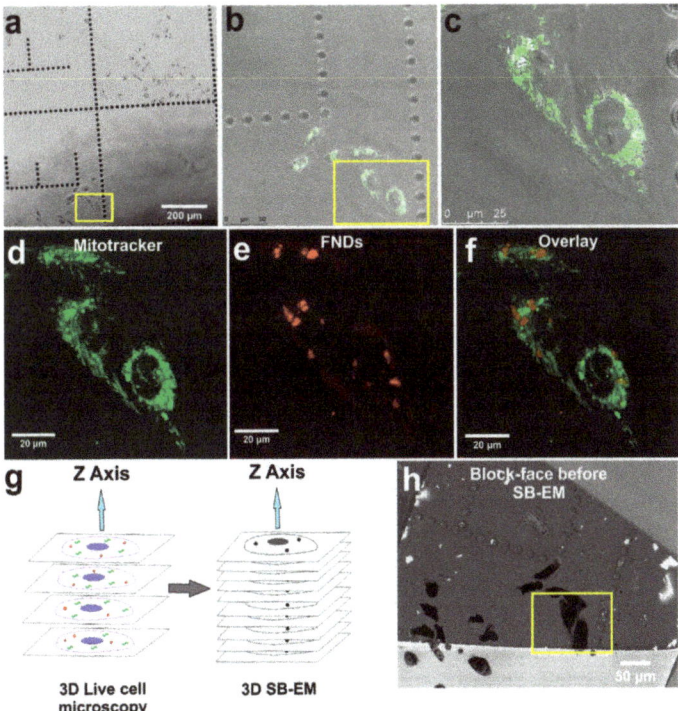

Figure 1. The 3D correlative light and electron microscopy workflow demonstrating the live-cell confocal microscopy to the serial block-face scanning electron microscopy (SB-EM). (**a**) Bright-field image of the living cells on a gridded glass-bottom dish. The cells selected for 3D CLEM are indicated by the yellow box. (**b**) MitoTracker signal from the stained selected cells (indicated by the yellow box). (**c**) Close-up view of the selected cells shown by an overlay of brightfield and MitoTracker images. (**d**) Maximum intensity z-projection image from the MitoTracker channel of the selected cells. (**e**) Maximum intensity z-projection image from the fluorescent nanodiamond (FND) channel of the selected cells. (**f**) Overlay of maximum intensity z-projections of MitoTracker and FND channels. (**g**) Schematic representation of 3D CLEM workflow with FNDs (red dots) and a standard organic fluorophore (green structures). (**h**) Localization of the selected cells on the EM block-face (near the letter E) for SB-EM. The yellow box indicates the same selected cells as in (**a**).

Correlation of the LM and SB-EM volume datasets was done using the eC-CLEM plugin on the Icy bioimage analysis platform [52,54]. First corresponding intracellular FNDs were identified in both datasets. FNDs aggregated in vesicles have a distinct appearance in SEM images (Supplementary Figure S1) and they are easily distinguished from morphological features of the cell. Figure 3 shows representative SB-EM and 3D LM image pairs (Figure 3a,b; Figure 3d,e) in which the corresponding FNDs are identified and marked.

Correlation of the two volume datasets was calculated using the identified FND position pairs as fiducials, and the accordingly transformed volume dataset of the fluorescence signal of interest (MitoTracker) was overlayed on the SB-EM stack. The FNDs facilitated mapping of the mitochondrial locations throughout the cell volume (Figure 4a–d) resulting in good colocalization of the MitoTracker signal with mitochondria seen in the EM image stack (Videos S4–S6 and Figure S2).

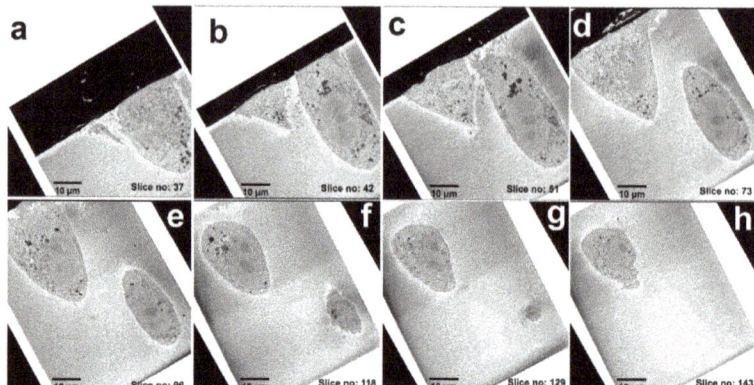

Figure 2. A collage of multi-plane images from the SB-EM 3D series. (**a–h**) Images from the 3D EM stack acquired from the selected cells are shown in the increasing order of the z-axis. The distance between the slices is 50 nm.

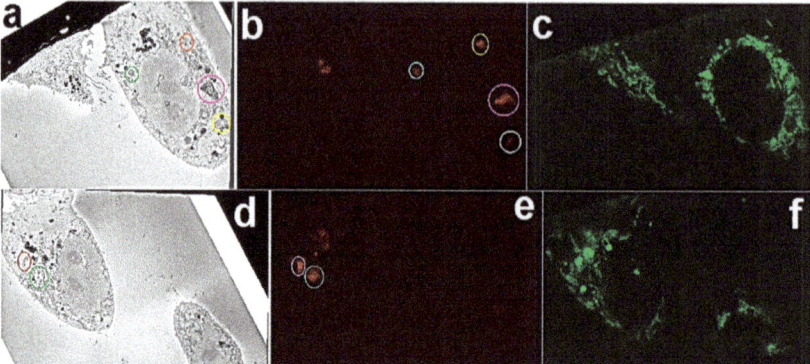

Figure 3. Overview of the corresponding FND aggregates in EM and LM. Corresponding FNDs (color-coded) were matched in respective EM and light microscopy (LM) sections. (**a,d**) SEM images with FND localized in vesicles (color-coded). (**b,e**) Respective FNDs (color-coded) in LM images were matched up. (**c,f**) corresponding MitoTracker channels.

Quite commonly in the literature, the multi-modal correlation is performed in absence of such a common landmark, and the process of 3D dataset correlation severely suffers from misalignment and errors in localizing critical information across 3D. However, in this type of CLEM approach, there can be multiple factors that could affect precise image correlation. The major challenge encountered in the CLEM experiment was inherently low axial (600 nm) and lateral (250 nm) resolution provided by confocal microscopes compared to the nanometer scale resolution provided by EM (Supplementary Figure S3). Currently, the limited resolution of confocal microscopy can result in the misalignment of details within large scale datasets. Sample autofluorescence, unspecific binding of fluorophores, and obtaining a bright FND signal with live-cell imaging are additional parameters that still must be optimized.

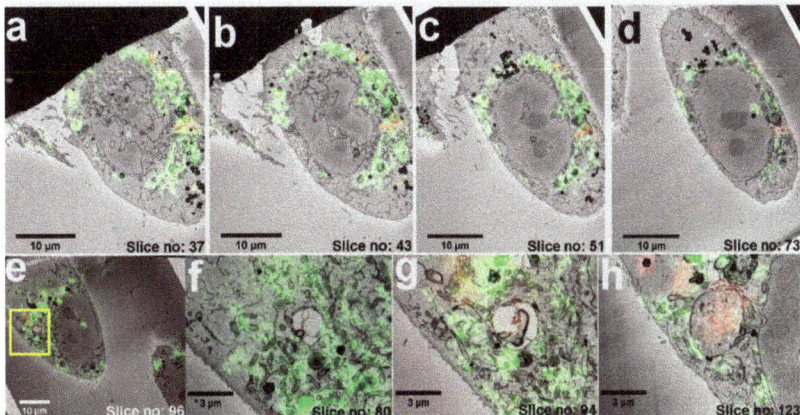

Figure 4. Volume-CLEM of living cells. (**a–d**) CLEM images of multiple planes in increasing z-axis. (**e**) ROI selected in CLEM image to demonstrate the correlation of LM over EM. (**f**) In slice no: 80, a single high-resolution image shows numerous mitochondria (green) and an empty vesicle. (**g**) In slice no: 94, FNDs (red), mitochondria (green), and a vesicle can be seen. (**h**) In slice no: 123, a vesicle filled with FNDs (red), and fewer mitochondria (green) can be seen. FNDs in the EM image are the dark dots inside the vesicle.

4. Discussion

We have introduced a novel FND enabled cell volume (3D) correlative microscopy method. The CLEM workflow is straightforward and can be performed without any dedicated CLEM imaging systems. We demonstrated that a standard organic fluorophore can be used for 3D CLEM experiments with the FND-based method without any special sample preparation requirements.

In general, organic fluorophores do not survive routine EM sample processing and are not electron dense molecules, and therefore are not detectable with EM. In contrast, the employed 35 nm FNDs were intracellularly detectable with both imaging modalities in our experiments, enabling the successful correlation of volume datasets for 3D CLEM. FNDs can offer multiple advantages over currently used CLEM fiducials as their internalization does not need chemical permeabilization, which has impacts on cellular morphology and ultrastructure. FNDs may be considered as a leading contender in the search for an exceptional CLEM probe because they are not prone to chemical degradation, have excellent photostability, and their nanoscale size facilitates their rapid internalization to cells.

In our CLEM workflow, confocal microscopy was chosen for 3D living cell imaging even if it offers a limited resolution. Pairing confocal with SB-EM imaging was a practical choice for our experiment because the specific instrument was available to us. However, the focused ion beam imaging (FIB-SEM) could be used as an alternative for automatically obtaining the serial section image stacks. However, SB-EM can manage larger sample volumes than FIB-SEM, but with more limited z resolution. Our next step is to explore the possibilities of performing FND-enabled CLEM with 3D super-resolution imaging.

Supplementary Materials: The following are available online at https://www.mdpi.com/2079-4991/11/1/14/s1. Figure S1: SEM imaging of vesicle aggregated FNDs; Figure S2: FND landmarks facilitated the alignment of 3D images; Figure S3: Single stacks image correlation; Video S1: 3D live cell confocal microscopy; Video S2: 3D reconstruction of FND distribution; Video S3: 3D SB-EM imaging of both cells; Video S4: 3D CLEM of both cells; Video S5: 3D CLEM of vesicle aggregated FND; Video S6: 3D CLEM of single cell. The video files referred to in the article as Videos S1–S6 are available on Zenodo at https://zenodo.org/record/4279702 (DOI:10.5281/zenodo.4279702).

Author Contributions: The manuscript was written and revised through the contributions of all authors. All authors agree to be accountable for all aspects of the work. Conceptualization, N.P. and M.P.; Funding acquisition, C.S. and J.M.R.; Investigation, N.P. and M.P.; Methodology, I.B.; Resources, H.-C.C., C.S., E.J. and J.M.R.; Software, X.H.; Supervision, H.-C.C., C.S., E.J. and J.M.R.; Writing—original draft, N.P.; Writing—review & editing, I.B., M.P., Xavier Heiligenstein, H.-C.C., C.S., E.J. and J.M.R. All authors have read and agreed to the published version of the manuscript.

Funding: Financial contribution from the Academy of Finland (Project No. 309374) and Sigrid Jusélius Foundation are greatly acknowledged. The authors also acknowledge Biocenter Finland for financial support.

Data Availability Statement: The data presented in this study are openly available in [Zenodo] at [doi.org/10.5281/zenodo.4384502].

Acknowledgments: The authors would like to acknowledge Jenni Laine and Kai-Lan Lin (Electron microscopy unit, University of Turku) for providing technical assistance with sample preparation for SEM and Mervi Lindman, the University of Helsinki for excellent technical assistance in the preparation of SB-EM specimens. Euro-BioImaging (www.eurobioimaging.eu) is acknowledged for providing access to 3D imaging technologies and services via the Finnish Advanced Light Microscopy Node (Helsinki, Finland). Helen Cooper is acknowledged for kindly providing mitochondrial staining reagents. We also thank Fen-Jen Hsieh for the preparation of 35 nm FNDs.

Conflicts of Interest: The authors declare no conflict of interest.

References

1. Mironov, A.A.; Beznoussenko, G.V. Correlative light-electron microscopy: A potent tool for the imaging of rare or unique cellular and tissue events and structures. *Methods Enzymol.* **2012**, *504*, 201–219. [CrossRef] [PubMed]
2. de Boer, P.; Hoogenboom, J.P.; Giepmans, B.N.G. Correlated light and electron microscopy: Ultrastructure lights up! *Nat. Methods* **2015**, *12*, 503–513. [CrossRef]
3. Sartori, A.; Gatz, R.; Beck, F.; Rigort, A.; Baumeister, W.; Plitzko, J.M. Correlative microscopy: Bridging the gap between fluorescence light microscopy and cryo-electron tomography. *J. Struct. Biol.* **2007**, *160*, 135–145. [CrossRef] [PubMed]
4. Polishchuk, E.V.; Polishchuk, R.S.; Luini, A. Correlative Light–Electron Microscopy as a Tool to Study in Vivo Dynamics and Ultrastructure of Intracellular Structures. In *Methods in Molecular Biology (Methods and Protocols)*; Taatjes, D., Roth, J., Eds.; Cell Imaging Techniques; Humana Press: Totowa, NJ, USA, 2012; Volume 931, pp. 413–422. [CrossRef]
5. Polishchuk, E.V.; Polishchuk, R.S. Pre-embedding labeling for subcellular detection of molecules with electron microscopy. *Tissue Cell* **2018**, *57*, 103–110. [CrossRef] [PubMed]
6. Watanabe, S.; Punge, A.; Hollopeter, G.; Willig, K.I.; Hobson, R.J.; Davis, M.W.; Hell, S.W.; Jorgensen, E.M. Protein localization in electron micrographs using fluorescence nanoscopy. *Nat. Methods* **2011**, *8*, 80–84. [CrossRef] [PubMed]
7. Kopek, B.G.; Shtengel, G.; Xu, C.S.; Clayton, D.A.; Hess, H.F. Correlative 3D superresolution fluorescence and electron microscopy reveal the relationship of mitochondrial nucleoids to membranes. *Proc. Natl. Acad. Sci. USA* **2012**, *109*, 6136–6141. [CrossRef]
8. Razi, M.; Tooze, S.A. Chapter 17 Correlative Light and Electron Microscopy. *Methods Enzymol.* **2009**, *452*, 261–275. [CrossRef]
9. Loussert Fonta, C.; Humbel, B.M. Correlative microscopy. *Arch. Biochem. Biophys.* **2015**, *581*, 98–110. [CrossRef]
10. Smith, C. Microscopy: Two microscopes are better than one. *Nature* **2012**, *492*, 293–297. [CrossRef]
11. van Rijnsoever, C.; Oorschot, V.; Klumperman, J. Correlative light-electron microscopy (CLEM) combining live-cell imaging and immunolabeling of ultrathin cryosections. *Nat. Methods* **2008**, *5*, 973–980. [CrossRef]
12. Ando, T.; Bhamidimarri, S.P.; Brending, N.; Colin-York, H.; Collinson, L.; De Jonge, N.; De Pablo, P.J.; Debroye, E.; Eggeling, C.; Franck, C.; et al. The 2018 correlative microscopy techniques roadmap. *J. Phys. D Appl. Phys.* **2018**, *51*, 443001. [CrossRef] [PubMed]
13. Johnson, E.; Seiradake, E.; Jones, E.Y.; Davis, I.; Grünewald, K.; Kaufmann, R. Correlative in-resin super-resolution and electron microscopy using standard fluorescent proteins. *Sci. Rep.* **2015**, *5*, 9583. [CrossRef] [PubMed]
14. Peddie, C.J.; Collinson, L.M. Exploring the third dimension: Volume electron microscopy comes of age. *Micron* **2014**, *61*, 9–19. [CrossRef] [PubMed]
15. Joosten, B.; Willemse, M.; Fransen, J.; Cambi, A.; van den Dries, K. Super-Resolution Correlative Light and Electron Microscopy (SR-CLEM) Reveals Novel Ultrastructural Insights into Dendritic Cell Podosomes. *Front. Immunol.* **2018**, *9*, 1908. [CrossRef] [PubMed]
16. Peddie, C.J.; Domart, M.-C.; Snetkov, X.; O'Toole, P.; Larijani, B.; Way, M.; Cox, S.; Collinson, L.M. Correlative super-resolution fluorescence and electron microscopy using conventional fluorescent proteins in vacuo. *J. Struct. Biol.* **2017**, *199*, 120–131. [CrossRef] [PubMed]
17. Wolff, G.; Hagen, C.; Grünewald, K.; Kaufmann, R. Towards correlative super-resolution fluorescence and electron cryo-microscopy. *Biol. Cell* **2016**, *108*, 245–258. [CrossRef]

18. Johnson, E.; Kaufmann, R. Preserving the photoswitching ability of standard fluorescent proteins for correlative in-resin super-resolution and electron microscopy. *Methods Cell Biol.* **2017**, *140*, 49–67. [CrossRef]
19. Hemelaar, S.R.; de Boer, P.; Chipaux, M.; Zuidema, W.; Hamoh, T.; Martinez, F.P.; Nagl, A.; Hoogenboom, J.P.; Giepmans, B.N.G.; Schirhagl, R.; et al. Nanodiamonds as multi-purpose labels for microscopy. *Sci. Rep.* **2017**, *7*, 720. [CrossRef]
20. Paez-Segala, M.G.; Sun, M.G.; Shtengel, G.; Viswanathan, S.; Baird, M.A.; Macklin, J.J.; Patel, R.; Allen, J.R.; Howe, E.S.; Piszczek, G.; et al. Fixation-resistant photoactivatable fluorescent proteins for CLEM. *Nat. Methods* **2015**, *12*, 215–218. [CrossRef]
21. Liv, N.; Zonnevylle, A.C.; Narvaez, A.C.; Effting, A.P.J.; Voorneveld, P.W.; Lucas, M.S.; Hardwick, J.C.; Wepf, R.A.; Kruit, P.; Hoogenboom, J.P. Simultaneous Correlative Scanning Electron and High-NA Fluorescence Microscopy. *PLoS ONE* **2013**, *8*, e55707. [CrossRef]
22. Biazik, J.; Vihinen, H.; Anwar, T.; Jokitalo, E.; Eskelinen, E.-L. The versatile electron microscope: An ultrastructural overview of autophagy. *Methods* **2015**, *75*, 44–53. [CrossRef]
23. Nathans, J.; Hopkins, J.; Shan Xu, C.; Hayworth, K.J.; Lu, Z.; Grob, P.; Hassan, A.M.; García-Cerdá, J.G.; Niyogi, K.K.; Nogales, E.; et al. Enhanced FIB-SEM systems for large-volume 3D imaging. *eLife* **2017**, *6*, e25916. [CrossRef]
24. Denk, W.; Horstmann, H. Serial Block-Face Scanning Electron Microscopy to Reconstruct Three-Dimensional Tissue Nanostructure. *PLoS Biol.* **2004**, *2*, e329. [CrossRef]
25. Knott, G.; Marchman, H.; Wall, D.; Lich, B. Serial section scanning electron microscopy of adult brain tissue using focused ion beam milling. *J. Neurosci.* **2008**, *28*, 2959–2964. [CrossRef]
26. Webb, R.; Webb, R. Quick Freeze Substitution Processing of Biological Samples for Serial Block-face Scanning Electron Microscopy. *Microsc. Microanal.* **2015**, *21*, 1115–1116. [CrossRef]
27. Ghosh, S.; Tran, K.; Delbridge, L.M.D.; Hickey, A.J.R.; Hanssen, E.; Crampin, E.J.; Rajagopal, V. Insights on the impact of mitochondrial organisation on bioenergetics in high-resolution computational models of cardiac cell architecture. *PLoS Comput. Biol.* **2018**, *14*, e1006640. [CrossRef]
28. Hussain, A.; Ghosh, S.; Kalkhoran, S.B.; Hausenloy, D.J.; Hanssen, E.; Rajagopal, V. An automated workflow for segmenting single adult cardiac cells from large-volume serial block-face scanning electron microscopy data. *J. Struct. Biol.* **2018**, *202*, 275–285. [CrossRef]
29. Kremer, A.; Lippens, S.; Bartunkova, S.; Asselbergh, B.; Blanpain, C.; Fendrych, M.; Goossens, A.; Holt, M.; Janssens, S.; Krols, M.; et al. Developing 3D SEM in a broad biological context. *J. Microsc.* **2015**, *259*, 80–96. [CrossRef]
30. Deerinck, T.J.; Shone, T.M.; Bushong, E.A.; Ramachandra, R.; Peltier, S.T.; Ellisman, M.H. High-performance serial block-face SEM of nonconductive biological samples enabled by focal gas injection-based charge compensation. *J. Microsc.* **2018**, *270*, 142–149. [CrossRef]
31. Russell, M.R.G.; Lerner, T.R.; Burden, J.J.; Nkwe, D.O.; Pelchen-Matthews, A.; Domart, M.-C.; Durgan, J.; Weston, A.; Jones, M.L.; Peddie, C.J.; et al. 3D correlative light and electron microscopy of cultured cells using serial blockface scanning electron microscopy. *J Cell Sci* **2017**, *130*, 278–291. [CrossRef]
32. Bosch, C.; Martínez, A.; Masachs, N.; Teixeira, C.M.; Fernaud, I.; Ulloa, F.; Pérez-Martínez, E.; Lois, C.; Comella, J.X.; DeFelipe, J.; et al. FIB/SEM technology and high-throughput 3D reconstruction of dendritic spines and synapses in GFP-labeled adult-generated neurons. *Front. Neuroanat.* **2015**, *9*, 60. [CrossRef]
33. Beckwith, M.S.; Beckwith, K.S.; Sikorski, P.; Skogaker, N.T.; Flo, T.H.; Halaas, Ø. Seeing a Mycobacterium-Infected Cell in Nanoscale 3D: Correlative Imaging by Light Microscopy and FIB/SEM Tomography. *PLoS ONE* **2015**, *10*, e0134644. [CrossRef]
34. Booth, D.G.; Beckett, A.J.; Molina, O.; Samejima, I.; Masumoto, H.; Kouprina, N.; Larionov, V.; Prior, I.A.; Earnshaw, W.C. 3D-CLEM Reveals that a Major Portion of Mitotic Chromosomes Is Not Chromatin. *Mol. Cell* **2016**, *64*, 790–802. [CrossRef]
35. Lucas, M.S.; Günthert, M.; Gasser, P.; Lucas, F.; Wepf, R. Bridging Microscopes: 3D Correlative Light and Scanning Electron Microscopy of Complex Biological Structures. In *Methods in Cell Biology*; Academic Press Inc.: Cambridge, MA, USA, 2012; Volume 111, pp. 325–356.
36. Lucas, M.S.; Guenthert, M.; Gasser, P.; Lucas, F.; Wepf, R. Correlative 3D imaging: CLSM and FIB-SEM tomography using high-pressure frozen, freeze-substituted biological samples. In *Methods in Molecular Biology*; Humana Press: Clifton, NJ, USA, 2014; Volume 1117, ISBN 9781627037354.
37. Hsieh, F.-J.; Chen, Y.-W.; Huang, Y.-K.; Lee, H.-M.; Lin, C.-H.; Chang, H.-C. Correlative Light-Electron Microscopy of Lipid-Encapsulated Fluorescent Nanodiamonds for Nanometric Localization of Cell Surface Antigens. *Anal. Chem.* **2018**, *90*, 1566–1571. [CrossRef]
38. Han, S.; Raabe, M.; Hodgson, L.; Mantell, J.; Verkade, P.; Lasser, T.; Landfester, K.; Weil, T.; Lieberwirth, I. High-Contrast Imaging of Nanodiamonds in Cells by Energy Filtered and Correlative Light-Electron Microscopy: Toward a Quantitative Nanoparticle-Cell Analysis. *Nano Lett.* **2019**, *19*, 2178–2185. [CrossRef]
39. Prabhakar, N.; Peurla, M.; Koho, S.; Deguchi, T.; Näreoja, T.; Chang, H.-C.; Rosenholm, J.M.; Hänninen, P.E. STED-TEM Correlative Microscopy Leveraging Nanodiamonds as Intracellular Dual-Contrast Markers. *Small* **2018**, *14*, 1701807. [CrossRef]
40. Schrand, A.M.; Hens, S.A.C.; Shenderova, O.A. Nanodiamond Particles: Properties and Perspectives for Bioapplications. *Crit. Rev. Solid State Mater. Sci.* **2009**, *34*, 18–74. [CrossRef]
41. Vlasov, I.I.; Shiryaev, A.A.; Rendler, T.; Steinert, S.; Lee, S.-Y.; Antonov, D.; Vörös, M.; Jelezko, F.; Fisenko, A.V.; Semjonova, L.F.; et al. Molecular-sized fluorescent nanodiamonds. *Nat. Nanotechnol.* **2014**, *9*, 54–58. [CrossRef]

42. Mochalin, V.N.; Shenderova, O.; Ho, D.; Gogotsi, Y. The properties and applications of nanodiamonds. *Nat. Nanotechnol.* **2011**, *7*, 11–23. [CrossRef]
43. Prabhakar, N.; Näreoja, T.; Von Haartman, E.; Karaman, D.Ş.; Jiang, H.; Koho, S.; Dolenko, T.A.; Hänninen, P.E.; Vlasov, D.I.; Ralchenko, V.G.; et al. Core-shell designs of photoluminescent nanodiamonds with porous silica coatings for bioimaging and drug delivery II: Application. *Nanoscale* **2013**, *5*, 3713–3722. [CrossRef]
44. Hui, Y.Y.; Cheng, C.-L.; Chang, H.-C. Nanodiamonds for optical bioimaging. *J. Phys. D Appl. Phys.* **2010**, *43*, 374021. [CrossRef]
45. Chang, H.-C.; Li, C.-L.; Cheng, C.-A.; Chang, C.-F.; Yeh, S.-H.; Fang, C.-Y.; Vaijayanthimala, V. The Exocytosis of Fluorescent Nanodiamond and Its Use as a Long-Term Cell Tracker. *Small* **2011**, *7*, 3363–3370. [CrossRef]
46. Vaijayanthimala, V.; Tzeng, Y.-K.; Chang, H.-C.; Li, C.-L. The biocompatibility of fluorescent nanodiamonds and their mechanism of cellular uptake. *Nanotechnology* **2009**, *20*, 425103. [CrossRef] [PubMed]
47. Prabhakar, N.; Khan, M.H.; Peurla, M.; Chang, H.-C.; Hänninen, P.E.; Rosenholm, J.M. Intracellular Trafficking of Fluorescent Nanodiamonds and Regulation of Their Cellular Toxicity. *ACS Omega* **2017**, *2*, 2689–2693. [CrossRef]
48. Prabhakar, N.; Rosenholm, J.M. Nanodiamonds for advanced optical bioimaging and beyond. *Curr. Opin. Colloid Interface Sci.* **2019**, *39*, 220–231. [CrossRef]
49. Su, L.-J.; Fang, C.-Y.; Chang, Y.-T.; Chen, K.-M.; Yu, Y.-C.; Hsu, J.-H.; Chang, H.-C. Creation of high density ensembles of nitrogen-vacancy centers in nitrogen-rich type Ib nanodiamonds. *Nanotechnology* **2013**, *24*, 315702. [CrossRef]
50. Deerinck, T.J.; Bushong, E.; THOR, A.; Ellisman, M.; Deerinck, T.; Thor, A.; Deerinck, T.; Bushong, E.; Thor, C.A.; Ellisman, M. NCMIR methods for 3D EM: A new protocol for preparation of biological specimens for serial block face scanning electron microscopy. *Microscopy* **2010**, *1*, 6–8.
51. Belevich, I.; Joensuu, M.; Kumar, D.; Vihinen, H.; Jokitalo, E. Microscopy Image Browser: A Platform for Segmentation and Analysis of Multidimensional Datasets. *PLoS Biol.* **2016**, *14*, e1002340. [CrossRef]
52. Paul-Gilloteaux, P.; Heiligenstein, X.; Belle, M.; Domart, M.-C.; Larijani, B.; Collinson, L.; Raposo, G.; Salamero, J. eC-CLEM: Flexible multidimensional registration software for correlative microscopies. *Nat. Methods* **2017**, *14*, 102–103. [CrossRef]
53. Prabhakar, N.; Peurla, M.; Shenderova, O.; Rosenholm, J.M. Fluorescent and Electron-Dense Green Color Emitting Nanodiamonds for Single-Cell Correlative Microscopy. *Molecules* **2020**, *25*, 5897. [CrossRef]
54. de Chaumont, F.; Dallongeville, S.; Chenouard, N.; Hervé, N.; Pop, S.; Provoost, T.; Meas-Yedid, V.; Pankajakshan, P.; Lecomte, T.; Le Montagner, Y.; et al. Icy: An open bioimage informatics platform for extended reproducible research. *Nat. Methods* **2012**, *9*, 690–696. [CrossRef] [PubMed]

MDPI
St. Alban-Anlage 66
4052 Basel
Switzerland
Tel. +41 61 683 77 34
Fax +41 61 302 89 18
www.mdpi.com

Nanomaterials Editorial Office
E-mail: nanomaterials@mdpi.com
www.mdpi.com/journal/nanomaterials